Drugs and the Pharmaceutical Science

Drugs and the Pharmaceutical Science

Editor: John Jensen

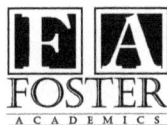

FOSTER
ACADEMICS

www.fosteracademics.com

www.fosteracademics.com

FA
FOSTER
ACADEMICS

Cataloging-in-Publication Data

Drugs and the pharmaceutical science / edited by John Jensen.
     p. cm.
Includes bibliographical references and index.
ISBN 978-1-63242-828-8
1. Drugs. 2. Pharmacology. 3. Materia medica. 4. Pharmacy.
5. Pharmaceutical industry. I. Jensen, John.
RM300 .D78 2019
615--dc23

Foster Academics,
118-35 Queens Blvd., Suite 400,
Forest Hills, NY 11375, USA

ISBN 978-1-63242-828-8 (Hardback)

Contents

Preface

The purpose of the book is to provide a glimpse into the dynamics and to present opinions and studies of some of the scientists engaged in the development of new ideas in the field from very different standpoints. This book will prove useful to students and researchers owing to its high content quality.

Any substance which causes a temporary physiological or psychological change in the body on being consumed, inhaled, smoked or absorbed is called a drug. Pharmaceutical drugs are the chemical substances which are used to prevent, diagnose, cure or treat diseases or to promote well-being. They can be used for limited period or on regular basis according to the diseases. They are produced from medicinal plants or by organic synthesis. The domain of pharmaceutical science is concerned with the design, delivery, disposition and action of such drugs. The topics included in this book on drugs and pharmaceutical sciences are of utmost significance and bound to provide incredible insights to readers. It strives to provide a fair idea about this discipline and to help develop a better understanding of the latest advances within this field. For all those who are interested in drugs and pharmaceutical sciences, this book can prove to be an essential guide.

At the end, I would like to appreciate all the efforts made by the authors in completing their chapters professionally. I express my deepest gratitude to all of them for contributing to this book by sharing their valuable works. A special thanks to my family and friends for their constant support in this journey.

Editor

Essential Oil from Flowers and Leaves of *Elaeagnus Angustifolia* (Elaeagnaceae): Composition, Radical Scavenging and General Toxicity Activities

Mohammadali Torbati[1], Solmaz Asnaashari[2], Fariba Heshmati Afshar[3]*

[1] *Department of Food Science and Technology, Faculty of Nutrition, Tabriz University of Medical Sciences, Tabriz, Iran.*
[2] *Biotechnology Research Center, Tabriz University of Medical Sciences, Tabriz, Iran.*
[3] *Department of Pharmacognosy, Faculty of Pharmacy, Tabriz University of Medical Sciences, Tabriz, Iran.*

Keywords:
· *Elaeagnus angustifolia* L.
· Essential oil
· Radical scavenging activity
· General toxicity
· E-ethyl cinnamate

Abstract

Purpose: The aim of this work was to identify the chemical composition of the essential oils obtained from the flowers and leaves of *Elaeagnus angostifolia* (Elaeagnaceae) along with evaluate the radical scavenging and general toxicity activities.

Methods: A combination of GC-MS and GC-FID were utilized for analyzing the chemical profile of the essential oils extracted by hydro-distillation from the leaves and flowers of *E. angustifolia*. The essential oils were subjected to general toxicity and radical scavenging assays using brine shrimp lethality test and DPPH method, respectively.

Results: In total, 53 and 25 components were identified and quantified in the essential oils of flowers and leaves, accounting for 96.59% and 98.97% of the oil, respectively. The both oils were observed to be rich in ester compounds. The most abundant components of the oil from flowers were E-ethyl cinnamate (60.00%), hexahydrofarnesyl acetone (9.99%), palmitic acid (5.20%) and phytol (3.29%). The major constituents of the oil from leaves were E-ethyl cinnamate (37.27%), phytol (12.08%), nonanal (10.74%) and Z-3-hexenyl benzoate (7.65%). Both oils showed moderate activity in DPPH assay; however, they exhibited potent tocixity in brine shrimp lethality test.

Conclusion: The remarkable toxicity effects of the oils are worthy to further investigation to find the probable mechanisms of action accountable for the noticeable toxic effect of these essential oils.

Introduction

In many countries, the representatives of the genus *Elaeagnus* have been studied in order to produce natural material for nutrition, agriculture and pharmaceuticals. The genus *Elaeagnus*, an important member of Elaeagnaceae family, is widely distributed from the northern areas of Asia to the Himalayas, as well as Europe.[1,2] Although this genus consists of around 40 species in the world, it is only represented by two species in the flora of Iran including *Elaeagnus angustifolia* L. and *E. orientalis* with their common names of "silver berry, Russian olive, oleaster or oleander".[3,4] *E. angustifolia*, with its Persian name "Senjed", is a perennial deciduous tree or large multi-stemmed shrub with flexible branches that can reach 12 m in height. The leaves are alternate and petiolate and the whole leaves, stems, buds and fruits are densely covered by silvery scales. The flowers are fragrant, 3- to 12-mm long, with four-lobed creamy yellow calyx, in small axillary clusters. The plant also possesses the edible fruits which are berry-like or drupe-, oval-shaped, between 1 and 2 cm long as well as deep or extensive roots, with various well-developed laterals.[1,4-6] *E. angustifolia* have been used for centuries as a herbal remedies for the treatment of various diseases in Iran's traditional medicine.[7] Some of them were proven to exhibit anti-inflammatory,[1,8] muscle relaxant activity,[9] anti-ulcerogenic,[10] antimicrobial,[11-14] antinociceptive,[15,16] antitumor,[17,18] and antioxidant effects.[11,12,14,19-21] Likewise, the whole fruit and medulla powder of *E. angustifolia* showed positive effect in improving pain, stiffness and physical function in women with osteoarthritis of the knee.[22,23] In Azarbaijan province folk medicine, the fruit and flower preparations have been used for healing jaundice, asthma, flatulence, vomiting and nausea.[24] Phytochemical studies on different extracts from fruits and flowers of *E. angustifolia* indicated the presence of polysaccharides, flavonoids, coumarins, phenolcarboxylic acids, amino acids, saponins, carotenoids, vitamins, and tannins as secondary metabolites.[12,13,25] Besides mentioned secondary metabolites, this plant also contains volatile oils that may be useful as a source of nutrition or pharmaceutical compounds.[26-28] To the best of our knowledge, the essential oil composition of the Iranian *E. angustifolia*

***Corresponding author:** Fariba Heshmati Afshar, Emails: heshmatif@live.com, fariba.afshar@ubc.ca*

has not been investigated; therefore, based on the prevalent food and medicinal uses of this plant, the present study was conducted to analyze the chemical composition of the essential oils hydrodistilled from the leaves and flowers of *E. angustifolia* as well as their general toxicity and radical scavenging activities.

Materials and Methods
Plant Material
Flowers and leaves of *E. angustifolia* L. were collected from a garden near Toramin, Ilkhchi, Tabriz, East Azarbaijan province, Iran, in May 2015. The identity of the plant was botanically confirmed by morphological examination in comparison to the herbarium specimens. Voucher specimens (no: Tbz-fph-763) is deposited in the Herbarium of faculty of Pharmacy, Tabriz University of Medical Sciences, Tabriz, Iran.

Essential oil Isolation
The air-dried leaves and flowers of *E. angustifolia* L. (65 and 73 g, respectively) were separately submitted to hydro-distillation for 4 h, in a Clevenger type apparatus using hexane (2ml) as collector solvent. The pale yellow colored essential oils were dried over anhydrous sodium sulfate, and then the solvent was evaporated, and the oil stored in sealed vials before chemical analyses.

GC-MS and GC-FID analysis
The analysis of the essential oils were performed on a Shimadzu GCMS-QP5050A gas chromatograph coupled to a Mass Spectrometer detector (GC-MS) equipped with a fused methyl silicon DB-1 column (1% phenylmethylpolysiloxane, 60 m × 0.25 mm i.d., 0.25 μm film thickness), working with the following temperature program: 3 min at 50°C, subsequently at 3°C/min up to 270°C, and held for 4 min; Helium was used as carrier gas at a flow rate of 1.3 mL/min. The injector temperature was 250°C and split ratio was adjusted at 1:24. The injection volume was 1 μL. The transfer line temperature was 280°C. All mass spectra were acquired in electron-impact (EI) mode with an ionization voltage of 70 eV with other operating parameters as follow: ion source temperature 280°C; quadrupole temperature 100°C; solvent delay 8.0 min; resolution 2000 amu/s and scan time 78 min; scan range 30-600 amu; EM voltage 3000 volts. Moreover, flame ionization detector (FID) which was operated in ionization potential mode at 70 eV and used the same program reported above, was applied for quantification purpose for calculating the relative area percentage (area %) without the use of correction factors. The mixture of *n*-alkanes (C8-C20) was then injected using the above temperature program in order to calculate the retention indices of each volatile component.

Identification of the compounds
The components of the oils were identified based on GC retention times, retention indices relative to *n*-alkanes and computer matching with the NIST10, NIST 21, NIST 69 and Wiley 229 library data, as well as by comparison of the mass spectra with those reported in the literature.[29,30] Relative area percentages of the volatile constituents were obtained electronically from the GC-FID response without any correction factor.

Free-Radical-Scavenging Activity
The ability of the essential oils to scavenge radicals was assessed by the method based on the reduction of DPPH (molecular formula $C_{18}H_{12}N_5O_6$) solutions in the presence of a hydrogen donating antioxidant. DPPH (8 mg) was dissolved in chloroform (100 ml) to obtain a concentration of 80 μg/ml. The essential oil were dissolved in chloroform to provide a concentration of 1 mg/ml. Dilutions were made to obtain different concentrations of essential oils and then diluted solutions (5 ml each) were mixed with DPPH (5ml). After a 30 minute incubation period at room temperature, the absorbance was read against a blank at 517 nm with a Shimadzu UV/Visible Spectrophotometer 160A (USA). The percentage reduction was plotted against the sample oils concentration in order to calculate RC_{50} values which is the oil concentration providing 50% loss of DPPH activity. Trolox® was used as positive control and all tests were conducted in triplicate.[31,32]

General toxicity assay (Brine shrimp lethality test)
The general toxicity of the essential oils was evaluated by the brine shrimp lethality test presented by Meyer *et al.*[33] with some modifications.[34,35] Brine shrimps were hatched using brine shrimp eggs (*Artemia salina*, Sera brand, Aquarium and Fish shop, Khaghani Avenue, Tabriz, Iran) in a conical shaped vessel, filled with 200 mL filtered sterile seawater (Prepared from commercial sea salt, 38g/L, Aqua Marine, Thailand). The vessel was kept in a water bath (29-30°C) under a bright light and constant aeration for 48 hours. Stock solutions were prepared by dissolving essential oils in DMSO and diluted with seawater so that the final DMSO concentration did not exceed 1%. Seven different concentrations of essential oils were derived through serial dilution. After hatching, ten nauplii (hatched brine shrimp) were transferred to each test and control (containing DMSO and seawater) tubes. Then, the volume was adjusted with sterile seawater and the tubes were left uncovered under the lamp. Three replicates were prepared for each essential oil. After 24 h after introducing the shrimps, the number of dead and surviving nauplii in each tube were counted and recorded. LD_{50} values were determined from the best-fit line plotted concentration versus percentage lethality. Podophyllotoxin was used as a positive control.

Statistical analysis
All experiments were carried out in triplicate measurements and presented as the mean ± standard deviation. Data were analyzed by using Excel 2010 Microsoft. The RC_{50} and LD_{50} values were calculated from linear regression analysis.

Results and Discussion

The hydro-distillation from the flowers and leaves of *E. angustifolia* L. exuded pale yellow oils with a yield of 0.10% and 0.05% W/W, respectively, based on the dry mass. The list of the components in order of their elution from a DB-1 column, the percentage of the individual compounds and their retention indices are compiled in Table 1. A total of 53 volatile components were identified in the essential oil of the flowers, corresponding to 96.59% of the total oil while 3.41% of the essential oil remained unidentified. Oxygenated compounds especially aromatic esters (65.75%) had the highest contribution and represented 91.90% of the oil (Figure 1). The major components were E-ethyl cinnamate (60.00%), hexahydrofarnesyl acetone or phytone (9.99%), hexadecanoic acid or palmitic acid (5.20%) and phytol (3.29%). The remaining constituents (n=49) present in small quantities, most of them existing at contents lower than 3%. With respect to the leaves, 25 components were identified, accounting for 98.97% of the total oil. Also in this case oxygenated compounds furnished the major contribution of the oil (95.95%), with E-ethyl cinnamate (37.27%), phytol (12.08%), nonanal (10.74%) and Z-3-hexenyl benzoate (7.65%) as the most prevalent. Apart from the major volatiles reported about oil of leaves, only hexadecanoic acid (3.33%) and 9,12,15-octadecatrienal (5.43%) exceeded a content of 3% of the total oil, whilst the remaining volatiles (n=19) were present in low amounts. As depicted in Figure 1, among oxygen-containing components, esters were the most abundant by percentage of 65.75% and 49.12 % of the flowers and leaves oil, respectively. Conversely, the hydrocarbons were relatively poor and constituted 4.69% and 3.02%, respectively. To the best of our knowledge, the essential oil of Iranian *E. angustifolia* has so far never been studied, while there are a few studies about the chemical composition of the same species from other countries.[26-28] With respects to the previous investigation which considered the essential oil from flowers of *E. angustifolia* growing in Romania, limonene, anethol, E-ethyl cinnamate, 2-phenyl ethyl benzoate, 2-phenyl ethyl isovalerate, nerolidole, squalene and acetophenone were identified as the main components.[27] However, the oil studied in China in 2011 represented E-ethyl cinnamate (77.36%), (E)-2-methoxy-4-(1-propenyl) phenol (3.03%), acetal (2.70%), Z-ethyl cinnamate (1.09%) and ethyl benzenacetate (1.06%) as the main components.[28] According to the other report by Zhaolin et al, E-ethyl cinnamte (78.88%) constitutes the principle components of the flowers oil.[26] The comparison of our results with previous literatures shows remarkable similarities and also differences in terms of chemical composition of the flower oil. Presence of E-ethyl cinnamate as the principle constituent is the main similarity of the previous oils[26-28] with our examined flower oil (60.00%). Conversely, anethol, limonene, β-myrcene, squalene and acetophenone were detected at in considerable amounts in previous works,[14,27] whereas it was not found in our

tested sample. Moreover, it is notable that hexahydrofarnesyl acetone (phytone), palmitic acid and phytol were found at a relatively high level in our examined flower oil whereas it was not detected in considerable quantities in the oil of previous studies. A variety of factors such as geographical location, climatic condition, altitude, extraction methods and sample collection season might attribute in observed variations in the flower oils composition.[34,35] In regard to leaves, as shown in Table 1 and Figure 1, the essential oil was again characterized by E-ethyl cinnamate (37.27%), however, in this case, aliphatic alcohols and aldehyds reached higher levels in comparison with flowers by percentages of 12.80% and 21.73%, respectively. They were represented by phytol (12.08%) and nonanal (10.74%). The comparison of our results with literature exhibited remarkable differences in terms of chemical composition. According to the report by Incilay, l-limonen, β-myrcene and E-2-hexanal were the main components of leaves essential oil.[14]

The radical scavenging activity of the essential oils from flowers and leaves of *E. angostifolia* was evaluated using DPPH method. From results reported in Table 2, the both essential oils exhibited moderate radical scavenging activity with RC_{50} values of 3.48 ± 0.70 mg/ml (flower oil) and 1.50 ± 0.50 mg/ml (leaves) compared with the values reported for Trolox (0.002 ± 0.20 mg/ml) used as a reference. The more potent activity of the essential oil obtained from leaves can be related to the higher proportion of oxygenated compounds especially alcohols and aldehydes, known to possess antioxidant activity due to their O-atoms. The presence of a hydroxyl moiety on a hydrocarbon skeleton causes that the compound easily oxidizes and shows antioxidant properties; therefore, the possibility that the higher radical scavenging activity by the essential oil of leaves would be due to the presence of higher amount of phytol in leaves (12.08%) could not be excluded. Previous investigations demonstrated that phytol, as a natural linear diterpene alcohol, showed antioxidant activity in different assays[36,37] as well as it is utilized in manufactoring synthetic vitamins E and K.[38] The general toxicity of essential oils was assessed by brine shrimp lethality test which represent a quick, inexpensive and efficient method for evaluating extracts and essential oils toxicity and most of the time correlates fairly well with anti-proliferative and antitumor activities.[34,35] In this assay, compared with the positive control (Podophyllotoxin, LD_{50}= 2.69 ± 0.30 µg/ml) , the essential oils of flowers and leaves showed potent toxicity against brine shrimps with LD_{50} values of 2.25 ± 0.60 and 11.00 ± 5.19 µg/ml, respectively. As can be seen in Figure 2, the toxicity of the oils raised by increasing in the concentration of the essential oil and exposure duration. The general toxicity effects of flower oils were a little more potent than podophyllotoxin. As illustrated above, the essential oil of flowers and leaves are both noticeably rich in ester compounds especially E-ethyl cinnamate; hence, the potent toxicity activity of these oils might be ascribed to this compounds in high proportion. Preceding studies demonstrated that E-ethyl cinnamate revealed a remarkable insecticidal, nematocidal and antifeedant activities;[39-42] thus, the strong toxicity effect of flowers oil might be attributed to the presence of considerable amount of E-ethyl cinnamate. It is notable that oral and topical administration of extracts containing high amount of E-ethyl cinnamate caused neither fatality nor significant differences or irritation in the body;[40] so, it might be considered as a safe product for human beings or mammals when applied for insecticidal or anti fungal purposes.

Table 1. Composition of the essential oils isolated from the flowers and leaves of *E. angustifolia*

Compound name and class [a]	RI	Flowers (%)	Leaves (%)	Identification method [b]	Compound name and class [a]	RI	Flowers (%)	Leaves (%)	Identification method [b]
Heptanal	877	0.41	-	GC/MS, I$_b$	2-Hexyl-1-octanol	1669	0.19	-	GC/MS, I$_s$
Benzaldehyde	928	0.06	-	GC/MS, I$_s$	Hexadecanal(Palmitaldehyde)	1696	0.42	4.09	GC/MS, I$_s$
Benzeneacetaldehyde(Hyacinthin)	1007	0.25	-	GC/MS, I$_s$	2-Methylhexadecan-1-ol	1723	0.58	-	GC/MS, I$_s$
Nonanal	**1083**	**1.36**	**10.74**	GC/MS, I$_s$	Tetradecanoic acid (Myristic acid)	1744	0.36	-	GC/MS, I$_s$
Linalool	1185	-	0.17	GC/MS, I$_s$	n-Octadecane	1800	0.13	-	GC/MS, I$_s$
Decanal	1185	0.20	0.45	GC/MS, I$_s$	2-Phenylethyl benzoate	1819	0.39	1.89	GC/MS, I$_s$
4-Ethylphenyl acetate	1213	0.40	-	GC/MS, I$_s$	6,10,14-trimethyl-2-pentadecanone	1831	-	2.01	GC/MS, I$_s$
(-)-Myrtenyl acetate	1273	-	1.83	GC/MS, I$_s$	**Hexahydrofarnesyl acetone(phytone)**	**1835**	**9.99**	-	GC/MS, I$_s$
Undecanal	1287	0.35	-	GC/MS, I$_s$	1-Octadecene	1864	0.12	0.45	GC/MS, I$_s$
Theaspirane A	1293	-	0.99	GC/MS, I$_s$	9,12,15-Octadecatrienal	1869	0.22	5.43	GC/MS, I$_s$
Theaspirane B	1307	-	0.98	GC/MS, I$_s$	Farnesyl acetone	1895	0.16	-	GC/MS, I$_s$
Ethyl dihydrocinnamate	1319	0.08	-	GC/MS, I$_s$	n-Nonadecane	1900	0.21	0.54	GC/MS, I$_s$
Methyl cinnamate	1352	1.38	-	GC/MS, I$_s$	9-Hexadecenoic acid	1921	0.40	-	GC/MS, I$_s$
E-β-Damascenone	1364	0.17	0.72	GC/MS, I$_s$	**Hexadecanoic acid (Palmitic acid)**	**1950**	**5.20**	3.33	GC/MS, I$_s$
n-Decanoic acid	1366	0.07	-	GC/MS, I$_s$	Hexadecanoic acid, ethyl ester	1978	0.22	-	GC/MS, I$_s$
n-Dodecanal (Lauraldehyde)	1389	0.23	-	GC/MS, I$_f$	E-15-Heptadecenal	2104	0.1	-	GC/MS, I$_f$
Trimethyl-tetrahydronaphthalene	1398	0.4	-	GC/MS, I$_s$	**Phytol**	**2108**	**3.29**	**12.08**	GC/MS, I$_s$
β-Caryophyllene	1420	-	2.14	GC/MS, I$_s$	Methyl linolenate	2117	1.11	-	GC/MS, I$_s$
Neryl acetone	1430	-	0.73	GC/MS, I$_s$	9-Octadecenoic acid (Oleic acid)	2146	0.37	-	GC/MS, I$_s$
E-Ethyl cinnamate	**1435**	**60.00**	**37.27**	GC/MS, I$_s$	(E)-Ethyl- 9-octadecenoate	2151	1.06	-	GC/MS, I$_s$
Oxacyclotetradeca-4,11-diyne	1457	0.47	-	GC/MS, I$_s$	Octadecanoic acid, ethyl ester	2177	0.13	-	GC/MS, I$_s$
2,3,5,8-tetramethyl-decane	1461	0.16	-	GC/MS, I$_s$	Docosane	2200	0.18	-	GC/MS, I$_b$
β- Ionone	1466	-	1.80	GC/MS, I$_s$	1-Docosene	2271	0.47	-	GC/MS, I$_b$
4,6-Dimethyl-dodecane	1468	1.77	-	GC/MS, I$_s$	n-Tricosane	2300	0.37	-	GC/MS, I$_b$
Germacrene D	1483	0.1	-	GC/MS, I$_s$	Eicosanoic acid, ethyl ester	2339	0.1	-	GC/MS, I$_b$
Tridecanal	1493	0.32	-	GC/MS, I$_s$	1-Docosanol (Behenic alcohol)	2388	0.7	-	GC/MS, I$_b$
γ-Cadinene	1517	-	0.34	GC/MS, I$_s$	n-Pentacosane	2500	0.12	-	GC/MS, I$_b$
Isobutylcinnammate	1540	0.68		GC/MS, I$_s$	n-Heptacosane	2700	0.51	-	GC/MS, I$_b$
Z-3-Hexenyl benzoate	**1546**	**0.12**	**7.65**	GC/MS, I$_s$	n-Octacosane	2800	0.15	-	GC/MS, I$_b$
Nerolidole B	1550	0.20	-	GC/MS, I$_s$					
2-Phenylethyl tiglate	1555	0.28	0.52	GC/MS, I$_s$	Total compounds		53	25	
(+)- Spathulenol	1568	-	0.55	GC/MS, I$_s$	Total identified		96.59	98.97	
Caryophyllene oxide	1575	-	1.70	GC/MS, I$_s$	Not identified		3.41	1.03	
Tetradecanal (Myristaldehyde)	1594	**0.08**	0.57	GC/MS, I$_s$	Hydrocarbons		4.69	3.02	
Elemicin	1613	0.08	-	GC/MS, I$_s$	Oxygenated compounds		91.9	95.95	

a) Compounds are listed in order of their elution from a DB-1 column. Their nomenclature is in accordance with Adams [29]. b) Identification Method (Is = Kovats retention indices as determined on DB-1 column using homologous series of C$_8$-C$_{20}$, Ib = Kovats retention indices according to Literature published by Adams [29] and/or listed in the NIST08 mass-spectral library [30].

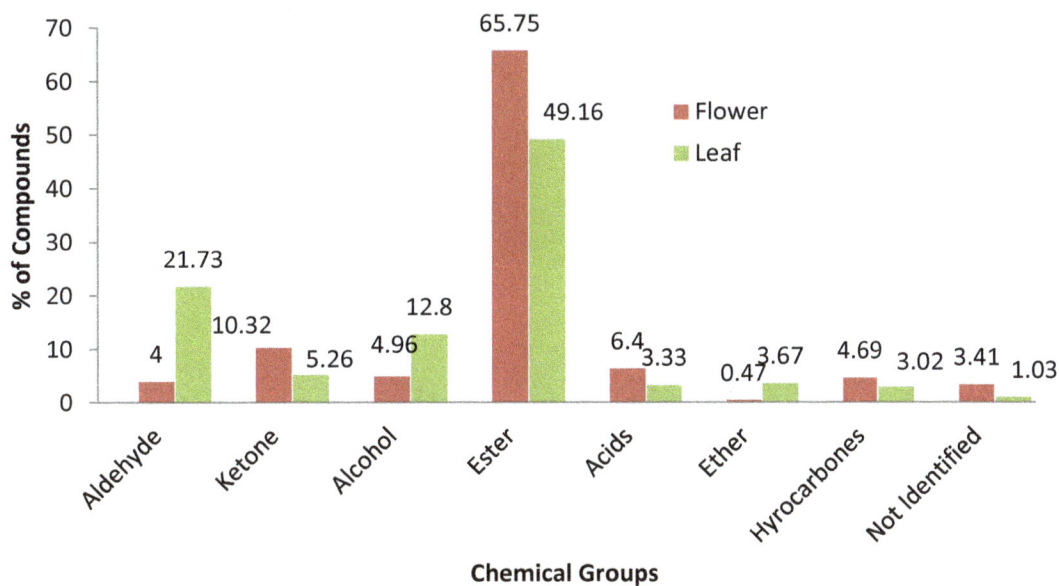

Figure 1. Identified chemical groups from the essential oils of the flowers and leaves of *Elaeagnus angustifolia* L.

Table 2. Radical scavenging and general toxicity activities of the essential oils obtained from leaves and flowers of *E. angustifolia* L.

	DPPH assay (RC$_{50}$, mg/ml)	General toxicity (LD$_{50}$, μg/ml)
Essential oil of flowers	3.48 ± 0.70	2.25 ± 0.60
Essential oil of leaves	1.50 ± 0.50	11.00 ± 5.19
Trolox®	0.002 ± 0.20	-
Podophyllotoxin	-	2.69 ± 0.30

RC$_{50}$, the concentration of compound that affords a 50% reduction in the assay, LD$_{50}$, the required dose of compound that kills 50% of a population of brine shrimps

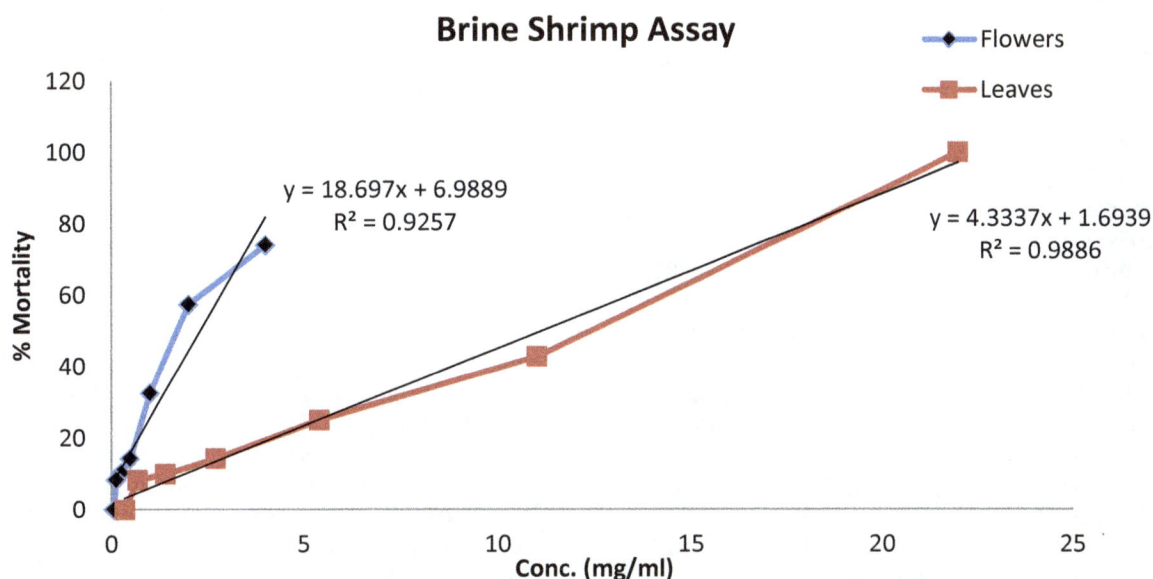

Figure 2. Brine shrimp lethality assay of the essential oils obtained from the flowers and leaves of *Elaeagnus angustifolia* L. against *Artemia salina*

Conclusion

To sum up, the present study reported the chemical profile of the essential oils obtained from the leaves and flowers of Iranian *E. angustifolia* for the first time, and also assessed the radical scavenging and general toxicity activities of the oils. On the basis of the chemical composition and bioactivity results, we can declare that the oils of this plant might be considered as preservative agents in food industry as well as natural insecticides in agriculture.

Acknowledgments

This study was financially supported by grant no. 5.97.516 from Faculty of Nutrition, Tabriz University of Medical Sciences, Tabriz, Iran.

Ethical Issues

Not applicable.

Conflict of Interest

The authors report no conflicts of interest.

References

1. Ahmadiani A, Hosseiny J, Semnanian S, Javan M, Saeedi F, Kamalinejad M, et al. Antinociceptive and anti-inflammatory effects of *Elaeagnus angustifolia* fruit extract. *J Ethnopharmacol* 2000;72(1-2):287-92. doi: 10.1016/S0378-8741(00)00222-1

2. Zargari A. Medicinal Plant. Vol. 1. Iran: Tehran University Press; 1990.

3. Mozaffarian V. Trees and shrubs of Iran. 1st ed. Iran: Tehran, Farhang Moaser; 2004.

4. Mozaffarian V. A dictionary of Iranian plant names. 5th ed. Iran: Tehran, Farhang Moaser; 2007.

5. Klich MG. Leaf variations in *Elaeagnus angustifolia* related to environmental heterogeneity. *Environ Exp Bot* 2000;44(3):171-83. doi: 10.1016/s0098-8472(00)00056-3

6. Ayaz FA, Bertoft E. Sugar and phenolic acid composition of stored commercial oleaster fruits. *J Food Compost Anal* 2001;14(5):505-11. doi: 10.1006/jfca.2001.1004

7. Mehrabani Natanzi M, Pasalar P, Kamalinejad M, Dehpour AR, Tavangar SM, Sharifi R, et al. Effect of Aqueous Extract of *Elaeagnus angustifolia* Fruit on Experimental Cutaneous Wound Healing in Rats. *Acta Med Iran* 2012;50(9):589-96.

8. Farahbakhsh SH, Arbabian S, Emami F, Moghadam BR, Ghoshooni H, Noroozzadeh A, et al. Inhibition of cyclooxygenase type 1 and 2 enzyme by aqueous extract of *Elaeagnus angustifolia* in mice. *Basic Clin Neurosci* 2011;2(2):31-7.

9. Hosseinzadeh H, Ramezani M, Namjo N. Muscle relaxant activity of *Elaeagnus angustifolia* L. fruit seeds in mice. *J Ethnopharmacol* 2003;84(2-3):275-8. doi: 10.1016/S0378-8741(02)00331-8

10. Khodakarm-Tafti A, Mehrabani D, Homafar L, Farjanikish G. Healing effects of *Elaeagnus angustifolia* extract in experimentally induced ulcerative colitis in rats. *J Pharmacol Toxicol* 2015;10(1):29-35. doi: 10.3923/jpt.2015.29.35

11. Okmen G, Turkcan O. A study on antimicrobial, antioxidant and antimutagenic activities of *Elaeagnus angustifolia* L. leaves. *Afr J Tradit Complement Altern Med* 2014;11(1):116-20. doi: 10.4314/ajtcam.v11i1.17

12. Farzaei MH, Bahramsoltani R, Abbasabadi Z, Rahimi R. A comprehensive review on phytochemical and pharmacological aspects of *Elaeagnus angustifolia* L. *J Pharm Pharmacol* 2015;67(11):1467-80. doi: 10.1111/jphp.12442

13. Okmen G, Turkcan O. The antibacterial activity of *Elaeagnus angustifolia* L. against mastitis pathogens and antioxidant capacity of the leaf methanolic extracts. *J Anim Vet Adv* 2013;12(4):491-6. doi: 10.3923/javaa.2013.491.496

14. Incilay G. Volatile composition, antimicrobial and antioxidant properties of different parts from *Elaeagnus angustifolia* L. *J Essent Oil Bear Plants* 2014;17(6):1187-202. doi: 10.1080/0972060X.2014.929044

15. Ramezani M, Hosseinzadeh H, Daneshmand N. Antinociceptive effect of *Elaeagnus angustifolia* fruit seeds in mice. *Fitoterapia* 2001;72(3):255-62. doi: 10.1016/S0367-326X(00)00290-2

16. Karimi G, Hosseinzadeh H, Rassoulzadeh M, Razavi BM, Taghiabadi E. Antinociceptive effect of *Elaeagnus angustifolia* fruits on sciatic nerve ligated mice. *Iran J Basic Med Sci* 2010;13(3):97-101.

17. Ya W, Shang-Zhen Z, Chun-Meng Z, Tao G, Jian-Ping M, Ping Z, et al. Antioxidant and antitumor effect of different fractions of ethyl acetate part from *Elaeagnus angustifolia* L. *Adv J Food Sci Technol* 2014;6(5):707-10.

18. Wang Y, Fan M, Li J, Guo T. Antitumor effect of edible part of *Elaeagnus angustifolia* L. in vivo and in vitro. *J Chin Inst Food Sci Technol* 2013;13(6):26-31.

19. Yalcin G, Sogut O. Antioxidant capacity of *Elaeagnus angustifolia* L. and investigation of eosin y as the fluorescent probe in ORAC method. *J Food Agric Environ* 2014;12(2):51-4.

20. Cansev A, Sahan Y, Celik G, Taskesen S, Ozbey H. Chemical properties and antioxidant capacity of *Elaeagnus angustifolia* L. Fruits. *Asian J Chem* 2011;23(6):2661-5.

21. Caliskan E, Elmastas M, Gokce I. Evaluation of antioxidant properties of *Elaeagnus angustifolia* flowers. *Asian J Chem* 2010;22(4):2840-8.

22. Ebrahimi AA, Nikniaz Z, Ostadrahimi A, Mahdavi R, Nikniaz L. The effect of *Elaeagnus angustifolia* L. whole fruit and medulla powder on women with osteoarthritis of the knee: A randomized controlled clinical trial. *Eur J Integr Med* 2014;6(6):672-9. doi: 10.1016/j.eujim.2014.07.016

23. Nikniaz Z, Ostadrahimi A, Mahdavi R, Ebrahimi AA, Nikniaz L. Effects of *Elaeagnus angustifolia* L. supplementation on serum levels of inflammatory

cytokines and matrix metalloproteinases in females with knee osteoarthritis. *Complement Ther Med* 2014;22(5):864-9. doi: 10.1016/j.ctim.2014.07.004

24. Asadiar LS, Rahmani F, Siami A. Assessment of genetic diversity in the Russian olive (*Elaeagnus angustifolia*) based on ISSR genetic markers. *Rev Cienc Agron* 2012;44(2):310-16. doi: 10.1590/S1806-66902013000200013

25. Abizov EA, Tolkachev ON, Mal'tsev SD, Abizova EV. Composition of biologically active substances isolated from the fruits of Russian olive (*Elaeagnus angustifolia*) introduced in the European part of Russia. *Pharm Chem J* 2008;42(12):696-8. doi: 10.1007/s11094-009-0203-5

26. Zhaolin L, Ning C, Dunyuan X, Haiquan L, Yaozu C. Study on Chemical Constituents of Volatile Oil of Fresh Flowers of *Elaeagnus angustifolia* L. *Chem J Chin Univ* 1989;10(8):804-8.

27. Bucur L, Stanciu G, Istudor V. The GC-MS analysis of *Elaeagnus angustifolia* L. flowers essential oil. *Rev Chim* 2007;58(11):1027-9.

28. Qiao HJ ,Yang JT, Yang X, Zhao LB, Li TH. GC-MS analysis of chemical composition of volatile oil from flowers of *Elaeagnus angustifolia* L. *Food Sci* 2011;32(16):233-5.

29. Adams RP. Identification of Essential Oil Components by Gas Chromatography/Mass Spectroscopy. Carol Stream, Ill. : Allured Pub. Corp; 2001.

30. NIST 08. Mass spectral library (NIST/EPA/NIH). Gaithersburg, MD: National Institute of Standards and Technology; 2008.

31. Afshar FH, Delazar A, Janneh O, Nazemiyeh H, Pasdaran A, Nahar L, et al. Evaluation of antimalarial, free-radical-scavenging and insecticidal activities of *Artemisia scoparia* and *A. spicigera*, Asteraceae. *Braz J Pharmacog* 2011;21(6):986-90. doi: 10.1590/S0102-695X2011005000144

32. Takao T, kitatani F, Watanabe N, Yagi I, Sakata K. A Simple Screening Method for Antioxidants and Isolation of Several Antioxidants Produced by Marine Bacteria from Fish and Shellfish. *Biosci Biotechnol Biochem* 1994;58(10):1780-3. doi: 10.1271/bbb.58.1780

33. Meyer BN, Ferrigni NR, Putnam JE, Jacobsen LB, Nichols DE, McLaughlin JL. Brine Shrimp: A Convenient General Bioassay for Active Plant Constituents. *Planta Med* 1982;45(5):31-4. doi: 10.1055/s-2007-971236

34. Mojarrab M, Delazar A, Esnaashari S, Heshmati Afshar F. Chemical composition and general toxicity of essential oils extracted from the aerial parts of *Artemisia armeniaca* Lam. and *A. incana* (L.) Druce growing in Iran. *Res Pharm Sci* 2013;8(1):65-9.

35. Nikbakht MR, Esnaashari S, Heshmati Afshar F. Chemical composition and general toxicity of essential oil extracted from the stalks and flowers of *Rheum ribes* L. growing in Iran. *J Rep Pharm Sci* 2013;2(2):76-81.

36. Miguel MG. Antioxidant and anti-inflammatory activities of essential oils: A short review. *Molecules* 2010;15(12):9252-87. doi: 10.3390/molecules15129252

37. Venditti A, Bianco A, Nicoletti M, Quassinti L, Bramucci M, Lupidi G, et al. Characterization of secondary metabolites, biological activity and glandular trichomes of *Stachys tymphaea* HAUSSKN. from the Monti Sibillini National Park (Central Apennines, Italy). *Chem Biodivers* 2014;11(2):245-61. doi: 10.1002/cbdv.201300253

38. Maggi F, Tirillini B, Vittori S, Sagratini G, Papa F. Analysis of the Volatile Components of *Onosma echioides* (L.) L. var. columnae Lacaita Growing in Central Italy. *J Essent Oil Res* 2009;21(5):441-7. doi: 10.1080/10412905.2009.9700213

39. Abdelgaleil SA, Abbassy MA, Belal AS, Abdel Rasoul MA. Bioactivity of two major constituents isolated from the essential oil of *Artemisia judaica* L. *Bioresour Technol* 2008;99(13):5947-50. doi: 10.1016/j.biortech.2007.10.043

40. Choi IH, Park JY, Shin SC, Park IK. Nematicidal activity of medicinal plant extracts and two cinnamates isolated from *Kaempferia galanga* L. (Proh Hom) against the pine wood nematode, *Bursaphelenchus xylophilus*. *Nematology* 2006;8(3):359-65. doi: 10.1163/156854106778493402

41. Park IK, Park JY, Kim KH, Choi KS, Chio IH, Kim CS, et al. Nematicidal activity of plant essential oils and components from garlic (*Allium sativum*) and cinnamon (*Cinnamomum verum*) oils against the pine wood nematode (*Bursaphelenchus xylophilus*). *Nematology* 2005;7(5):767-74. doi: 10.1163/156854105775142946

42. Oka Y, Nacar S, Putievsky E, Ravid U, Yaniv Z, Spiegel Y. Nematicidal activity of essential oils and their components against the root-knot nematode. *Phytopathology* 2000;90(7):710-15. doi: 10.1094/PHYTO.2000.90.7.710

2

Pharmacological Properties of *Vochysia Haenkeana* (Vochysiaceae) Extract to Neutralize the Neuromuscular Blockade Induced by Bothropstoxin-I (Lys49 Phospholipase A₂) Myotoxin

Carolina Harder[1], Akila Lara de Oliveira[2], Andreia Borges Scriboni[3], Adélia Cristina Oliveira Cintra[4], Raphael Schezaro-Ramos[5], Márcio Galdino dos Santos[6], Karina Cogo-Müller[7], Regina Yuri Hashimoto Miura[1], Rafael Stuani Floriano[5], Sandro Rostelato-Ferreira[1], Yoko Oshima-Franco[2]*

[1] *Institute of Health Sciences, Universidade Paulista (Unip), Av. Independência 210, 18087-100, Sorocaba, SP, Brazil.*

[2] *University of Sorocaba (Uniso), Rodovia Raposo Tavares km 92.5, 18023-000, Sorocaba, SP, Brazil.*

[3] *Department of Pharmacology, Piracicaba Dental School, State University of Campinas (UNICAMP), Av. Limeira 901, 13414-903, Piracicaba, SP, Brazil.*

[4] *Faculty of Pharmaceutical Sciences, Department of Clinical and Toxicological Analysis and Bromatology, São Paulo University (USP), Via do Café S/N, 14040-903, Ribeirão Preto, SP, Brazil.*

[5] *Department of Pharmacology, Faculty of Medical Sciences, State University of Campinas (UNICAMP), Rua Tessália Vieira de Camargo 126, 13083-887, Campinas, SP, Brazil.*

[6] *Tocantins Federal University (UFT), Av. NS 15, ALC NO14, 109 Norte, 77001-090, Palmas, TO, Brazil.*

[7] *Faculty of Pharmaceutical Sciences, State University of Campinas (UNICAMP), Rua Cândido Portinari, 200, 13083-871, Campinas, SP, Brazil.*

Keywords:
· Antimicrobial activity
· Antiophidian activity
· Bothropstoxin-I
· Myotoxicity
· Neurotoxicity
· *V. haenkeana* extract

Abstract

Purpose: *Bothrops* snakes are responsible for more than 70 % of snakebites every year in Brazil and their venoms cause severe local and systemic damages. The pharmacological properties of medicinal plants have been widely investigated in order to discover new alternative treatments for different classes of diseases including neglected tropical diseases as envenomation by snakebites. In this work, we have investigated the ability of *Vochysia haenkeana* stem barks extract (VhE) to neutralize the neuromuscular effects caused by Bothropstoxin-I (BthTX-I), the major phospholipase A₂ (PLA₂) myotoxin from *B. jararacussu* venom.

Methods: The biological compounds of VhE were analysed under thin layer chromatography (TLC) and its neutralizing ability against BthTX-I was assessed through twitch-tension recordings and histological analysis in mouse phrenic nerve-diaphragm (PND) preparations. The antimicrobial activity of VhE was assessed against *S. aureus, E. coli* and *P. aeruginosa* strains. The aggregation activity of VhE was analysed under protein precipitation assay.

Results: VhE showed the presence of phenolic compound visualized by blue trace under TLC. VhE abolished the neuromuscular blockade caused by BthTX-I applying the pre-toxin incubation treatment and partially neutralized the BthTX-I action under post-toxin incubation treatment; VhE contributed slightly to decrease the myotoxicity induced by BthTX-I. The neutralizing mechanism of VhE may be related to protein aggregation. VhE showed no antimicrobial activity.

Conclusion: *V. haenkeana* extract which has no antimicrobial activity exhibited neutralizing ability against the neuromuscular blockade caused by BthTX-I and also contributed to decrease its myotoxicity. Protein aggregation involving phenolic compounds may be related in these protective effects.

Introduction

In Brazil, *Bothrops* snakes comprise more than 30 species distributed throughout the country and they are responsible for approximately 70 % of snakebites every year; the World Health Organization (WHO) has considered snakebites as a neglected tropical disease due to the numerous cases and difficulties in specific regions to reach antivenom therapy.[1-5]

Bothrops venoms induce severe local and systemic damages due to their high enzymatic action basically mediated by proteases and phospholipases A₂ (PLA₂).[6,7]

In envenomation by *Bothrops* venoms, the local effects

---

*Corresponding author: Yoko Oshima-Franco, Email: yoko.franco@prof.uniso.br

are marked by intense necrosis accompanied by edema, equimosis and acute inflammatory activity. In addition, local infections caused by gram-negative anaerobic bacteria derived from oral flora of snakes are considered an important clinical complication in victims of snakebites.[4,8] Snakebites are conventionally treated through antivenom serum therapy; however, based on popular practices, the pharmacological properties of medicinal plants have been widely investigated in order to discover new alternative treatments for different classes of diseases including neglected tropical diseases as envenomation by snakebites.[9] Recent investigations have shown that plant extracts exhibit antimicrobial and antiophidian activities.[10-12]

Bothrops jararacussu snake, popularly known as Jararacuçu, is widely distributed in Southeast region of Brazil[6] and its venom is composed by enzymatic and non-enzymatic proteins, carbohydrates, peptides, lipids, biogenic amines and inorganic components, similarly to other *Bothrops* venoms.[13] Bothropstoxin-I (BthTX-I) is a non-enzymatic Lys49 PLA_2 isolated from *B. jararacussu* venom which induces irreversible neuromuscular blockade in vertebrate neuromuscular preparations *in vitro* characterized by intense myonecrosis, increase in creatine kinase release, muscle contracture and membrane depolarization.[14-17]

Vochysia haenkeana (Vochysiaceae), plant popularly known in Brazil as "escorrega-macaco", "pau-amarelo" and/or "cambarazinho", comes from semidecidual broadleaf forest common in Mato Grosso do Sul, Mato Grosso and Goiás Brazilian States; *V. haenkeana* exhibits a great variety of secondary metabolites such as tannins, saponins, phenolic compounds, flavonoids and coumarins and it has been cited in ethnobotanical studies related to treatment of respiratory diseases.[18-20] However, its pharmacological activities have been poorly investigated.[21]

In this work, we have assessed the neutralizing ability of *V. haenkeana* hydroalcoholic extract against the main PLA_2-myotoxin (BthTX-I) from *B. jararacussu* venom in mouse nerve-diaphragm preparations and its antimicrobial activity against *Staphyloccus aureus*, *Escherichia coli* and *Pseudomonas aeruginosa* strains.

Materials and Methods
Reagents and BthTX-I
All salts for the physiological solution were of analytical grade. BthTX-I was provided by Dra Adélia Cristina Oliveira Cintra from São Paulo University (USP, Ribeirão Preto, SP, Brazil).

Animals
Male Swiss mice (25–30 g) obtained from Multidisciplinary Center for Biological Investigation (CEMIB/Unicamp) were housed at a maximum of 10 mice per cage at 23 °C on a 12 h light/dark cycle. The animals had free access to food and water *ad libitum*.

Plant material
The hydroalcoholic extract from stem barks of *V. haenkeana* was provided by Dr Márcio Galdino dos Santos from Tocantins Federal University (UFT, Palmas, TO, Brazil). The full description about the origin of the extract has been shown elsewhere.[18] The plant exsiccate was deposited in the Herbarium of the Tocantins Federal University (UFT, Porto Nacional, TO, Brazil) as voucher specimen #10.074 by Solange de Fátima Lolis according to the International Code of Botanical Nomenclature (ICBN).

Solubilisation of V. haenkeana extract
In order to find out the ideal solvent for *V. haenkeana* extract (VhE) without affecting the basal twitch responses recorded in mammalian nerve-muscle preparations, polyethylene glycol 400 (PEG 400, Synth®), dimethyl sulfoxide (DMSO, Sigma®) and ethanol (Synth®) were selected to be tested. Ethanol (30 μL) showed be the best solvent to solubilize VhE; ethanol 70 % did not change the twitch responses in control experiments recorded from mouse phrenic nerve-diaphragm (PND) preparations.[22]

Thin layer chromatography (TLC)
For TLC, it was used aluminium plates coated with silica gel 60 (0.20 mm thick) containing the fluorescent indicator UV254 (Macherey-Nagel GmbH & Co., Bethlehem, PA, USA) and phytochemical standard in methanol (1 %) (Sigma-Aldrich Co., St. Louis, MO, USA) including quercetin (1), rutin (2), caffeic acid (3), tannic acid (4), coumarin (5), gallic acid (6) and VhE (7); a purposeful empty lane was maintained for observing the solvent race (8). The solvent system (mobile phase, 10 mL) consisted of ethyl acetate, formic acid, acetic acid and water (100:11:11:27), as described elsewhere.[23] The chromatograms were initially stained with diphenylboric acid 2-aminoethyl ester solution (5 % in ethanol) (Sigma-Aldrich Co., St. Louis, MO, USA) followed by polyethylene glycol 4000 solution (5 % in ethanol) (Sigma-Aldrich Co., St. Louis, MO, USA), with visualization under UV light at 360 nm. The retention factor (*Rf*) and sample colours were visually compared to phytochemical standards.

Antimicrobial activity of VhE
The following bacterial strains were purchased from American Type Culture Collection (ATCC): *Escherichia coli* ATCC 25922, *E. coli* ATCC 10536, *Pseudomonas aeruginosa* ATCC 25922, *S. aureus* ATCC 29213, methicillin-resistant *S. aureus* (MRSA) ATCC 33591, and methicillin/oxacillin resistant *S. aureus* (MRSA/ORSA) ATCC 43300. The cultures were stored at -80 °C in Tryptic soy broth (TSB; Difco Laboratories, Detroit MI, USA) containing 40 % (v/v) glycerol and were routinely cultured in Tryptic soy agar (TSA; Difco Laboratories) under aerobic conditions at 37 °C.
Antimicrobial activity of the extract was tested by using the broth microdilution method according to the guidelines

from the Clinical and Laboratory Standards Institute (CLSI), protocol M07-A9. Briefly, four to five colonies were harvested from pure cultures growing on TSA and were used to prepare a bacterial inoculum. Colonies were transferred into tubes containing 5 mL of TSB and cultured at 37 °C until reaching turbidity equivalent to 0.1 at 660 nm (approximately 1.5×10^8 CFU/mL). Two-fold dilutions of the VhE (from 1000 to 0.4 μg/mL) were made in 96-well plates with 100 μL of Mueller Hinton Broth (MHB; Difco) per well. Then, the bacterial suspension (100 μL) was inoculated, and the plates were incubated for 24 h at 37 °C. The lowest concentration with any visible bacterial growth was taken as the minimum inhibitory concentration (MIC). In addition, bacterial growth was assessed by optical density measurement (660 nm).

Mouse phrenic nerve-diaphragm (PND) preparation
PND preparations were obtained from male Swiss mice killed with isoflurane (Fortvale®, Vinhedo, SP, Brazil). The preparations were mounted under a resting tension of 5 g in a 5 mL organ bath containing aerated (95 % O_2/5 % CO_2) Tyrode solution (composition, in mM: NaCl 137, KCl 2.7, $CaCl_2$ 1.8, $MgCl_2$ 0.49, NaH_2PO_4 0.42, $NaHCO_3$ 11.9 and glucose 11.1, pH 7.0) at 37 °C as described elsewhere.[24] The preparations were stimulated indirectly (5–7 V, 0.1 Hz, 0.2 ms) with supramaximal stimuli being delivered from a stimulator (Model ESF-15D, Ribeirão Preto, SP, Brazil) via bipolar electrodes positioned on the nerve. Muscle twitches were recorded using a force displacement transducer coupled to a two-channel Gemini recorder (both from Ugo Basile®, Varese, Italy). After stabilization for 20 min, VhE and BthTX-I (a single concentration per experiment) was added to the preparations and left in contact for 120 min or until complete blockade. For neutralization assays, we applied two types of protocols, as suggested elsewhere:[25] 1) pre-toxin incubation; BthTX-I was maintained under incubation with VhE for 30 min before twitch tension experiments) and 2) post-toxin incubation (VhE was added into the recording chamber 10 min later than BthTX-I).

Protein precipitation measurement
The protein precipitation induced by VhE extract was evaluated as previously described elsewhere.[26,27] Albumin and BthTX-I (10 μg) was incubated separately with VhE (150 μg) following the protocols: 1) pre-toxin incubation with VhE: BthTX-I (50 μg/mL) was maintained under incubation with VhE (0.4 mg/mL) for 30 min at room temperature (23-25 °C) and then for 60 min at 37 °C; 2) without pre-toxin incubation with VhE: BthTX-I (50 μg/mL) was maintained incubated with VhE (0.4 mg/mL) for 60 min directly at 37 °C. In both of protocols, the mixture was centrifuged at 5,000 rpm for 15 min and the protein concentration in supernatant was measured as essentially described elsewhere.[28] The absorbance obtained was compared with tubes containing only protein (albumin or BthTX-I) to assess the % of protein precipitation. Ethanol (solvent for VhE)

was tested alone to verify its influence on the protein precipitation. Tubes containing the same amount of VhE or ethanol, in absence of albumin or BthTX-I, were used as blanks.

Quantitative histological study
The preparations from the preincubation and post toxin assays were analysed by a quantitative morphometric method and compared to Tyrode control, VhE and BthTX-I. At the end of each experiment (after 120 min), three preparations of each group were fixed by a formalin 10 % solution, and processed by routine morphological techniques. Cross-sections (5 μm thick) of diaphragm muscle were stained with 0.5 % (w/v) hematoxylin-eosin, for microscopy examination. Tissue damage (edema, intense myonecrosis characterized by atrophy of the muscle fibers, hyaline aspect, sarcolemmal disruption and lysis of the myofibrils) was verified by three different trained people and it was expressed as a myotoxicity index (MI), i.e., the percentage of damaged muscle cells number divided by the total number of cells in three non-overlapping, non-adjacent areas of each preparation.[29]

Statistical analysis
Changes in the twitch-tension responses of PND preparations were expressed as a percentage relative to baseline (time zero) values and morphological alterations measured based on myotoxicity index (MI, in %). The results were expressed as the mean ± SEM and statistical comparisons were done using Student's t-test with $p < 0.05$ indicating significance. All data analyses were done using Microcal Origin 8 SR4 v.8.0951 (Microcal Software Inc., Northampton, MA, USA) software.

Results and Discussion
Based on popular medicinal practices, stem barks from *Vochysia haenkeana* (a plant variety of the Vochysiaceae family widely distributed in semidecidual broadleaf forest from west central region of Brazil) has been selected in this work to be investigated in terms of its neutralizing ability against the effects induced by snake venoms and antimicrobial activity. *V. haenkeana* is popularly known as "escorrega-macaco" and shows long plump trunk and smooth barks.

V. haenkeana contains secondary metabolites such as tannins, saponins, phenolic compounds, flavonoids and coumarins.[21] Here, we selected a sample *V. haenkeana* extract (VhE) to be subjected to Thin Layer Chromatography which revealed the presence of phenolic compounds characterized by a blue spot not matched with caffeic, tannic nor gallic acids; a weak yellow spot (indicated by an arrow) can be also seen in the chromatogram profile suggesting the presence of flavonoids not related to quercetin or rutin (Figure 1).

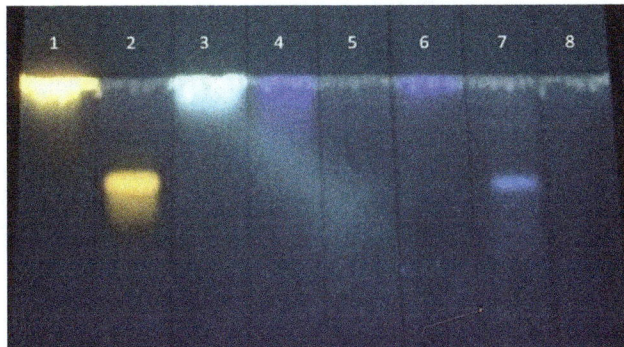

Figure 1. Thin layer chromatography (TLC) of phytochemical standards [quercetin (1), rutin (2), caffeic acid (3), tannic acid (4), coumarin (5), gallic acid (6), VhE (7) and solvent alone (8)]. Solvent: ethyl acetate, formic acid, acetic acid and water (100:11:11:27, respectively). Stain: NP – diphenylboric acid 2-aminoethyl ester, PEG – polyethylene glycol 4000. Arrow: yellow spot weekly revealed indicating an eventual presence of flavonoids in VhE.

We have not observed the presence of coumarin in VhE under TLC system; our data were inconclusive to justify the involvement of this compound eventually present in VhE with treatment of respiratory diseases, as suggested by popular practices.[19,20] However, it has already shown that commercial coumarin alone does not protect the neuromuscular blockade induced by *B. jararacussu* or *Crotalus durissus terrificus* venoms *in vitro*.[30] Orange and blue compounds visualized by TLC in plant extracts are suggestive of flavonoids and polyphenol compounds. Oshima-Franco and Dal Belo[31] reviewed antineurotoxic polyphenol plants, such as: *Camellia sinensis* L., *Casearia sylvestris* Sw., *Casearia gossypiosperma* Briquet, *Curcuma zedoaroides* A. Chaveerach & T. Tanee, *Dipteryx alata* Vogel, *Galactia glaucescens* Kunth., *Hypericum brasiliense* Choisy, *Jatropha elliptica* (Pohl) Oken., *Mikania laevigata* Sch. Bip. ex Baker, *Plathymenia reticulata* Benth., *Terminalia fagifolia* Mart., and *Vellozia flavicans* Mart. ex Schult. As showed in this work, *V. haenkeana* also has *in vitro* antineurotoxic effect, by an *in vitro* interaction.

Vochysia haenkeana has been poorly studied and its pharmacological properties are still unknown and need to be further explored. It has been shown that VhE does exhibit antitumoral activity in rats with induced Erlich tumor.[18] In addition, our data have shown that VhE also does not promote antimicrobial action against *S. aureus*, *E. coli* and *P. aeruginosa* strains. Investigations about antimicrobial activities of plant extracts associated to local effects induced by snake venoms show potentially useful to indicate alternative methods to treat snakebites since infections caused by bacteria from snake's mouth is often associated to snakebites.[32]

Before subjecting VhE to neutralization assays in PND preparations, we have verified whether the extract by itself could cause changes in twitch responses; a concentration-response experiment was carried out using 0.2, 0.4 and 0.8 mg of VhE/mL; the concentrations of 0.2 and 0.4 mg/mL did not cause changes in PND preparations during 120 min incubation ($p > 0.05$)

whereas 0.8 mg of VhE/mL induced a slight decrease in twitch tension from 50 min incubation ($p < 0.05$ compared to Tyrode solution alone). We have selected the VhE concentration of 0.4 mg/mL to be used in those protocols with neutralization of BthTX-I-induced neuromuscular blockade (50 µg/mL; concentration enough to produce complete neuromuscular blockade in PND preparations) (Figure 2).

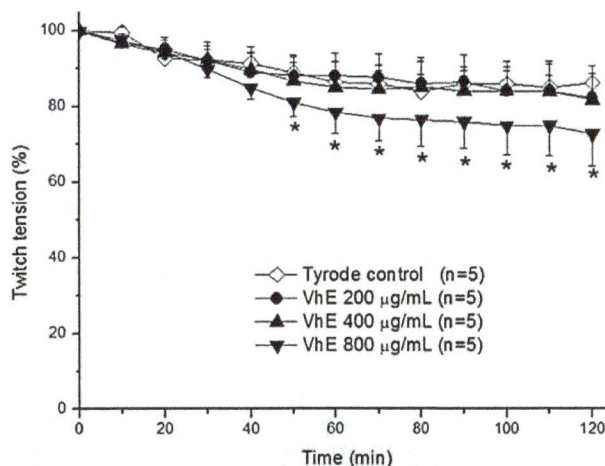

Figure 2. Neuromuscular responses of VhE (0.2–0.8 mg/mL) on mouse phrenic nerve-diaphragm (PND) preparation maintained under indirect stimulation. The points are the mean ± SEM (n = 5). *$p < 0.05$ compared to Tyrode control. VhE: *Vochysia haenkeana* extract.

BthTX-I induces irreversible neuromuscular blockade and myonecrosis *in* vitro similarly to effects caused by crude venom of *Bothrops jararacussu* from where it comes from.[16,17] The ability of this toxin to reproduce the neuromuscular effects seen with crude venom becomes it the main myotoxin from *B. jararacussu* venom. We have applied two different protocols to assess the neutralizing ability of VhE: pre-toxin incubation (BthTX-I was maintained under incubation for 30 min with VhE prior experiments in PND preparations) and post-toxin incubation (VhE was added into the record chamber 10 min after toxin addition). Under pre-toxin incubation, VhE neutralized completely the neuromuscular blockade caused by BthTX-I; on the other hand, VhE was not able to avoid the blockade by BthTX-I when added after toxin although it has been noticed a slight attenuation over 120 min (Figure 3).

Oshima-Franco et al.[15] studied the presynaptic nature of BthTX-I. Thus, the preincubation of toxin with VhE observed in pre-toxin experiments can be related to ability of VhE to avoid the presynaptic trigger of myotoxin; which, in turn, once triggered VhE was unable of repairing (post-toxin experiments).

Table 1 compares the level of myotoxicity induced BthTX-I to those ones reached by VhE under pre- and post-toxin incubation protocols. The pool of BthTX-I used in this work caused low myotoxicity when compared to other data shown in previous investigations, where 20 µg of toxin/mL induced 67 ± 2.3 % of damage cell in PND preparations.[33] Here, we have used 50 µg of toxin/mL to obtain complete muscle paralysis. Under pre- and post-toxin incubation protocols, VhE contributed to decrease in ~50 % the cell damage caused by BthTX-I.

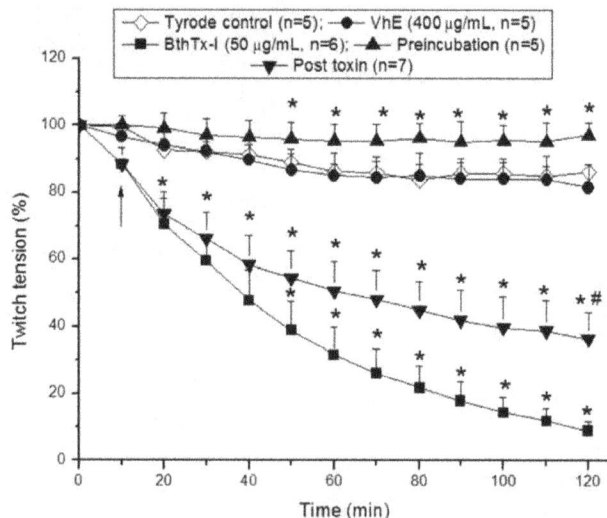

Figure 3. Effect of VhE on the neuromuscular blockade induced by BthTX-I on mouse phrenic nerve-diaphragm (PND) preparations maintained under indirect stimulation. Note that VhE prevented the BthTX-I blockade-induced under pre-toxin incubation. The points are the mean ± SEM (n = 5–7). *$p < 0.05$ compared to Tyrode control. #$p < 0.05$ compared to BthTX-I alone. BthTX-I: Bothropstoxin-I; VhE: *Vochysia haenkeana* extract. Arrow indicates the exact moment in which VhE was added for post-toxin incubation protocols.

Table 1. Morphological analysis of diaphragm muscle expressed as Myotoxicity Index (MI, in %)

Muscles resulting from Pharmacological assays	MI (%)
Tyrode control	8.04 ± 5
VhE	7.85 ± 5
BthTX-I	26.7 ± 16
Pre-toxin incubation	14.4 ± 10
Post-toxin incubation	14.8 ± 11

The neutralizing ability of VhE against the neuromuscular blockade caused by BthTX-I *in vitro* may be related to its capacity to induced protein aggregation as seen in our experiments in protein precipitation assay (Figure 4). The incubation with VhE promoted the precipitation of BthTX-I reducing the toxin-concentration in 70.5 ± 7.1 %. The incubation of VhE with albumin has also been evaluated as positive control showing 79.4 ± 6.7 % of precipitation. Ethanol (solvent for VhE) alone was assessed under protein precipitation assay as negative control in order to refute its influence in that protein aggregation seen with VhE; it did not promote protein aggregation in both of compounds albumin and BthTX-I.

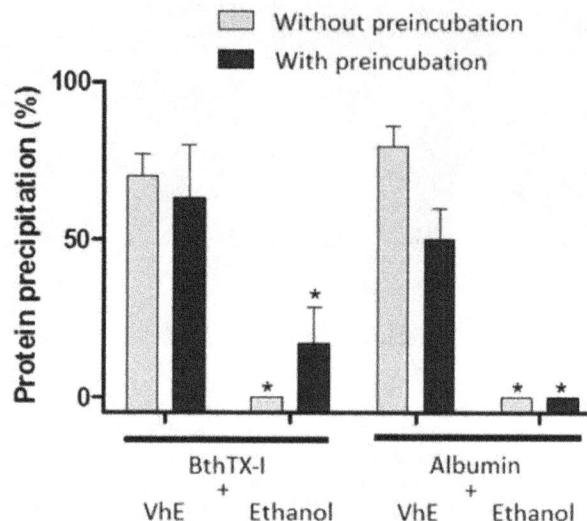

Figure 4. Protein precipitation induced by VhE. Note that VhE caused significant precipitation of BthTX-I and albumin; ethanol (used for solubilizing the VhE) had no activity on these effects. *$p < 0.05$. VhE: *V. haenkeana* extract.

The pharmacological action of plant extracts to neutralize the neuromuscular activity of snake venoms and their toxins *in vitro* shows still unknown but it is frequently associated with protein precipitation, proteolytic degradation, enzyme inactivation, metal chelation and antioxidant action.[30] Flavonoids and tannins are the main components related with those activities and both of them were previously observed in VhE.[21,27,34] Although we have not found evidence for tannic acid in this extract, responsible for antiophidian mechanism of plant extracts as suggested by Melo et al.,[30] the protein precipitation promoted by VhE may be related to its neutralizing effect against BthTX-I.

Conclusion

V. haenkeana stem barks extract abolished the neuromuscular blockade caused by BthTX-I under pre-toxin incubation treatment; however, it was not efficient to neutralize the toxin-induced neuromuscular blockade under post-toxin treatment. In both of treatments VhE contributed to decrease the myotoxicity caused by toxin. These effects may be related to protein aggregation involving phenolic compounds which represent the major constituent of VhE, as shown by TLC. VhE showed no antimicrobial activity against *S. aureus*, *E. coli* and *P. aeruginosa* strains.

Acknowledgments

This work was supported by Conselho Nacional de Desenvolvimento Científico e Tecnológico (Pibic/CNPq, Brazil,) and Fundação de Amparo à Pesquisa do Estado de São Paulo (FAPESP, Brazil, grant numbers: 04/09705-8; 07/53883-6; 08/52643-4; 12/08271-0; 15/01420-9). CH was supported by scientific initiation scholarship from Santander in partnership with Paulista University (UNIP, Brazil).

Ethical Issues

This study was approved by the institutional Ethics Committee on Animal Use (CEUA/UNISO, protocol no. 054/2015) and the experiments were carried out according to the guidelines established by the Brazilian Society of Laboratory Animal Science (SBCAL).

Conflict of Interest

The authors declare that they have no competing interests.

References

1. Bernarde PS. Anfíbios e répteis: introdução ao estudo da herpetofauna brasileira. Curitiba: *Analisbooks*; 2012.

2. Motta YP. Aspectos clínico, laboratorial e histopatológico da intoxicação experimental pelos venenos das serpentes *Bothrops jararaca* e *Crotalus durissus terrificus* em ratos Wistar tratados com antiveneno e *Mikania glomerata*. Botucatu: Universidade Estadual Paulista (UNESP); 2008.

3. Palacio TZ. Isolamento e caracterização bioquímica e funcional de um inibidor de metaloproteases presente no soro de serpente *Bothrops alternatus*. Ribeirão Preto: Universidade de São Paulo; 2014.

4. Cardoso JLC, Fan HW, Málaque CMS, Haddad Jr V. Animais peçonhentos no Brasil, Biologia, clínica e terapêutica dos acidentes. 2nd ed. São Paulo: *Sarvier*; 2009.

5. Incidência de casos de acidentes por serpentes por 100.000 habitantes entre. Brasil: Grandes Regiões e Unidades Federadas; 2000 – 2013.

6. Silveira ACP. Atividade antimicrobiana da BthTX-I e seu uso como melhorador de desempenho alternativo na avicultura. Uberlândia: Universidade Federal de Uberlândia; 2013.

7. Sacoman TM. Efeito da interação entre Bothropstoxina-I e Crotapotina na junção neuromuscular de camundongos "*in vitro*": estágio em iniciação científica. Brazil: Universidade Estadual Paulista; 2008.

8. Martines MS. Efeito da fitoterapia na injuria renal aguda induzida pela peçonha de *Bothrops jararaca*. Dissertação apresentada à Faculdade de Medicina da Universidade de São Paulo para obtenção de título de Mestrado em Ciências. São Paulo: 2013.

9. Rodrigues L, Cunha DB, Leite GB, Borja-Oliveira CR, Cintra ACO, Rodrigues-Simioni L, et al. Ação da heparina contra a atividade neurotóxica da miotoxina bothropstoxina-I. *Saúde Rev* 2004;6(4):19-29.

10. Moura VM, Mourão RHV, Santos MCD. Acidentes ofídicos na Região Norte do Brasil e o uso de espécies vegetais como tratamento alternativo e complementar à soroterapia. *Scientia Amazonia* 2015;4(1):2-12.

11. Vilar JC, Carvalho CM, Furtado MFD. Ofidismo e plantas utilizadas como antiofídicas. *Biol Geral Exper* 2005;6(1):3-36.

12. Collaço RCO, Junior-Rocha DS, Silva MG, Cogo JC, Oshima-Franco Y, Randazzo-Moura P. Propriedade antiofídica do extrato metanólico de *Mikania laevigata* sobre as ações biológicas induzidas pelo veneno de *Philodryas olfersii* na junção neuromuscular. *REU* 2010;36(2):105-13.

13. Elífio-Esposito SL, Hess PL, Moreno AN, Lopes Ferreira M, Ricart CAO, Souza MV, et al. A C-type lectin from *Bothrops jararacussu* venom can adhere to extracellular matrix proteins and induce the rolling of leukocytes. *J Venom Anim Toxins incl Trop Dis* 2007;13(4):782-99.

14. Dos Santos JI, Cardoso FF, Soares AM, dal Pai Silva M, Gallacci M, Fontes MR. Structural and functional studies of a bothropic myotoxin complexed to rosmarinic acid: new insights into Lys49-PLA(2) inhibition. *Plos One* 2011;6(12):e28521. doi: 10.1371/journal.pone.0028521

15. Oshima-Franco Y, Leite GB, Belo CA, Hyslop S, Prado-Franceschi J, Cintra AC, et al. The presynaptic activity of bothropstoxin-I, a myotoxin from *Bothrops jararacussu* snake venom. *Basic Clin Pharmacol Toxicol* 2004;95(4):175-82. doi: 10.1111/j.1742-7843.2004.pto_950405.x

16. Rostelato-Ferreira S, Leite GB, Cintra AC, Cruz-Höfling MA, Rodrigues-Simioni L, Oshima-Franco Y. Heparin at low concentration acts as antivenom against *Bothrops jararacussu* venom and bothropstoxin-I neurotoxic and myotoxic actions. *J Venom Res* 2010;1:54-60.

17. Heluany NF, Homsi-Brandeburgo MI, Giglio JR, Prado-Franceschi J, Rodrigues-Simioni L. Effects induced by bothropstoxin, a component from *Bothrops jararacussu* snake venom, on mouse and chick muscle preparations. *Toxicon* 1992;30(10):1203-10.

18. Cezari EJ. Plantas medicinais: atividade antitumoral do extrato bruto de sete plantas do cerrado e o uso por povos tradicionais. Dissertação (Mestrado) – Universidade Federal do Tocantins, Programa de Pós-Graduação em Ciências do Ambiente. Palmas: UFT; 2010.

19. Pasa MC. Saber local e medicina popular: a etnobotânica em Cuiabá, Mato Grosso, Brasil. Universidade Federal de Mato Grosso. Brasil: Rondonópolis, Mato Grosso; 2011.

20. Lima CP, Santos MG, Calabrese KS, Silva ALA, Almeida F. Evaluation of the leishmanicidal activity of plant species of the Brazilian savanna. *Rev Patol Trop* 2015;44(1):45-55. doi: 10.5216/rpt.v44i1.34800

21. Rizzi ES, Pereira KCL, Abreu CAA, Silva BCFL, Fernandes RM, Oliveira AKM, et al. Allelopathic potential and phytochemistry of cambarazinho (*Vochysia haenkeana* (Spreng.) Mart.) leaves in the germination and development of lettuce and tomato. *Biosci J* 2015;32(1):98-107.

22. Collaço RCO, Cogo JC, Rocha T, Oshima-Franco Y, Randazzo-Moura P. Protection by *Mikania laevigata* (guaco) extract against the toxicity of *Philodryas olfersii* snake venom. *Toxicon* 2012;60(4):614-22. doi: 10.1016/j.toxicon.2012.05.014

23. Costa KN, Gomes RM, Farrapo NM, Oshima-Franco Y. Validação farmacológica de fitoquímicos comerciais sob o parâmetro da junção neuromuscular (JNM) e do perfil cromatográfico. In: Oliveira-Junior JM, et al, editors. *Os Múltiplos Olhares na Área da Pesquisa – da Observação ao Conhecimento.* Brazil: Eduniso; 2011. PP. 11-29.

24. Bülbring E. Observation on the isolated phrenic nerve diaphragm preparation of the rat. *Br J Pharmacol* 1946;1:38-61.

25. Tribuiani N, Silva AM, Ferraz MC, Silva MG, Bentes APG, Graziano TS, et al. *Vellozia flavicans* Mart. ex Schult. hydroalcoholic extract inhibits the neuromuscular blockade induced by *Bothrops jararacussu* venom. *BMC Complement Altern Med* 2014;14:48. doi: 10.1186/1472-6882-14-48

26. Ambikabothy J, Ibrahim H, Ambu S, Chakravarthi S, Awang K, Vejayan J. Efficacy evaluations of *Mimosa pudica* tannin isolate (MPT) for its anti-ophidian properties. *J Ethnopharmacol* 2011;137(1):257-62. doi: 10.1016/j.jep.2011.05.013

27. Félix-Silva J, Souza T, Menezes YA, Cabral B, Câmara RB, Silva-Junior AA, et al. Aqueous leaf extract of *Jatropha gossypiifolia* L. (Euphorbiaceae) inhibits enzymatic and biological actions of *Bothrops jararaca* snake venom. *PLoS One* 2014;9(8):e104952. doi: 10.1371/journal.pone.0104952

28. Lowry OH, Rosebrough NJ, Farr AL, Randall RJ. Protein measurement with the Folin phenol reagent. *J Biol Chem* 1951;193(1).265-75.

29. Ferraz MC, Parrilha LAC, Moraes MSD, Filho JA, Cogo JC, Santos MG, et al. The effect of lupane triterpenoids (*Dipteryx alata* Vogel) in the *in vitro* neuromuscular blockade and myotoxicity of two snake venoms. *Curr Org Chem* 2012;16(22):2717-23. doi: 10.2174/138527212804004481

30. Melo RS, Farrapo NM, Rocha-Junior DS, Silva MG, Cogo JC, Dal Belo CA, et al. Antiophidian mechanisms of medicinal plants. In: Keller RB, editor. *Flavonoids: Biosynthesis, Biological Effects and Dietary Sources.* New York: Nova Science; 2009. PP. 249-62.

31. Oshima-Franco Y, Dal Belo CA. Recognizing antiophidian plants using the neuromuscular junction apparatus. *Int J Complement Alt Med* 2017;5(5):00165.

32. Ministério da Saúde: Textos Básicos de Saúde (Cadernos de Atenção Básica; n. 22). Brasil: Health surveillance:zoonoses; 2009.

33. Oshima-Franco Y, Rosa LJR, Silva GAA, Amaral Filho J, Silva MG, Lopes PS, et al. Antibothropic action of *Camellia sinensis* extract against the neuromuscular blockade by *Bothrops jararacussu* snake venom and its main toxin, bothropstoxin-I. Croatia: Intech; 2012.

34. Mors WB, Nascimento MC, Pereira BM, Pereira NA. Plant natural products active against snake bite-the molecular approach. *Phytochemistry* 2000;55(6):627-42.

3

Legionella Pneumophila and Dendrimers-Mediated Antisense Therapy

Roghiyeh Pashaei-Asl[1,2,3], Khodadad Khodadadi[4], Fatima Pashaei-Asl[5], Gholamreza Haqshenas[6], Nasser Ahmadian[7], Maryam Pashaiasl[8,9]*, Reza Hajihosseini Baghdadabadi[1]*

[1] *Department of Biology, Payame Noor University, Tehran, Iran.*
[2] *Department of Anatomy, Medical School, Iran University of Medical Science, Tehran, Iran.*
[3] *Cellular and Molecular Research Center, Iran University of Medical Sciences, Tehran, Iran.*
[4] *Genetic Theme, Murdoch Children's Research Institute, Royal Children's Hospital, The University of Melbourne, Melbourne, Australia.*
[5] *Molecular Biology Laboratory, Biotechnology Research Center, Tabriz University of Medical Sciences, Tabriz, Iran.*
[6] *Microbiology Department, Biomedical Discovery Institute, Monash University, Melbourne, Australia.*
[7] *Transplantation Center, Department of Curative Affairs, Ministry of Health and Medical Education, Tehran, Iran.*
[8] *Drug Applied Research Center, Tabriz University of Medical Sciences, Tabriz, Iran.*
[9] *Department of Anatomical Sciences, Faculty of Medicine, Tabriz University of Medical Sciences, Tabriz, Iran.*

Keywords:
· Legionella pneumophila
· DrrA (SidM)
· LepA and LepB
· Intracellular replication
· Rab
· Vesicular trafficking

Abstract

Finding novel and effective antibiotics for treatment of *Legionella disease* is a challenging field. Treatment with antibiotics usually cures *Legionella* infection; however, if the resultant disease is not timely recognized and treated properly, it leads to poor prognosis and high case fatality rate. *Legionella pneumophila* DrrA protein (Defects in Rab1 recruitment protein A)/also known as SidM affects host cell vesicular trafficking through modification of the activity of cellular small guanosine triphosphatase (GTPase) Rab (Ras-related in brain) function which facilitates intracellular bacterial replication within a supporter vacuole. Also, *Legionella pneumophila* LepA and LepB (Legionella effector protein A and B) proteins suppress host-cell Rab1 protein's function resulting in the cell lysis and release of bacteria that subsequently infect neighbour cells. Legionella readily develops resistant to antibiotics and, therefore, new drugs with different modes of action and therapeutic strategic approaches are urgently required among antimicrobial drug therapies;gene therapy is a novel approach for *Legionnaires disease* treatment. On the contrary to the conventional treatment approaches that target bacterial proteins, new treatment interventions target DNA (Deoxyribonucleic acid), RNA (Ribonucleic acid) species, and different protein families or macromolecular complexes of these components. The above approaches can overcome the problems in therapy of Legionella infections caused by antibiotics resistance pathogens. Targeting Legionella genes involved in manipulating cellular vesicular trafficking using a dendrimer-mediated antisense therapy is a promising approach to inhibit bacterial replication within the target cells.

Introduction

Legionnaires' disease is a serious form of pneumonia and lung inflammation, which is caused by intracellular bacterium Legionella. Although early therapeutic intervention using antibiotics usually cures Legionnaires' disease, some patients experience complications that could lead to death.[1] Legionella rapidly develops resistance to commonly used antibacterial agents.[2] Therefore, there is an urgent demand for discovery of new antibacterial targets to overcome the resistance problem. Bacterial pathogens deliver effector proteins which interfere with host cell physiological functions and hijack their target cell machinery leading to specific clinical symptoms.[3,4] To escape degradation by its host cells, a Legionella-containing vacuole (LCV) is formed and protects the bacterium from cell immune defense, possibly through secretion of bacterial proteins into the host cytosol.[5] Therefore, specific antibiotics with high levels of permeability are required to pass cell membrane barrier and reach the bacterium within the cells.[6] This review describes different gene therapy approaches including antisense therapy mediated by dendrimers to target and eliminate or disarm pathogen, novel method for specific targeting of effective types of antibiotics to intracellular *L. pneumophila* (Legionella pneumophila). We also describe antisense therapy for *L. pneumophila* treatment targeting bacterial protein synthesis aiming to disturb host trafficking pathway through interference with phagosome and lysosome fusion in macrophages, therefore targeting bacteria in the cytoplasm by different methods such as RNA interference type would be an

Corresponding authors: Maryam Pashaiasl and Reza Hajihosseini Baghdadabadi, Email: pashaim@tbzmed.ac.ir, r.hajihosseini@shargh.tpnu.ac.ir

alternative option to prevent bacterial growth and prevent the clinical symptoms.

Legionella pneumophila a medically important intracellular pathogen

The most recent major outbreak of *L. pneumophila*, or Legionnaires' disease happened in Portugal in 2014, and was referred to one of the biggest in European history. If this relatively rare infection is not timely recognized and properly treated, it can have poor prognosis and present a high case fatality rate.[7]

L. pneumophila is a gram-negative intracellular bacterium[8] that causes Legionnairesis in humans. The natural host of *L. pneumophila* is unicellular protozoa and it infects human alveolar macrophages.[9,10] Despite progress in the antimicrobial treatment, pneumonia is still one of the important infectious diseases, causing death in the developed countries.[11-13] *L. pneumophila* co-infection with influenza could lead to influenza infection with possibly lethal prognosis.[14]

Following inhalation, *L. pneumophila* infects and replicates in alveolar macrophages, which contribute to inflammation and progress of the disease. *L .pneumophila*, with ability to deliver above 300 proteins to the host cell through its Type IVB, Icm/Dot (the intracellular multiplication/defective organelle trafficking) translocation system conserves the major recognized set of translocated substrates between all bacterial pathogens.[15] Inside host cells, *L. pneumophila* avoids phagosome-lysosome fusion and influences host cell procedures to form a particular phagosome which is proper for intracellular replication.[3,8,16] The Icm/Dot system is used by the bacterium to translocate its effectors.[4,15]

Legionella pathogenesis

The lungs are the main site of infection, where bacteria grow inside the lung macrophages.[16-19] In the extra pulmonary forms of disease, organs such as heart, CNS, liver and intestines are involved and heart is the most common organ involved in the hospitalized patient. Recipients of organ transplant and patients with diabetes mellitus and chronic lung disease as well as aged people and cigarette smokers are suitable candidate for this disease.[20]

L. pneumophila Life Cycle

Intracellular pathogens use different mechanisms to manipulate the host cell system for intracellular replication. For example, *L. pneumophila* as an intracellular bacterial pathogen hijacks host vesicle trafficking pathway to stop phagosome and lysosome fusion inside the cell.[4,21-23] Lysosomes are intracellular organelles with acidic pH in eukaryotic cells containing hydrolytic enzymes for digesting cellular waste products, bacteria and viruses. Normally when bacteria enter to cell by phagocytes, they are killed in lysosomes through digesting by the lysosomal enzymes.[23]

Host cells use the defense mechanism for limiting the intracellular infection.[23] Following cell infection by *L .pneumophila*, some immune system cells such as macrophages surround the bacteria but bacteria manipulate host cells using membrane trafficking pathway. Inside the macrophages, pathogen utilizes the host cell proteins mediating intracellular trafficking pathway. This forms an organelle termed *L. pneumophila* - containing vacuole (LCV) which supports bacteria replication (Figure 1).[9,16,21,23,24]

Type IV secretion system of *L. pneumophila* which is encoded by the Icm/Dot genes enables bacteria to transfer its proteins into host cytosol.[25-27] A number of different translocated substrates of Icm/Dot have been identified with similar functions to eukaryotic host cell proteins involving in vesicle trafficking pathway (Figure 1).[9,23,27-31]

Rab GTPase proteins in eukaryotic cells act as molecular switches and are important in cellular trafficking pathway. Following pathogen phagocytosis or endocytosis, host cell Rab GTPase proteins are essential for intracellular transportation. Bacterial effectors hijack Rab proteins at the molecular level act to escape degradation, be carried directly to specific intracellular locations, and control host vesicles carrying molecules requiring for a stable niche and/or bacterial development and differentiation.[4,32,33]

Development of antibacterial resistance by Legionella

The discovery and therapeutic use of antibiotics in the 1950s have certainly contributed to the one of the ultimate profits to human; however, because of the short life cycle and capacity to adjust rapidly to variations in the environmental condition, pathogenic bacteria continue to persevere by regularly overcoming the effect of drugs used to eliminate them. The growing drug resistance was the first problem resulting from the extensive, uncontrolled and inappropriate use of antibiotics. In spite of the entrance of new antibiotic into the market, drug resistance is detected in years or even months. At present, more than 70% of pathogenic bacteria are resistant to most antibiotics existing on the market and the mortality of some multi-resistant infections has extended to 50 - 80% and also the mortality rate as a result of bacterial infections is above 2 millions per year, worldwide.[34,35] Furthermore, nowadays, some environmental bacterial pathogens such as Legionella spp. as a result of artificial ecosystems are a main problematic issue in industrialized countries, associated with Other factors such as modern medications and lifestyles have been caused an increased incidence of unintended pathogens in the form of emerging pathogens.[36]

According to the different approaches especially bacterial resistance and action of antibacterial medications presently used, different targets such as cellular structures, the cell wall biosynthesis, protein biosynthesis, DNA, different RNA families, biosynthetic pathway, new protein families or macromolecular complexes of these components have been suggested by commercial antibacterial companies and scientists.[35,37] Therefore, targeting specific bacteria such as *L. pneumophila* which may present as Legionnaires'

diseases and cause case fatality rate of about 10% and even mortality rate higher than 25% in immune suppressed and nosocomial patients[11] requires to be paid more attention.

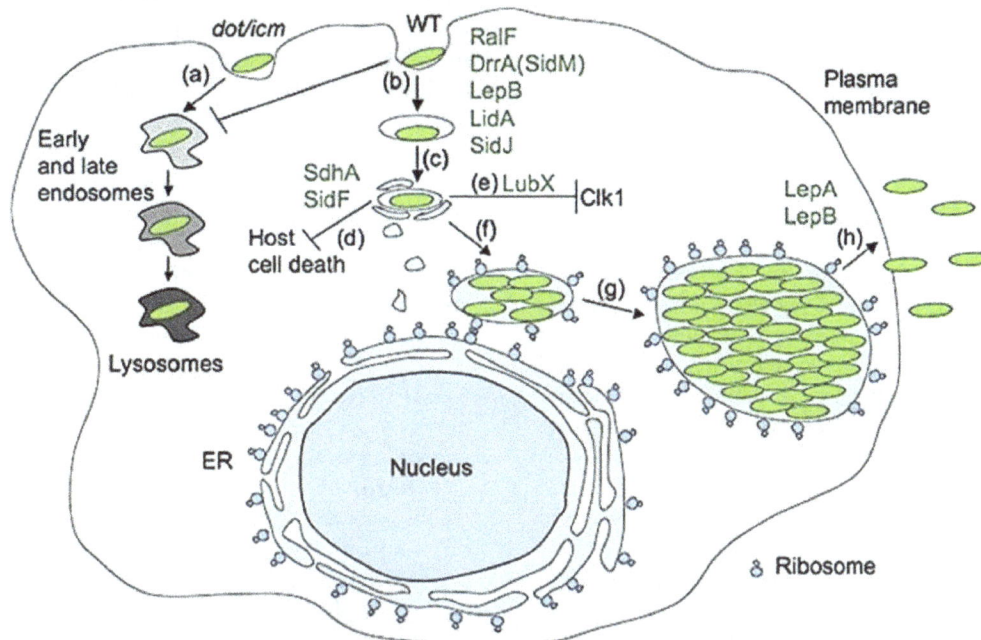

Figure 1. The replication of *Legionella pneumophila* inside the cell (Figure adapted from [23])
Wild-type and mutant form of Legionella use different ways for trafficking pathways(a) *dot/icm* mutants and trafficking pathway, (b) Wild-type of *Legionella Pneumophila*, the LCV formed and avoids endosomal fusion, (c) The Dot/Icm different effectors, (d) Host cell is prevented from death by the Dot/Icm effectors SdhA and Sid F, (e) the Dot/Icm effecter LubX effect the host cell factor Clk1, (f) the LCV was surrounded with Ribosomes, (g) Several cycle of *Legionella Pneumophila* replication,(h) *Legionella Pneumophila* Dot/Icm effectors LepA and B cause to *Legionella pneumophila* infect the other neighbour host cell Dot/Icm-translocated effectors is shown in green.[23]

Targeting *Legionella* proteins by antibacterial

Finding new and effective antibiotics is a challenging research area driven by novel approaches required to tackle unconventional targets. Intracellular grown Legionella is extremely resistant to antibiotics.[38,39] Although combination antibiotic therapy might be a choice in some conditions, it is not recommended for all patients and is a controversial and challenging issue.[40] *L. pneumophila* is able to manipulate vesicular trafficking by modification the activity of the small GTPase Rab1. *L .pneumophila* manipulates Rab1 function using some of its associate proteins such as DrrA (SidM). DrrA (SidM) has both guanine nucleotide exchange activity in Rab1 GDF (GDI dissociation factor) and Rab1 GEF (guanine nucleotide exchange factor).[19,41-43] Also there is another protein of *L. pneumophila* named LepB which manipulate and inactivate host-cell Rab1 protein's function.[33,41] Following growing inside the LCV, a bacterium lyses the host cell and release to infect the neighbour cells. Two effectors, LepA and LepB, which show a role in the non-lytic release of Legionella from protozoa, are translocated by the Icm/Dot TFSS (Type Four Secretion System).[42,44] Reduction of the Lep proteins through deletion of their genes contributes to better ability to lyse red blood cells. In contrast, overexpression of Lep-containing hybrid proteins seems to exactly block the activity of the Icm/Dot TFSS and

may stop the transfer of other effectors which are critical for intracellular multiplication.[33,42] Therefore, Legionella's effectors which hijack host protein to escape degradation and replicate intracellularly could be targeted in antibacterial treatment. In addition, the LepA and the LepB proteins in Legionella are the other targets to induce infection the neighbour cells in host cells.

Gene therapy approach for treatment of Legionella infection

Antibiotic resistance is a health threat, worldwide. In spite of good progresses in genome sequencing and genetic manipulation tools, there are still problems to be used for effective therapeutic aims.[45] Gene therapy is a technique which causes insertion, silencing or alteration of genes in a patient's cells to treat or prevent disease.[46] RNA regulators are developed to overcome various restrictions of protein regulators such as simple structures and mechanisms causing their behaviour in different conditions anticipated with software tools. Also they propagate signals directly and fast as RNAs.[47] The remodeling of RNA and DNA molecules with the aim of engineering antibiotic bunches to cause antibiotic overexpression is possible.[48] Recently, combination of CRISPR (Clusters regularly interspaced short palindromic repeats) and antisense RNA system in order to control bacterial gene expression is introduced.[47]

Through blocking genes that manipulate and inactivate host-cell Rab1 protein's function, Legionella can't form LCV to support bacteria inside LCV for replication.

CRISPR-Cas system: a novel tool for treatment of Legionellosis

Not only CRISPR-Cas component is important in the natural history and pathogenesis of Legionnaires' disease, but also *L. pneumophila Cas2* has a role that is unique from the main view of CRISPR-Cas function.[49] CRISPR , which were first discovered in bacteria in 1980s and then in archaea in 1990s, are a powerful genome editing tool. CRISPR function to facilitate adaptation of the organism to extreme environmental conditions and act as a part of bacterial immune system to defend against pathogens and harmful environment.[50,51] CRISPR/Cas systems are powerful and efficient genome modifying tool in comparison to other genome modifying tools like zinc-finger nucleases (ZFNs) and transcription activator-like effector nucleases (TALENs). The system includes a nuclease (Cas) and small guide RNA that recruits the Cas to cut at a specific place in the genome. This system is able to induce targeted specific gene deletion, correction or mutation via RNA guided DNA cleavage. Short palindromic repeat 36 base pair (bp) lengths in the genome associated with the (Cas) gene carry out targeted editing in the proposed genome. It works by binding a RNA stem-loop structure when attached to a short target sequence (22-33bp) to guide the Cas protein to a specific spot in the genome. These adaptable sequences together with non-contiguous direct repeat attached to Cas gene forming the CRISPR Cas systems.[52-57]

CRISPR type II, based on Cas9 is the primary system used to genetically modify mammalian cells. Cas9 function in CRISPR system is central part of the tool and is guided to the target sequence by a trans activating crRNA (tracrRNA) to cleave target DNA – Cas9 cleaves supercoiled, relaxed and linear DNA – cleavage occurs 3bp upstream of Pam motif.[54] This type of gene editing technology has been independently described by several groups and is termed RNA guided engineered nucleases (RGENs).[58]

CRISPR technology has some benefits over early methods of gene editing technology and is rapidly expanding in the area of genetic and biology research. It is a relatively rapid and cost effective genome editing technology that can be used to modify the genome in different organisms and various cell types. CRISPR Cas system target the bacterial lipoproteins transcript through dual RNA protein complexes (Figure 2).[59]

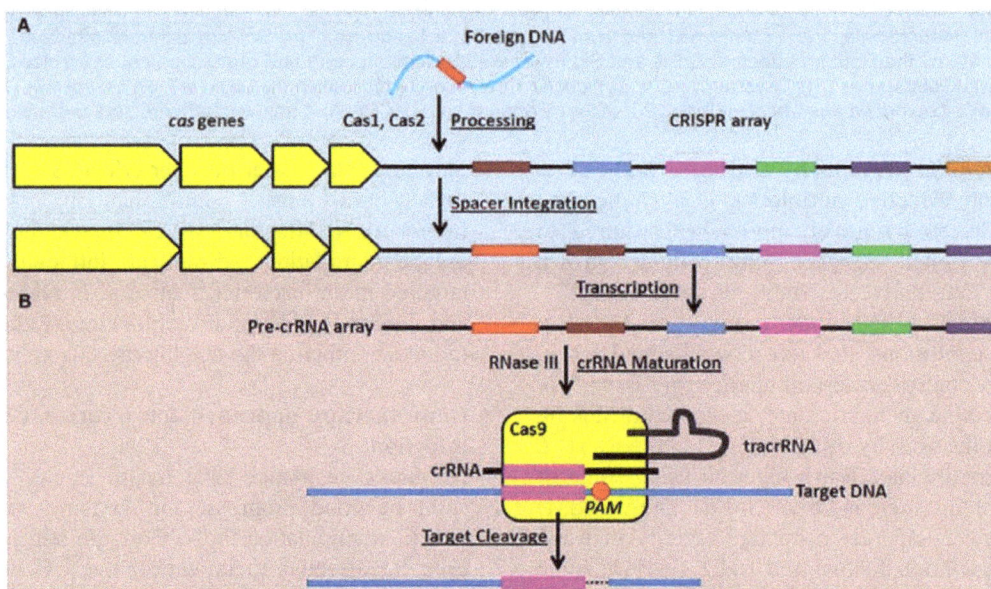

Figure 2. The Type II CRISPR-Cas system function in adaptive nucleic acid restriction (Figure adapted from[59])
(A) Invading DNA is located by Cas1 and Cas2 and take it as new spacer sequence inside CRISPR array (immune completion blue). **(B)** To stop invading DNA, the pro-crRNA in constructed and matured into small targeting crRNAs to associate with Cas9 and the sequence of spacer within the crRNA can hybridize the matching DNA. Cas9 then cleavages target DNA just 3bp downstream of PAM site and generates double stranded break on target DNA.[59]

Antisense therapy of Legionellosis

Gene expression could be down regulated by RNA interference and antisense oligonucleotides (AS-ODNs) through inducing enzyme-dependent degradation of targeted mRNA.[60] For treatment of different gene-specific diseases, oligonucleotide-based cure is a novel area of medicine to design new drugs. The antisense oligonucleotides and short interfering RNAs (siRNAs) are the more common forms, which often act against similar targets.[61] Using antisense and other gene silencing technologies provide an efficient alternative way of treatment for cancer, genetic disorders or infection.[62,63] The gene expression through changing mRNA splicing, arresting mRNA translation and inducing degradation of targeted mRNA are blocked through sequence-specific antisense oligonucleotides by

RNase H.[64] Antisense therapy is also convenient way of genetic alteration compare to more difficult methods such as generating gene knockout in cells and organisms. Antisense ODNs have been applied to efficiently block gene expression in eukaryotic cells and there is one antisense ODN-based product in the market and others in clinical trials.[65,66] This gene therapy method is common for silencing the abnormal gene to stop the human disease such as cancer progression[67-69] and neurodegenerative disorders[70] as well as pneumonia.[71]

Antisense transcription was first revealed in bacteria about 50 years ago. The significant amount of antisense transcription is an important feature of gene expression in eukaryotes. This technique mostly uses DNA or RNA to inactivate circular segment of bacterial genome resembling RNA interference and prevents duplication of bacterial cells or kills them;[62,71] however, antisense technology is not applied widely in prokaryotic systems. Gene regulations in prokaryotic cells have been done by antisense mechanisms of bacteria and also through increased antibiotic efficacy.[35,45,62,72] Former reports indicated short antisense and modified antisense oligodeoxynucleotide (AODNs) could inhibit gene expression in bacteria.[45,72,73] Others stated that gene expression in bacteria can be inhibited by peptide nucleic acid (PNA).[71,74] The transcriptomes of bacteria such as Escherichia coli, Synechocystis sp. strain PCC6803, Helicobacter pylori, Bacillus subtilis, Mycoplasma pneumoniae, Sinorhizobiummeliloti, Vibrio cholerae, Chlamydia trachomatis, Pseudomonas syringae, and Staphylococcus aureus have been stated to have antisense RNA (asRNA) transcripts.[35] The bacterial protein YidC is extremely preserved among pathogens and is necessary for membrane protein attachment and decrease of YidC production contributing to bacterial growth retardation. Therefore, it can be a novel potential target for therapeutic applications. Antisense RNA-mediated YidC down-expression in E. Colistrain resulted in identify antibacterial essential oils eugenol and carvacrol.[75] The influence of the antisense oligomer is extremely particular to the targeted gene's sequence, which is preserved in numerous bacterial types, and it does not have any noticeable toxicity against human cells.[45] The combined CRISPR and asRNA system, can be applied to reversibly repress or derepress multiple target genes concurrently, permitting for rational reprogramming of cellular functions. Gene target are repressed/derepressed by CRISPR system from Streptococcus pyogenes and synthetic antisense RNAs (asRNAs) in Escherichia coli strains. In fact, when the CRISPR system represses the target gene, it can be derepressed by expressing asRNA which hide away a small guide RNA (sgRNA). In addition, up to 95% of derepression can be attained through designing as RNAs which target various regions of a sgRNA and by changing the hybridization free energy of the sgRNA–asRNA complex.[47] RNA interference has been suggested to be an alternative method to prevent bacterial growth or demolish them. For this aim we suggest antisense therapy against type IV secretion system and Lep proteins synthesis in Legionella.

Dendrimers-based antisense delivery system approaches for treatment of Legionellosis

The important therapeutic aim in biotechnology is the capacity to safely and professionally transfer external DNA, RNA, antisense or drug[76] into cells.[63,77] The capability to deliver fragments of DNA or RNA to the required section of a cell is a challenging issue. Substrate-mediated transfection, which withstands the release of knocked DNA or vector/DNA complexes and provides cell growth, has been established to solve the problems associated with the extracellular obstacles in gene delivery system.[78] Rapid transfection which can achieve by viral carrier, immunological and oncologic side effects connected to these vectors have remained as controversial issues. Nowadays, non-viral gene delivery system to transfer genetic material to targeted cells such as natural/synthetic molecules or physical forces are preferred methods. They have some benefits such as targeting capability, simplicity of fabrication, possibility for repeat administration and low immune rejection.[79] There are different dendrimers such as peptide, and glycopeptide, has capability to bind bacterial polysaccharides representing interesting tools for both therapeutics and diagnostics applications. Nowadays, because of higher bacterial resistance for common antimicrobial drugs, discovery of new antibacterial medications and diagnostic tools are very important .[80] It has been reported that acid-triethylene glycol (GATG) dendrimers is valuable and versatile platform to develop a novel antimicrobial materials targeting microbial viability and/or virulence.[81,82] The anti-bacterial sequences (ABS) can be integrated into plasmids, viral, and other vectors and packaged in liposomes or cationic polymers such as polyethylenimine (PEL) to prevent or reduce the likelihood of infections leading to sepsis.[65] Dendrimers as non-viral gene delivery tools which can be utilized to deliver sequence of DNA or RNA as oligonucleotides to the certain part of cells are challenging experiments and novel method.[83,84] Dendrimers as Nano-sized synthetic polymers have positive charge with distinct, homogeneous, and monodisperse organization containing tree-like arms or branches.[85] Dendrimers are suitable and safe for the successful application in biomedicine such as imaging, drug delivery, gene delivery and photodynamic therapy.[86] The highest benefits are the progress in the antifungal properties and antibacterial action, for example decrease in toxicity, bioavailability, and target tissue which simplifies advanced therapeutic methods.[87,88]

Valuable effort is being performed to elucidate the techniques of using dendrimers for gene trafficking into the cells without any interference of damage to the cell's DNA. It is important to maintain DNA activity in the course of dehydration so dendrimer/DNA complexes need to be encapsulated and compressed in a water resolvable polymers, subsequently they are deposited on or inserted in functional polymer films with a fast degradation rate to facilitate gene transfection. Based on this method, for substrate-mediated gene delivery, Polyamidoamine (PAMAM) dendrimer/DNA complexes have been applied to encapsulate functional biodegradable polymers. Many reports have revealed that the fast-degrading functional polymer with excessive potential for localized transfection is a good tool.[78,86,89,90] Antisense has negative charge and conjugates with dendrimers as a positive charge polymer. We have established Epidermal growth factor receptor (EGFR) and c-Src antisense oligonucleotide encapsulated with PAMAM dendrimers in human colon cancer cell line and have showed its effects on signalling pathway.[63,68,91] To confirm entry of antisense to the cell, fluorescent microscope and Fluorescence-activated cell sorting (FACS) analysis have been carried out and showed that Fluorescein isothiocyanate (FITS) are conjugated effectively to dendrimers. Our studies evaluated the antisense dendrimers mediated transfer into cells and showed the effective antisense entry inside the cell; however, the antisense alone is not able to enter the cells. As a result, dendrimers could be safe and suitable tool to antisense delivery system for *L. pneumophila* treatment. Therefore, antisense against the type IV secretion system and Lep protein synthesis in Legionella encapsulated with dendrimers could be a novel approaches in Legionnaires' disease.

Conclusion
Vesicle trafficking pathway in L. *pneumophila* could be as a target for eliminating or disarming pathogens via antisense therapy. Antisense therapeutic application for bacterial protein synthesis has role in mediating the intracellular trafficking pathway to avoid phagosome and lysosome fusion in macrophages. Some of these proteins have been shown to participate in the trafficking of the Legionella phagosome. By reducing these proteins through antisense therapy, bacteria could not be able to hijack host vesicle trafficking pathway, therefore phagosome and lysosome fuse inside the cell and they are killed in lysosomes through digesting by the lysosomal enzymes. Nowadays, instead of proteins based targeting as potential drug action, drug companies and researchers are interested in utilizing different RNA species, DNA, new protein families or macromolecular complexes of these components to treat and eliminate antibiotics resistance pathogens.

Acknowledgments
The author thanks to Prof. Jamie Rossjohn and Associate Prof. Travis Beddoe at Monash University, Melbourne, Australia, for their attitude regarding *L. pneumophila*.

Ethical Issues
Not applicable.

Conflict of Interest
The authors report no conflicts of interest.

References
1. Massis LM, Assis-Marques MA, Castanheira FV, Capobianco YJ, Balestra AC, Escoll P, et al. Legionella longbeachae is immunologically silent and highly virulent in vivo. *J Infect Dis* 2017;215(3):440-51. doi: 10.1093/infdis/jiw560
2. Singh SB, Young K, Silver LL. What is an "ideal" antibiotic? Discovery challenges and path forward. *Biochem Pharmacol* 2017;133:63-73. doi: 10.1016/j.bcp.2017.01.003
3. Charpentier X, Gabay JE, Reyes M, Zhu JW, Weiss A, Shuman HA. Chemical genetics reveals bacterial and host cell functions critical for type iv effector translocation by Legionella pneumophila. *PLoS Pathog* 2009;5(7):e1000501. doi: 10.1371/journal.ppat.1000501
4. Stein MP, Muller MP, Wandinger-Ness A. Bacterial pathogens commandeer Rab gtpases to establish intracellular niches. *Traffic* 2012;13(12):1565-88. doi: 10.1111/tra.12000
5. Eisenreich W, Heuner K. The life stage-specific pathometabolism of Legionella pneumophila. *FEBS Lett* 2016;590(21):3868-86. doi: 10.1002/1873-3468.12326
6. Chahin A, Opal SM. Severe pneumonia caused by Legionella pneumophila: Differential diagnosis and therapeutic considerations. *Infect Dis Clin North Am* 2017;31(1):111-21. doi: 10.1016/j.idc.2016.10.009
7. Jacob M, Ramos HC, Morgado B. Severe Legionella pneumophila infection in an immunocompetent patient: A success story 300 kilometers away. *Cureus* 2016;8(12):e937. doi: 10.7759/cureus.937
8. Horwitz MA, Silverstein SC. Legionnaires' disease bacterium (Legionella pneumophila) multiples intracellularly in human monocytes. *J Clin Invest* 1980;66(3):441-50. doi: 10.1172/jci109874
9. Ensminger AW, Isberg RR. Legionella pneumophila dot/icm translocated substrates: A sum of parts. *Curr Opin Microbiol* 2009;12(1):67-73. doi: 10.1016/j.mib.2008.12.004
10. Fields BS. The molecular ecology of legionellae. *Trends Microbiol* 1996;4(7):286-90. doi: 10.1016/0966-842X(96)10041-X
11. Burillo A, Pedro-Botet ML, Bouza E. Microbiology and epidemiology of legionnaire's disease. *Infect Dis Clin North Am* 2017;31(1):7-27. doi: 10.1016/j.idc.2016.10.002
12. Lamoth F, Greub G. Amoebal pathogens as emerging causal agents of pneumonia. *FEMS Microbiol Rev* 2010;34(3):260-80. doi: 10.1111/j.1574-6976.2009.00207.x
13. Mandell LA, Wunderink RG, Anzueto A, Bartlett JG, Campbell GD, Dean NC, et al. Infectious diseases society of america/american thoracic society consensus guidelines on the management of community-acquired pneumonia in adults. *Clin Infect Dis* 2007;44 Suppl 2:S27-72. doi: 10.1086/511159

14. Magira EE, Zakynthinos S. Legionnaire's disease and influenza. *Infect Dis Clin North Am* 2017;31(1):137-53. doi: 10.1016/j.idc.2016.10.010

15. Urbanus ML, Quaile AT, Stogios PJ, Morar M, Rao C, Di Leo R, et al. Diverse mechanisms of metaeffector activity in an intracellular bacterial pathogen, Legionella pneumophila. *Mol Syst Biol* 2016;12(12):893. doi: 10.15252/msb.20167381

16. Horwitz MA. The legionnaires' disease bacterium (Legionella pneumophila) inhibits phagosome-lysosome fusion in human monocytes. *J Exp Med* 1983;158(6):2108-26. doi: 10.1084/jem.158.6.2108

17. Fraser DW, McDade JE. Legionellosis. *Sci Am* 1979;241(4):82-99. doi: 10.1038/scientificamerican1079-82

18. Fraser DW, Tsai TR, Orenstein W, Parkin WE, Beecham HJ, Sharrar RG, et al. Legionnaires' disease: Description of an epidemic of pneumonia. *N Engl J Med* 1977;297(22):1189-97. doi: 10.1056/nejm197712012972201

19. Ninio S, Roy CR. Effector proteins translocated by Legionella pneumophila: Strength in numbers. *Trends Microbiol* 2007;15(8):372-80. doi: 10.1016/j.tim.2007.06.006

20. Cunha BA, Burillo A, Bouza E. Legionnaires' disease. *Lancet* 2016;387(10016):376-85. doi: 10.1016/s0140-6736(15)60078-2

21. Heidtman M, Chen EJ, Moy MY, Isberg RR. Large-scale identification of Legionella pneumophila dot/icm substrates that modulate host cell vesicle trafficking pathways. *Cell Microbiol* 2009;11(2):230-48. doi: 10.1111/j.1462-5822.2008.01249.x

22. Mukherjee S, Liu X, Arasaki K, McDonough J, Galan JE, Roy CR. Modulation of Rab gtpase function by a protein phosphocholine transferase. *Nature* 2011;477(7362):103-6. doi: 10.1038/nature10335

23. Shin S, Roy CR. Host cell processes that influence the intracellular survival of Legionella pneumophila. *Cell Microbiol* 2008;10(6):1209-20. doi: 10.1111/j.1462-5822.2008.01145.x

24. Neild AL, Roy CR. Immunity to vacuolar pathogens: What can we learn from legionella? *Cell Microbiol* 2004;6(11):1011-8. doi: 10.1111/j.1462-5822.2004.00450.x

25. Berger KH, Isberg RR. Two distinct defects in intracellular growth complemented by a single genetic locus in Legionella pneumophila. *Mol Microbiol* 1993;7(1):7-19. doi: 10.1111/j.1365-2958.1993.tb01092.x

26. Hilbi H, Segal G, Shuman HA. Icm/Dot-dependent upregulation of phagocytosis by Legionella pneumophila. *Mol Microbiol* 2001;42(3):603-17. doi: 10.1046/j.1365-2958.2001.02645.x

27. Isberg RR, O'Connor TJ, Heidtman M. The Legionella pneumophila replication vacuole: Making a cosy niche inside host cells. *Nat Rev Microbiol* 2009;7(1):13-24. doi: 10.1038/nrmicro1967

28. Machner MP, Isberg RR. Targeting of host Rab gtpase function by the intravacuolar pathogen Legionella pneumophila. *Dev Cell* 2006;11(1):47-56. doi: 10.1016/j.devcel.2006.05.013

29. Murata T, Delprato A, Ingmundson A, Toomre DK, Lambright DG, Roy CR. The Legionella pneumophila effector protein DrrA is a Rab1 guanine nucleotide-exchange factor. *Nat Cell Biol* 2006;8(9):971-7. doi: 10.1038/ncb1463

30. Voth DE, Broederdorf LJ, Graham JG. Bacterial Type IV secretion systems: Versatile virulence machines. *Future Microbiol* 2012;7(2):241-57. doi: 10.2217/fmb.11.150

31. Michard C, Doublet P. Post-translational modifications are key players of the Legionella pneumophila infection strategy. *Front Microbiol* 2015;6:87. doi: 10.3389/fmicb.2015.00087

32. Grosshans BL, Ortiz D, Novick P. Rabs and their effectors: Achieving specificity in membrane traffic. *Proc Natl Acad Sci U S A* 2006;103(32):11821-7. doi: 10.1073/pnas.0601617103

33. Pfeffer S. Microbiology: Pathogen drop-kick. *Nature* 2007;450(7168):361-2. doi: 10.1038/450361a

34. Berdy J. Thoughts and facts about antibiotics: Where we are now and where we are heading. *J Antibiot (Tokyo)* 2012;65(8):385-95. doi: 10.1038/ja.2012.27

35. Rao CVS, De Waelheyns E, Economou A, Anne J. Antibiotic targeting of the bacterial secretory pathway. *Biochim Biophys Acta* 2014;1843(8):1762-83. doi: 10.1016/j.bbamcr.2014.02.004

36. Rivera-Perez JI, Gonzalez AA, Toranzos GA. From evolutionary advantage to disease agents: Forensic reevaluation of host-microbe interactions and pathogenicity. *Microbiol Spectr* 2017;5(1). doi: 10.1128/microbiolspec.EMF-0009-2016

37. Lange RP, Locher HH, Wyss PC, Then RL. The targets of currently used antibacterial agents: Lessons for drug discovery. *Curr Pharm Des* 2007;13(30):3140-54. doi: 10.2174/138161207782110408

38. Barker J, Scaife H, Brown MR. Intraphagocytic growth induces an antibiotic-resistant phenotype of Legionella pneumophila. *Antimicrob Agents Chemother* 1995;39(12):2684-8. doi: 10.1128/aac.39.12.2684

39. Jonas D, Engels I, Hartung D, Beyersmann J, Frank U, Daschner FD. Development and mechanism of fluoroquinolone resistance in Legionella pneumophila. *J Antimicrob Chemother* 2003;51(2):275-80. doi: 10.1093/jac/dkg054

40. Tangden T. Combination antibiotic therapy for multidrug-resistant gram-negative bacteria. *Ups J Med Sci* 2014;119(2):149-53. doi: 10.3109/03009734.2014.899279

41. Ingmundson A, Delprato A, Lambright DG, Roy CR. Legionella pneumophila proteins that regulate Rab1 membrane cycling. *Nature* 2007;450(7168):365-9. doi: 10.1038/nature06336

42. Muller MP, Peters H, Blumer J, Blankenfeldt W, Goody RS, Itzen A. The legionella effector protein DrrA AMPylates the membrane traffic regulator Rab1b. *Science* 2010;329(5994):946-9. doi: 10.1126/science.1192276

43. Tan Y, Luo ZQ. Legionella pneumophila SidD is a deAMPylase that modifies Rab1. *Nature* 2011;475(7357):506-9. doi: 10.1038/nature10307

44. Massip C, Descours G, Ginevra C, Doublet P, Jarraud S, Gilbert C. Macrolide resistance in Legionella pneumophila: The role of lpeab efflux pump. *J Antimicrob Chemother* 2017. doi: 10.1093/jac/dkw594

45. Ayhan DH, Tamer YT, Akbar M, Bailey SM, Wong M, Daly SM, et al. Sequence-specific targeting of bacterial resistance genes increases antibiotic efficacy. *PLoS biol* 2016;14(9):e1002552. doi: 10.1371/journal.pbio.1002552

46. Ermak G. Emerging medical technologies. World Scientific: 2015.

47. Lee YJ, Hoynes-O'Connor A, Leong MC, Moon TS. Programmable control of bacterial gene expression with the combined CRISPR and antisense RNA system. *Nucleic Acids Res* 2016;44(5):2462-73. doi: 10.1093/nar/gkw056

48. Guzman-Trampe S, Ceapa CD, Manzo-Ruiz M, Sanchez S. Synthetic biology era: Improving antibiotic's world. *Biochem Pharmacol* 2017;134:99-113. doi: 10.1016/j.bcp.2017.01.015

49. Gunderson FF, Cianciotto NP. The CRISPR-associated gene cas2 of Legionella pneumophila is required for intracellular infection of amoebae. *MBio* 2013;4(2):e00074-13. doi: 10.1128/mBio.00074-13

50. Mojica FJ, Diez-Villasenor C, Soria E, Juez G. Biological significance of a family of regularly spaced repeats in the genomes of Archaea, Bacteria and mitochondria. *Mol Microbiol* 2000;36(1):244-6. doi: 10.1046/j.1365-2958.2000.01838.x

51. Nakata A, Amemura M, Makino K. Unusual nucleotide arrangement with repeated sequences in the Escherichia coli K-12 chromosome. *J Bacteriol* 1989;171(6):3553-6. doi: 10.1128/jb.171.6.3553-3556.1989

52. Bolotin A, Quinquis B, Sorokin A, Ehrlich SD. Clustered regularly interspaced short palindrome repeats (CRISPRs) have spacers of extrachromosomal origin. *Microbiology* 2005;151(8):2551-61. doi: 10.1099/mic.0.28048-0

53. Horvath P, Barrangou R. CRISPR/Cas, the immune system of bacteria and archaea. *Science* 2010;327(5962):167-70. doi: 10.1126/science.1179555

54. Jinek M, East A, Cheng A, Lin S, Ma E, Doudna J. RNA-programmed genome editing in human cells. *eLife* 2013;2:e00471. doi: 10.7554/eLife.00471

55. Mojica FJ, Diez-Villasenor C, Garcia-Martinez J, Soria E. Intervening sequences of regularly spaced prokaryotic repeats derive from foreign genetic elements. *J Mol Evol* 2005;60(2):174-82. doi: 10.1007/s00239-004-0046-3

56. Pourcel C, Salvignol G, Vergnaud G. CRISPR elements in yersinia pestis acquire new repeats by preferential uptake of bacteriophage DNA, and provide additional tools for evolutionary studies. *Microbiology* 2005;151(Pt 3):653-63. doi: 10.1099/mic.0.27437-0

57. Weinberger AD, Gilmore MS. CRISPR-Cas: To take up DNA or not-that is the question. *Cell Host Microbe* 2012;12(2):125-6. doi: 10.1016/j.chom.2012.07.007

58. Kim H, Kim JS. A guide to genome engineering with programmable nucleases. *Nat Rev Genet* 2014;15(5):321-34. doi: 10.1038/nrg3686

59. Sampson TR, Weiss DS. CRISPR-Cas systems: New players in gene regulation and bacterial physiology. *Front Cell Infect Microbiol* 2014;4:37. doi: 10.3389/fcimb.2014.00037

60. Kole R, Krainer AR, Altman S. RNA therapeutics: Beyond RNA interference and antisense oligonucleotides. *Nat Rev Drug Discov* 2012;11(2):125-40. doi: 10.1038/nrd3625

61. Chi X, Gatti P, Papoian T. Safety of antisense oligonucleotide and siRNA-based therapeutics. *Drug Discov Today* 2017. doi: 10.1016/j.drudis.2017.01.013

62. Georg J, Hess WR. Cis-antisense RNA, another level of gene regulation in bacteria. *Microbiol Mol Biol Rev* 2011;75(2):286-300. doi: 10.1128/mmbr.00032-10

63. Najar AG, Pashaei-Asl R, Omidi Y, Farajnia S, Nourazarian AR. EGFR antisense oligonucleotides encapsulated with nanoparticles decrease EGFR, MAPK1 and STAT5 expression in a human colon cancer cell line. *Asian Pac J Cancer Prev* 2013;14(1):495-8. doi: 10.7314/APJCP.2013.14.1.495

64. Burnett JC, Rossi JJ. RNA-based therapeutics: Current progress and future prospects. *Chem Biol* 2012;19(1):60-71. doi: 10.1016/j.chembiol.2011.12.008

65. Chen Y, Tan XX. Nucleotides for prevention and treatment of bacterial and fungal pathologies. *US 8889397 B2*; 2014.

66. Uhlmann E. Oligonucleotide technologies: Synthesis, production, regulations and applications. 29-30th November 2000, Hamburg, Germany. *Expert Opin Biol Ther* 2001;1(2):319-28. doi: 10.1517/14712598.1.2.319

67. Gleave ME, Monia BP. Antisense therapy for cancer. *Nat Rev Cancer* 2005;5(6):468-79. doi: 10.1038/nrc1631

68. Nourazarian AR, Najar AG, Farajnia S, Khosroushahi AY, Pashaei-Asl R, Omidi Y. Combined EGFR and c-Src antisense oligodeoxynucleotides encapsulated with PAMAM denderimers inhibit HT-29 colon cancer cell proliferation. *Asian Pac J Cancer Prev*

2012;13(9):4751-6. doi: 10.7314/APJCP.2012.13.9.4751

69. Posey KL, Coustry F, Veerisetty AC, Hossain M, Gattis D, Booten S, et al. Antisense reduction of mutant COMP reduces growth plate chondrocyte pathology. *Mol Ther* 2017;25(3):705-14. doi: 10.1016/j.ymthe.2016.12.024

70. Evers MM, Toonen LJ, van Roon-Mom WM. Antisense oligonucleotides in therapy for neurodegenerative disorders. *Adv Drug Deliv Rev* 2015;87:90-103. doi: 10.1016/j.addr.2015.03.008

71. Cazzola M, Matera MG, Page CP. Novel approaches to the treatment of pneumonia. *Trends Pharmacol Sci* 2003;24(6):306-14. doi: 10.1016/s0165-6147(03)00129-9

72. Simons RW, Kleckner N. Biological regulation by antisense RNA in prokaryotes. *Annu Rev Genet* 1988;22:567-600. doi: 10.1146/annurev.ge.22.120188.003031

73. Gasparro FP, Edelson RL, O'Malley ME, Ugent SJ, Wong HH. Photoactivatable antisense DNA: Suppression of ampicillin resistance in normally resistant escherichia coli. *Antisense Res Dev* 1991;1(2):117-40.

74. Good L, Nielsen PE. Antisense inhibition of gene expression in bacteria by PNA targeted to mRNA. *Nat Biotechnol* 1998;16(4):355-8. doi: 10.1038/nbt0498-355

75. Patil SD, Sharma R, Srivastava S, Navani NK, Pathania R. Downregulation of yidC in escherichia coli by antisense RNA expression results in sensitization to antibacterial essential oils eugenol and carvacrol. *PLoS One* 2013;8(3):e57370. doi: 10.1371/journal.pone.0057370

76. Fathi M, Entezami AA, Pashaei-Asl R. Swelling/deswelling, thermal, and rheological behavior of PVA-g-NIPAAm nanohydrogels prepared by a facile free-radical polymerization method. *J Polym Res* 2013;20(5):125. doi: 10.1007/s10965-013-0125-5

77. Luo D, Saltzman WM. Synthetic DNA delivery systems. *Nat Biotechnol* 2000;18(1):33-7. doi: 10.1038/71889

78. Fu HL, Cheng SX, Zhang XZ, Zhuo RX. Dendrimer/DNA complexes encapsulated functional biodegradable polymer for substrate-mediated gene delivery. *J Gene Med* 2008;10(12):1334-42. doi: 10.1002/jgm.1258

79. Madaan K, Kumar S, Poonia N, Lather V, Pandita D. Dendrimers in drug delivery and targeting: Drug-dendrimer interactions and toxicity issues. *J Pharm Bioallied Sci* 2014;6(3):139-50. doi: 10.4103/0975-7406.130965

80. Sebestik J, Niederhafner P, Jezek J. Peptide and glycopeptide dendrimers and analogous dendrimeric structures and their biomedical applications. *Amino Acids* 2011;40(2):301-70. doi: 10.1007/s00726-010-0707-z

81. Leire E, Amaral SP, Louzao I, Winzer K, Alexander C, Fernandez-Megia E, et al. Dendrimer mediated clustering of bacteria: Improved aggregation and evaluation of bacterial response and viability. *Biomater Sci* 2016;4(6):998-1006. doi: 10.1039/c6bm00079g

82. Sousa-Herves A, Novoa-Carballal R, Riguera R, Fernandez-Megia E. GATG dendrimers and PEGylated block copolymers: From synthesis to bioapplications. *AAPS J* 2014;16(5):948-61. doi: 10.1208/s12248-014-9642-3

83. Bae Y, Rhim HS, Lee S, Ko KS, Han J, Choi JS. Apoptin gene delivery by the functionalized polyamidoamine dendrimer derivatives induces cell death of U87-MG glioblastoma cells. *J Pharm Sci* 2017. doi: 10.1016/j.xphs.2017.01.034

84. Dufes C, Uchegbu IF, Schatzlein AG. Dendrimers in gene delivery. *Adv Drug Deliv Rev* 2005;57(15):2177-202. doi: 10.1016/j.addr.2005.09.017

85. Sampathkumar SG, Yarema KJ. Dendrimers in cancer treatment and diagnosis. In: Kumar CS, editor. Nanotechnologies for the Life Sciences. Germany: Wiley; 2007.

86. Abbasi E, Aval SF, Akbarzadeh A, Milani M, Nasrabadi HT, Joo SW, et al. Dendrimers: Synthesis, applications, and properties. *Nanoscale Res Lett* 2014;9(1):247. doi: 10.1186/1556-276x-9-247

87. Voltan AR, Quindos G, Alarcon KPM, Fusco-Almeida AM, Mendes-Giannini MJS, Chorilli M. Fungal diseases: Could nanostructured drug delivery systems be a novel paradigm for therapy? *Int J Nanomedicine* 2016;11:3715-30. doi: 10.2147/ijn.s93105

88. Winnicka K, Wroblewska M, Wieczorek P, Sacha PT, Tryniszewska EA. The effect of PAMAM dendrimers on the antibacterial activity of antibiotics with different water solubility. *Molecules* 2013;18(7):8607-17. doi: 10.3390/molecules18078607

89. Fu HL, Cheng SX, Zhang XZ, Zhuo RX. Dendrimer/DNA complexes encapsulated in a water soluble polymer and supported on fast degrading star poly(DL-lactide) for localized gene delivery. *J Control Release* 2007;124(3):181-8. doi: 10.1016/j.jconrel.2007.08.031

90. Sarisozen C, Pan J, Dutta I, Torchilin VP. Polymers in the co-delivery of siRNA and anticancer drugs to treat multidrug-resistant tumors. *J Pharma Investig* 2017;47(1):37-49. doi: 10.1007/s40005-016-0296-2

91. Nourazarian AR, Pashaei-Asl R, Omidi Y, Najar AG. C-Src antisense complexed with PAMAM denderimes decreases of c-Src expression and EGFR-dependent downstream genes in the human HT-29 colon cancer cell line. *Asian Pac J Cancer Prev* 2012;13(5):2235-40. doi: 10.7314/APJCP.2012.13.5.2235

4

Spectroscopic and Spectrometric Methods Used for the Screening of Certain Herbal Food Supplements Suspected of Adulteration

Cristina Mateescu[1], Anca Mihaela Popescu[1,2]*, Gabriel Lucian Radu[2], Tatiana Onisei[1], Adina Elena Raducanu[1]

[1] *National Office for Medicinal, Aromatic Plants and Bee Products - National Research and Development Institute for Food Bioresources – IBA Bucharest, 6 Dinu Vintila Str., 021102, Bucharest, Romania.*
[2] *Faculty of Applied Chemistry and Materials Science - University Politehnica of Bucharest, 1-7 Polizu Str., 011061, Bucharest, Romania.*

Keywords:
· Fourier transform infrared
· GC-MS
· Herbal food supplements
· PDE-5 inhibitors
· Raman spectroscopy

Abstract

Purpose: This study was carried out in order to find a reliable method for the fast detection of adulterated herbal food supplements with sexual enhancement claims. As some herbal products are advertised as "all natural", their "efficiency" is often increased by addition of active pharmaceutical ingredients such as PDE-5 inhibitors, which can be a real health threat for the consumer.

Methodes: Adulterants, potentially present in 50 herbal food supplements with sexual improvement claims, were detected using 2 spectroscopic methods - Raman and Fourier Transform Infrared - known for reliability, reproductibility, and an easy sample preparation. GC-MS technique was used to confirm the potential adulterants spectra.

Results: About 22% (11 out of 50 samples) of herbal food supplements with sexual enhancement claims analyzed by spectroscopic and spectrometric methods proved to be "enriched" with active pharmaceutical compounds such as: sildenafil and two of its analogues, tadalafil and phenolphthalein. The occurence of phenolphthalein could be the reason for the non-relevant results obtained by FTIR method in some samples. 91% of the adulterated herbal food supplements were originating from China.

Conclusion: The results of this screening highlighted the necessity for an accurate analysis of all alleged herbal aphrodisiacs on the Romanian market. This is a first such a screening analysis carried out on herbal food supplements with sexual enhancement claims

Introduction

During the last period, the consumption of herbal food supplements meant to improve sexual performance has seen a considerable increase. Most consumers trust "100% Natural" advertised products considering them as safe and side effects free.[1] In spite of consumers'belief, this category of herbal supplements could be "tainted" with legal drugs such as: sildenafil, tadalafil, vardenafil, as well as their analogues. Unfortunately, all these substances were not tested from pharmacological or pharmacokinetic point of view.[2,3]

Phosphodiesterase type 5 inhibitors (PDE-5 inhibitors), namely sildenafil, tadalafil, vardenafil are drugs commonly used to treat erectile dysfunction and can be consumed only on medical prescription.[4-6] PDE-5 inhibitors are not recommended for patients on specific prescriptions as: organic nitrates (e.g. nitroglycerin, isosorbide dinitrate, isosorbide mononitrate, amyl nitrite, or nitrate used for the treatment of diabetes, hypertension, hyperlipidemia and ischemic heart disease), as they can cause serious and unpredictable blood pressure falls. These blood pressure falls are often accompanied by other specific symptoms among which: headache, flushing, dyspepsia, nasal congestion,

dizziness, myalgia, back pain, and abnormal vision, are but a few to be mentioned.[7-9]

A number of efficient analytical methods such as: TLC, GC-MS, LC/MS/MS, LC-HR/MS, HPLC-DAD, HPLC-MS, NMR have been developed in order to detect the PDE-5 inhibitors adulteration of food supplements.[1,10-15] Attia et al., have determined the vardenafil hydrocholorides as pure active ingredients in drugs using the TAI (thermal analysis investigation).[16]

However, all these methods require a laborius sample preparation and analysis while being very expensive from financial point of view. Therefore, for a quality screening of adulterated food supplements, a new approach was required: a non-destructive procedure, less laborious in respect of sample preparation and analysis, a faster and more efficient method involving minimal costs. Among such methods, Raman and Infrared spectroscopy proved to be the most efficient. According to specialized literature, these methods have been applied for various purposes: Kim et al. performed quality control of active pharmaceutical ingredients in drugs (capsules) using Raman spectroscopy; Olds used Spatially Offset Raman Spectroscopy (SORS) to identify

---

*Corresponding author: Anca Mihaela Popescu, Email: anca.popescu@bioresurse.ro

concealed substances from a multi-layered postal package. Other identifications were performed for capsules with antibiotics in plastic blister packs and drug dissolved in clear solvents bottled in opaque plastic vials. De Veij et al., detected counterfeit Viagra tablets using Raman while Trefi et al., using Raman spectroscopy and NMR (Nuclear Magnetic Resonance) identified counterfeit Cialis tablets illegally sold on the internet.[17-20] Fourier Transform Infrared Spectroscopy with Attenuated Total Reflectance (ATR-FTIR) and IR Spectroscopy were used to detect counterfeit drugs like Viagra and Cialis type by Ortiz et al., and Custers et al.[21,22] Using the same techniques, Champagne et al., detected sildenafil and tadalafil in raw materials used as ingredients in food supplements.[23] Chuang et al., and Yang et al., used near-infrared spectroscopy (NIR) to analyze bioactive compounds in herbs and herbal medicines, respectively.[24,25]

As consumers show an increasing demand for natural products (supplements), quality control, adequate risk assessment and clear regulation for botanicals and botanical preparations are highly required. While adulteration could be "economically motivated", occurrence of such pharmacological active compounds in herbal supplements may become a serious health threat for consumers.

In this study, a qualitative screening of 50 herbal food supplements samples collected from the local market, was carried out. Raman spectroscopy and Fourier Transform Infrared Spectroscopy were used as rapid screening methods. These analytical methods are complementary and cheaper and can be used to identify several chemical functional groups. They are less time consuming in both sample preparation and analysis. As soon as the adulteration was detected, the GC-MS technique was applied to confirme the adulterants spectra in the respective samples.

Materials and Methods

Chemicals

Reference standards of sildenafil (with purity of 98,8%) and tadalafil (with purity of 99,9%) were purchased from European Directorate for the Quality of Medicines & HealthCare, European Pharmacopoeia (Strasbourg, France). Acetone and methanol used as solvents were provided by Merck, Germany.

Commercial formulations of dietary supplements

A total number of 50 herbal food supplements promoted to improve sexual performance were analyzed. The samples were encoded from Hfsd1 up to Hfsd50. A number of 45 products were provided by the National Office for Medicinal, Aromatic Plants and Bee Products, 4 products were purchased on line while one product was bought from a local drugstore. The analyzed herbal supplements originated from different countries and were marketed as: capsules, tablets, liquids in vials, sachets, powders.

Raman measurements

Raman spectra were recorded by a NXR FT-Raman Module with InGaAs (Inidium-Gallium Arsenide) detector and CaF_2 beam splitter. The power of laser beam at the surface of the sample was about 0.3 mW. Each spectrum consisted of 64 co-added scans at a spectral resolution of 4 cm^{-1} in the field of 3701-100 cm^{-1}. Omnic software version 8 (Nicolet Instrument Co. Madison, USA) was used to determine the spectra.

ATR-FTIR measurements

A Nicolet 6700 FT-IR Spectrometer (Nicolet Instrument Co., Madison, USA) with DTGS (Deuterated Triglycine Sulphate) detector was used to record the absorbtion spectra.

A single bounce ZnSe – diamond crystal was used in the attenuated total reflectance (ATR) sampling system. A small amount of each homogenized sample was directly applied and pressed on the diamond crystal. The same pressure value was applied to all samples. Each spectrum was measured at a spectral resolution of 4 cm^{-1} and consisted of 64 co-added scans. Recordings were performed in the range of 3701-100 cm^{-1}. The crystal was cleaned in acetone and dried in open air, at room temperature following each measurement. To avoid possible contamination of the crystal, the background spectrum using identical instrumental conditions was measured after each acetone cleaning.

GC-MS analysis

For analytical screening and confirmation of the adulterated herbal food supplements, GC-MS was applied. The GC-MS system consisted of an Agilent HP6890N Gas Chromatograph and a HP5973N Mass Spectrometer. 1 μL volume was injected using splitless mode on the 250° C injector port with helium flow at 1.0 mL/min. A TR-5MS (30 m x 0.25 mm i.d. 0.25 μm film thickness) capillary column (5% phenyl polysilphenylene-siloxane) was used. The interface temperature was set at 290° C. The oven ramping temperature was programmed at 135-200° C (1 min hold) at a rate of 13°C/min, and 200-315°C at a rate of 6° C/min, at 315° C holds for 20 min. The screening was performed on selected ion monitoring mode at m/z 99, 404 for sildenafil and m/z 389, 262 for tadalafil, respectively. Adulterant identification was done on full scan mode (50-500 a.m.u), Man et al., adapted method.[26]

Sample preparation

The sample required minimal preparation. Each solid sample consisted of: the content of one capsule, a tablet (that was crushed) or the contents of a sachet. The powder obtained from each sample was homogenized using a mortar and pestle. For Raman analysis the obtained homogenized powder was inserted into a 6 mm diameter vial, that was further inserted in the equipment. Liquid samples did not require previously preparation.

GC-MS analysis
Stock solutions of sildenafil and tadalafil
For stock solutions preparation, 1 mg of high purity reference standards (sildenafil and tadalafil, respectively) was each dissolved in 1 ml absolute methanol. To get the reference ion chromatogram for each adulterant, a 1:10 dilution was performed.

Samples
Each 100 mg of homogene fine powder/sample (from a sachet, by emptying a capsule or crushing a tablet) was disolved in 1 ml of absolute methanol. For the liquid products, 2 ml/sample were taken and dilluted in 1 ml absolute methanol. Samples were thoroughly vortexed, followed by 15 minutes of sonication and 5 minutes centrifugation at 4000 rpm. The supernatant was collected and filtered by 0,2 μm membrane filters for GC-MS analysis.

Results and Discussion
Raman spectroscopy
The high purity reference standards of sildenafil and tadalafil were analyzed.
The specific bands corresponding to the characteristic functional groups of sildenafil were identified at 1698 cm^{-1} (band that can be attributed to stretching vibrations of the group C=O) as well as at the doublet 1580/1563 cm^{-1} (which is specific to C=C bond). For bonds containing nitrogen, Raman bands were present at 1529 cm^{-1}, due to v(N-C=N) and at 1238 cm^{-1}, respectively,

due to v(C=N). Raman bands registered at 1170 cm^{-1} and 648 cm^{-1} are attributed to the symmetrical group v(SO2), as well as to the stretching vibrations v(C-S), respectively.[19]
Specific responses for tadalafil occurred in the 3100-3000 cm^{-1} range and 1700-1500 cm^{-1} range, respectively. The characteristic spectral bands are consistent with the literature data.[20] These bands correspond to the vibrations of unsaturated or aromatic C-H bond and to the vibrations of unsaturated C=C bond, respectively.
The Raman spectra for all the 50 samples of dietary supplements that were registered according to the same procedure used for the reference standards.
As seen in Table 1 (A), four herbal supplements adulterated with sidenafil were identified. Almost all characteristic bands of high purity reference standard were present in the spectra of Hfsd50 sample (1170 cm^{-1} band was missing) and Hfs48 sample (1238 cm^{-1} was missing), while two or three bands were absent in the spectra of Hfsd4 and Hfsd49 samples.
As shown in Table 1 (B), other seven samples of herbal food supplements adulterated with tadalafil were also detected. Hfsd30 sample showed all the characteristic spectral bands of tadalafil, while in the spectra of Hfsd12 and Hfsd29 samples, one specific band was missing. In the spectra of Hfsd27 and Hfsd32 samples two and three bands, respectively, were missing. It has also been noticed that the spectra of the examined samples were of poor quality.

Table 1. Characteristic Raman bands of sildenafil and tadalafil detected in the analyzed samples

(A) Pure Sildenafil - reference standard/ Wave number (cm^{-1})	Sample						
	Hfsd4	Hfsd48	Hfsd49	Hfsd50	-	-	-
1698	1689 1583 1555	1682	-	1701			
1580	-	1595	1579	1580			
1563	-	-	1566 1539	1563			
1529	1175	1524	-	1529			
1238	632	1237	-	1239			
1170		1164	648	-			
648		652		647			

(B) Pure Tadalafil – reference standard/ Wave number (cm^{-1})	Sample						
	Hfsd12	Hfsd27	Hfsd28	Hfsd29	Hfsd30	Hfsd31	Hfsd32
3066	3056	3046	3055	3098	3095	-	3066
3002	-	-	-	3028	3074	-	-
1672	1685	1697	-	-	3057	-	-
1596	1592 1544	-	1591	1597	1643	1594	1591
1567		1567	-	1566	1611	1571	-
		1528			1580	1520	1525
		1514			1564		

In the Hfsd28 and Hfsd31 samples spectra only a part of the characteristic bands of tadalafil were detected. As the Raman spectra of the Hfsd28 and Hfsd31 samples were not enough relevant a clear conclusion on their tadalafil adulteration could not be drawn.

Raman spectroscopy used to screen the 50 herbal food supplements with sexual enhancement claims, detected 9 adulterated samples among which 4 products with sildenafil and 5 products with tadalafil. As already mentioned, two samples suspected to be adulterated with tadalafil showed no relevant spectra, missing three specific bands of the reference standard.

ATR-FTIR spectroscopy

The FTIR spectra for the 50 samples of herbal food supplements were also analysed against the sildenafil and tadalafil reference standards.

Absorption peaks characteristic for PDE-5 inhibitors were registerd in the 1800-525 cm^{-1} range. According to Champagne et al., this spectral range includes the 1720-1150 cm^{-1} domain, important for the detection of PDE-5 inhibitors analogues and homologues, respectively.[23]

The sildenafil spectrum (Figure 1a) showed significant absorption peaks at: 1698 cm^{-1} (characteristic to carbonyl groups (C=O)); 1579 cm^{-1} (specific to N-H bonds, occurring in the range of 1650-1500 cm^{-1}); 1489 cm^{-1} (resulted from C=C bonds in the benzene ring). C-N bonds from the functional group O=C-N is absorbed at 1400 cm^{-1} (but in this experiment the absorbtion value was 1391 cm^{-1}). Anzanello et al. reported that C-H aromatic out-of-plane deformation occurred at 939 cm^{-1}, which resulted in addition of new peaks at 1172, 758, 619, 587 cm^{-1}.[27]

The specific tadalafil absorption peaks of FTIR spectrum (Figure 1b) were registered at 1675 cm^{-1} (characteristic of amides C=O), 1646 cm^{-1} (C=C aromatic). The band of 1435 cm^{-1} belongs to the stretching vibration C-N, and the band 746 cm^{-1} is representative for benzene.[27]

Comparing the spectrum of sildenafil reference standard with all spectra of the 50 analyzed samples of herbal food supplements, the occurence of sildenafil adulteration of four samples (Hfsd4, Hfsd48, Hfsd49, Hfsd50) was noted (Table 2 (A)).

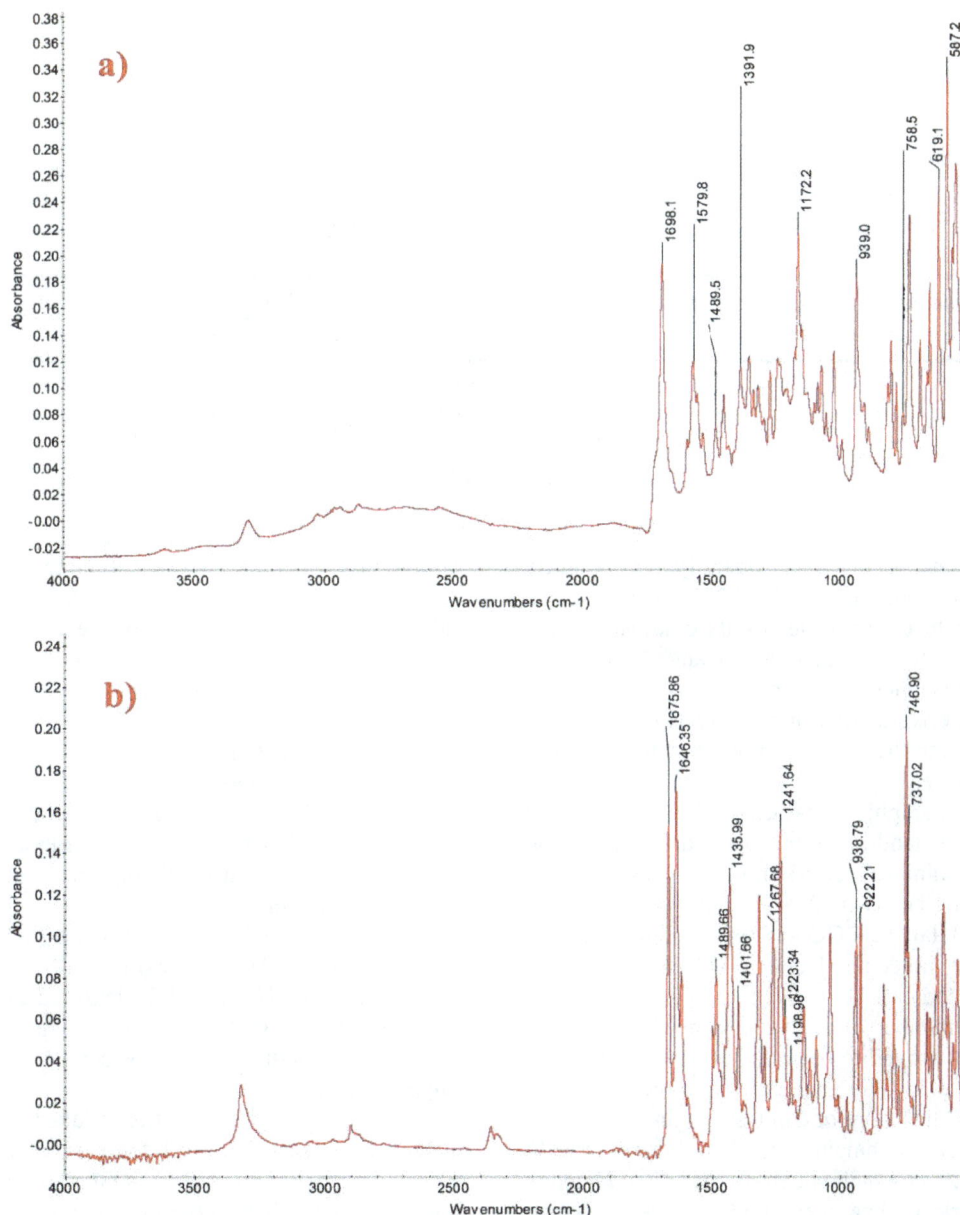

Figure 1. FTIR spectra for high purity reference substances: a) sildenafil and b) tadalafil

All characteristic absorption peaks for sildenafil were identified in the spectrum of Hfsd50 sample. The Hfsd48 sample spectrum did not show, the characteristic absorption peaks for: 1579 cm^{-1}, 1172 cm^{-1}, and 758 cm^{-1}. In the spectrum of Hfsd49 sample the four bands: 1579 cm^{-1}, 1489 cm^{-1}, 1391 cm^{-1} and 758 cm^{-1}, respectively, were absent. Hfsd4 sample showed a very poor spectrum (6 bands were missing: 1698 cm^{-1}, 1391 cm^{-1}, 1172 cm^{-1}, 758 cm^{-1}, 619 cm^{-1} and 587 cm^{-1}, respectively). This last result is not relevant if the adulteration with sildenalfil is to be considered.

Out of the total analyzed samples, seven herbal food supplements (Hfsd12, Hfsd27, Hfsd28, Hfsd29, Hfsd30,

Hfsd31, Hfsd32) were identified as adulterated with tadalafil (Table 2 (B)). All spectra of the adulterated samples showed the same absorption peaks as the tadalafil reference spectrum. Thus, FTIR analysis confirmed that Hfsd28 sample was adulterated with tadalafil while application of Raman spectroscopy to the mentioned sample could not detect this adulteration.

The screening of 50 herbal food supplements with sexual enhancement claims performed by ATR-FTIR spectroscopic method had as result the detection of a number of 10 adulterated samples with sildenafil (3 products) and tadalafil (7 products).

Table 2. Characteristic FTIR bands of sildenafil and tadalafil detected in the analyzed samples

(A) Pure Sildenafil - reference standard/ Wave numbers (cm^1)	Sample						
	Hfsd4	Hfsd48	Hfsd49	Hfsd50	-	-	-
1698	-	1687	1698	1700			
1579	1580	-	-	1581			
1489	1463	1488	-	1490			
1391	-	1397	-	1392			
1172	-	—	1172	1171			
939	934	932	939	939			
758	-	—	-	758			
619	-	617 583	619	619			
587	-		588	588			
(B) Pure Tadalafil – reference standard/ Wave numbers (cm^1)	Sample						
	Hfsd12	Hfsd27	Hfsd28	Hfsd29	Hfsd30	Hfsd31	Hfsd32
1675	1674	1675	1675	1675	1675	1675	1675
1646	1645	1646	1646	1646	1646	1645	1648
1435	1433	1436	1436	1435	1436	1435	1435
746	746	745	745	747	746	746	748

GC-MS

Due to its capacity to separate, quantify and identify unknown organic compounds, GC-MS was used as a sensitive method to confirm the results obtained by the two spectroscopic techniques (Raman and FTIR). The advantage of this method is related to the sample preparation (no derivatization or hydrolysis procedure is needed) as well as to the detection time (much shorter) of adulterant substances.

A good chromatographic separation of sildenafil and tadalafil reference standards was obtained at a retention time of 38.66 minutes, 36.63 minutes, respectively. Identification of the two PDE-5 inhibitors (namely sildenafil and tadalafil) by GC-MS was facilitated by the presence of their molecular ion m/z 474 (for sildenafil) and m/z 389 (for tadalafil).

Out of the total number of analyzed samples, 11 herbal food supplements proved to be adulterated with sildenafil or tadalafil (Table 3). The adulterated products (91% of the analyzed samples) were of Chinese origin.

Surprisingly, phenolphthalein was detected in Hfsd48 sample (Figure 2), in which sildenafil was also detected. It has to be noticed that phenolphthalein is a banned substance both in Europe and in USA since 1997 because of its potential carcinogenic effects. We suppose that

phenolphthalein was introduced in the herbal food supplement with the intention to conceal the presence of sildenafil and thus to prevent the detection of the adulterant (PDE-5 inhibitor) by spectroscopic analysis.

The occurence of phenolphthalein could be the reason for the non-relevant results obtained by FTIR method in Hfsd48 sample.

GC-MS technique proved to be more sensitive than spectroscopic methods Raman and ATR-FTIR: in Hfsd4, Hfsd49 and Hfsd50 samples, sildenafil was identified togeher with other two unknown compounds with similar fragmentation pattern (probably analogues of sildenafil) as it could be seen in Figure 3.

We suppose that sildenafil analogues (detected in Hfsd4, Hfsd49 and Hfsd50 samples) as well as phenolphthalein (detected in Hfsd48 sample) identified by GC-MS could be responsible for the low quality spectra recorded by ATR-FTIR method used to screen the herbal food supplements.

Using GC-MS analysis, the adulterant tadalafil was detected in seven herbal food supplements (Hfsd12, Hfsd27, Hfsd28, Hfsd29, Hfsd30, Hfsd31, and Hfsd32 samples). The chromatograms of all samples showed a common significant peak for tadalafil at the retention time at 37.4 min (see Figure 4).

Table 3. Characterization of analyzed herbal food supplements

| Sample | Product description | Country of origin | Identified adulterants | | | Analytical methods used | | |
			Sildenafil	Tadalafil	Others	Raman	FT-IR	GC-MS
Hfsd 4	flask with 60 capsules	China	+	-	Two analogues	+	Not relevant spectrum	+
Hfsd 12	flask with 15 capsules	China	-	+	-	+	+	+
Hfsd 27	Box of 1 blister with 4 capsules	China	-	+	-	+	+	+
Hfsd 28	Box of 1 blister with 4 capsules	China	-	+		Not relevant spectrum	+	+
Hfsd 29	Box of 1 blister with 4 capsules	China	-	+	-	+	+	+
Hfsd 30	Box of 1 blister with 4 capsules	China	-	+	-	+	+	+
Hfsd 31	Box of 1 blister with 4 capsules	China	-	+	-	Not relevant spectrum	+	+
Hfsd 32	Box of 1 blister with 4 capsules	China	-	+	-	+	+	+
Hfsd 48	Box of 1 blister with 2 capsules	USA	+	-	Phenolphthalein	+	+	+
Hfsd 49	Foil with 2 capsules	China	+	-	Two analogues	+	+	+
Hfsd 50	Box of 1 blister with 4 tablets	China	+	-	Two analogues	+	+	+

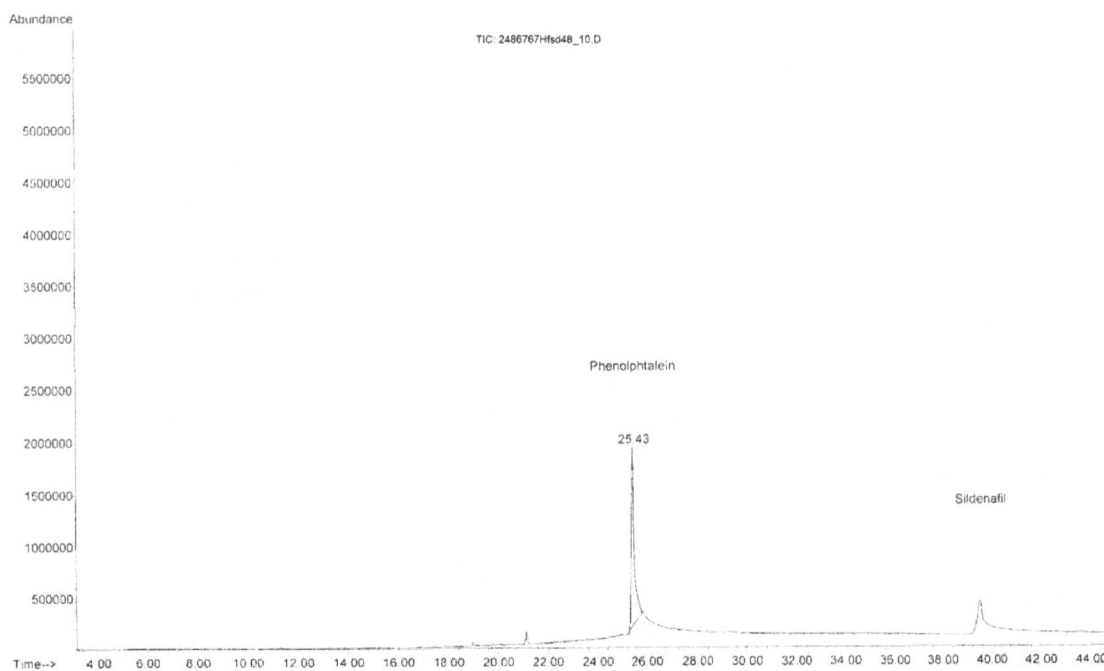

Figure 2. Total ion chromatogram of Hfsd48 sample adulterated with sildenafil and phenolphthalein

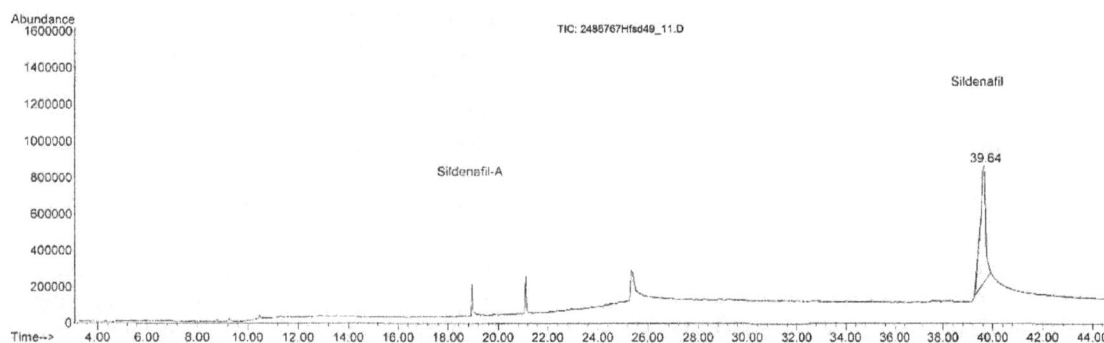

Figure 3. Total ion chromatogram of Hfsd49 sample adulterated with sildenafil and two similar compounds

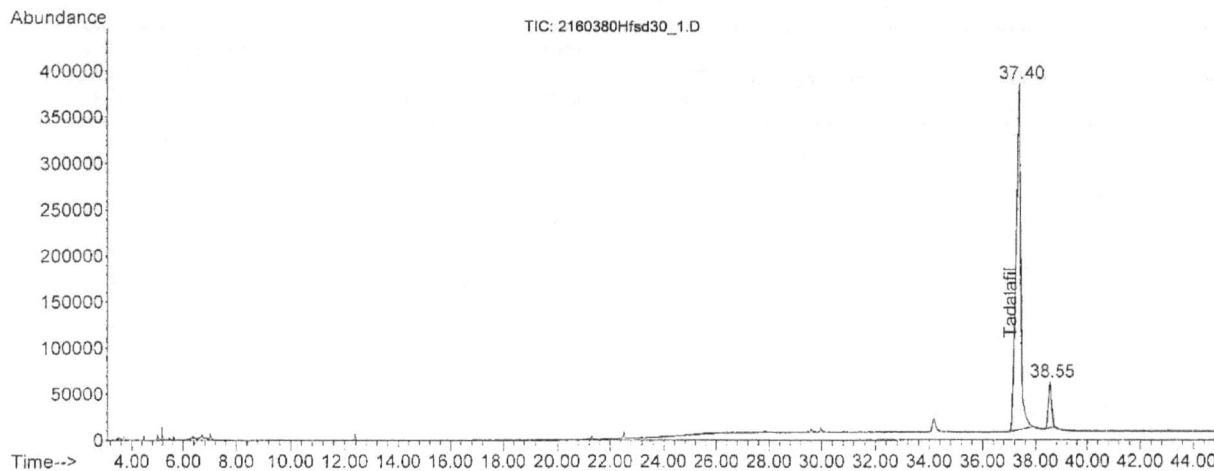

Figure 4. Total ion chromatogram of Hfsd30 sample adulterated with tadalafil

The GC-MS method used to confirm the results of the spectroscopic methods applied for same samples showed that tadalafil could be detected more specific as compared to Raman technique (Hfsd28 and Hfsd31 samples were relevant examples).

About 22% of herbal food supplements with sexual enhancement claims analyzed by spectroscopic and spectrometric methods proved to be "enriched" with active pharmaceutical compounds such as: sildenafil and two of its analogues, tadalafil and phenolphthalein.

All these adulterants were detected in similar alleged herbal aphrodisiacs by different researchers (see literature data).[13-15]

Conclusion

The screening performed on a total number of 50 herbal food supplements promoted as natural aphrodisiacs emphasised that 11 samples (22% of the analyzed products) were adulterated with pharmaceuticals compounds (PDE-5 inhibitors and their analogues) or chemical substances (phenolphthalein).

The adulterated food supplements are a real health threat for the consumers, due to the misleading labelling ("100% natural products") and undeclared pharmaceutical substances hidden in their composition. The consumption of these adulterated herbal food supplements can seriously harm health as PDE-5 inhibitors and their analogues the most frequent adulterants in sexual enhancement products) could interact with nitrates based drugs and result in side effects or adverse reactions. As adulteration could affect not only the safety of end products but also the raw materials used by manufacturers, the fast screening spectroscopic methods could have more applications in the market control and surveillance of natural products.

In this study, the detection of adulterants using spectroscopic methods (Raman and Fourier transform infrared) was confirmed by gas chromatography coupled with mass spectrometry (GC-MS).

The minimal sample preparation required by spectroscopic methods as well as the very short analysis time (about 5 minutes/sample) and minimal costs (no special reagents are needed) are the main advanteges when a huge number of samples have to be screened. Thus, spectroscopic methods proved to be a very useful tool for the control and surveillance of the herbal food supplements market.

The screening of the products suspected to be adulterated could be rapidly performed. As soon as non-compliant products are identified, the adulterants can be detected by GC-MS techniques, which proved to be a very sensitive key method able to confirm the spectroscopic results.

The preliminary results obtained by the screening of 50 herbal food supplements with sexual enhancement claims, highlighted the necessity for an accurate analysis of all alleged herbal aphrodisiacs commercialized on the Romanian market, due to their potential risk profile.

Acknowledgments

The work has been funded by the Sectoral Operational Programme Human Resources Development 2007-2013 of the Romanian Ministry of Labour, Family and Social Protection through the Financial Agreement POSDRU/107/1.5/S/76903.

Ethical Issues

Not applicable.

Conflict of Interest

The authors declare no conflict of interests.

References

1. Venhuis BJ, Blok-Tip L, de Kaste D. Designer drugs in herbal aphrodisiacs. *Forensic Sci Int* 2008;177(2-3):e25-7. doi: 10.1016/j.forsciint.2007.11.007
2. Göker H, Coşkun M, Alp M. Isolation and identification of a new acetildenafil analogue used to adulterate a dietary supplement: dimethylacetildenafil. *Turk J Chem* 2010;34:157-63. doi: 10.3906/kim-1002-25
3. Singh S, Prasad B, Savaliya AA, Shah RP, Gohil VM, Kaur A. Strategies for characterizing sildenafil, vardenafil, tadalafil and their analogues in herbal dietary supplements, and detecting counterfeit

products containing these drugs. *TrAC, Trends Anal Chem* 2009;28(1):13-28. doi: 10.1016/j.trac.2008.09.004

4. Zou P, Oh SS, Hou P, Low MY, Koh HL. Simultaneous determination of synthetic phosphodiesterase-5 inhibitors found in a dietary supplement and pre-mixed bulk powders for dietary supplements using high-performance liquid chromatography with diode array detection and liquid chromatography-electrospray ionization tandem mass spectrometry. *J Chromatogr A* 2006;1104(1-2):113-22. doi: 10.1016/j.chroma.2005.11.103

5. Gratz SR, Flurer CL, Wolnik KA. Analysis of undeclared synthetic phosphodiesterase-5 inhibitors in dietary supplements and herbal matrices by LC-ESI-MS and LC-UV. *J Pharm Biomed Anal* 2004;36(3):525-33. doi: 10.1016/j.jpba.2004.07.004

6. Ge X, Low MY, Zou P, Lin L, Yin SO, Bloodworth BC, et al. Structural elucidation of a PDE-5 inhibitor detected as an adulterant in a health supplement. *J Pharm Biomed Anal* 2008;48(4):1070-5. doi: 10.1016/j.jpba.2008.08.019

7. Gratz SR, Zeller M, Mincey DW, Flurer CL. Structural characterization of sulfoaildenafil, an analog of sildenafil. *J Pharm Biomed Anal* 2009;50(2):228-31. doi: 10.1016/j.jpba.2009.04.003

8. Kostis JB, Jackson G, Rosen R, Barrett-Connor E, Billups K, Burnett AL, et al. Sexual Dysfunction and Cardiac Risk (the Second Princeton Consensus Conference). *Am J Cardiol* 2005;96(2):313-21. doi: 10.1016/j.amjcard.2005.03.065

9. Wespes E, Amar E, Hatzichristou D, Hatzimouratidis K, Montorsi F, Pryor J, et al. EAU Guidelines on Erectile Dysfunction: An Update. *Eur Urol* 2006;49(5):806-15. doi: 10.1016/j.eururo.2006.01.028

10. Miller GM, Stripp R. A study of western pharmaceuticals contained within samples of Chinese herbal/patent medicines collected from New York City's Chinatown. *Leg Med (Tokyo)* 2007;9(5):258-64. doi: 10.1016/j.legalmed.2007.04.001

11. Popescu AM, Radu GL, Onisei T, Raducanu AE, Niculae CG. Detection by gas chromatography-mass spectrometry of adulterated food supplements. *Rom Biotechnolog Lett* 2014;19(4):9485-92.

12. Radu GL, Popescu AM, Niculae CG, Raducanu AE, Onisei T. Identification by Liquid Chromatography-Mass Spectrometry of Herbal Food Supplements Adulterated with PDE-5 Inhibitors. *Rev Chim* 2015;66(1):1-5.

13. Tseng MC, Lin JH. Determination of sildenafil citrate adulterated in a dietary supplement capsule by LC/MS/MS. *J Food Drug Anal* 2002;10(2):112-9.

14. Kim SH, Kim HJ, Son J, Jeon BW, Jeong ES, Cha EJ, et al. Simultaneous Determination of Synthetic Phosphodiesterase-5 Inhibitors in Dietary Supplements by Liquid Chromatography-High Resolution/Mass Spectrometry. *Mass Spectrom Lett* 2012;3(2):50-3. doi: 10.5478/MSL.2012.3.2.50

15. Venhuis BJ, Zomer G, de Kaste D. Structure elucidation of a novel synthetic thiono analogue of sildenafil detected in an alleged herbal aphrodisiac. *J Pharm Biomed Anal* 2008;46(4):814-7. doi: 10.1016/j.jpba.2007.12.007

16. Attia AK, Souaya ER, Soliman EA. Thermal analysis investigation of dapoxetine and vardenafil hydrochlorides using molecular orbital calculations. *Adv Pharm Bull* 2015;5(4):523-9. doi: 10.15171/apb.2015.071

17. Kim J, Noh J, Chung H, Woo YA, Kemper MS, Lee Y. Direct, non-destructive quantitative measurement of an active pharmaceutical ingredient in an intact capsule formulation using Raman spectroscopy. *Anal Chim Acta* 2007;598(2):280-5. doi: 10.1016/j.aca.2007.07.049

18. Olds WJ, Jaatinen E, Fredericks P, Cletus B, Panayiotou H, Izake EL. Spatially offset Raman spectroscopy (SORS) for the analysis and detection of packaged pharmaceuticals and concealed drugs. *Forensic Sci Int* 2011;212(1-3):69-77. doi: 10.1016/j.forsciint.2011.05.016

19. de Veij M, Deneckere A, Vandenabeele P, de Kaste D, Moens L. Detection of counterfeit Viagra® with Raman spectroscopy. *J Pharm Biomed Anal* 2008;46(2):303-9. doi: 10.1016/j.jpba.2007.10.021

20. Trefi S, Routaboul C, Hamieh S, Gilard V, Malet-Martino M, Martino R. Analysis of illegally manufactured formulations of tadalafil (Cialis®) by ^{1}H NMR, 2D DOSY ^{1}H NMR and Raman spectroscopy. *J Pharm Biomed Anal* 2008;47(1):103-13. doi: 10.1016/j.jpba.2007.12.033

21. Ortiz RS, de Cassia Mariotti K, Fank B, Limberger RP, Anzanello MJ, Mayorga P. Counterfeit Cialis and Viagra fingerprinting by ATR-FTIR spectroscopy with chemometry: Can the same pharmaceutical powder mixture be used to falsify two medicines? *Forensic Sci Int* 2013;226(1-3):282-9. doi: 10.1016/j.forsciint.2013.01.043

22. Custers D, Vandemoortele S, Bothy JL, De Beer JO, Courselle P, Apers S, et al. Physical profiling and IR spectroscopy: simple and effective methods to discriminate between genuine and counterfeit samples of Viagra® and Cialis®. *Drug Test Anal* 2016;8(3-4):378-87. doi: 10.1002/dta.1813

23. Champagne AB, Emmel KV. Rapid screening test for adulteration in raw materials of dietary supplements. *Vib Spectrosc* 2011;55(2):216-23. doi: 10.1016/j.vibspec.2010.11.009

24. Chuang YK, Yang IC, Lo YM, Tsai CY, Chen S. Integration of independent component analysis with near-infrared spectroscopy for analysis of bioactive components in the medicinal plant Gentiana scabra Bunge. *J Food Drug Anal* 2014;22(3):336-44. doi: 10.1016/j.jfda.2014.01.021

25. Yang IC, Tsai CY, Hsieh KW, Yang CW, Ouyang F, Lo YM, et al. Integration of SIMCA and near-infrared spectroscopy for rapid and precise

identification of herbal medicines. *J Food Drug Anal* 2013;21(3):268-78. doi: 10.1016/j.jfda.2013.07.008

26. Man CN, Nor NM, Lajis R, Harn GL. Identification of sildenafil, tadalafil and vardenafil by gas chromatography-mass spectrometry on short capillary column. *J Chromatogr A* 2009;1216(47):8426-30. doi: 10.1016/j.chroma.2009.10.016

27. Anzanello MJ, Ortiz RS, Limbergerb RP, Mayorga P. A multivariate-based wavenumber selection method for classifying medicines into authentic or counterfeit classes. *J Pharm Biomed Anal* 2013;83:209-14. doi: 10.1016/j.jpba.2013.05.004

5

Two Active Compounds From *Caesalpinia sappan* L. In Combination With Cisplatin Synergistically Induce Apoptosis And Cell Cycle Arrest On WiDr Cells

Sri Handayani[1,2], Ratna Asmah Susidarti[2], Riris Istighfari Jenie[2], Edy Meiyanto[2]*

[1] *Research Center for Chemistry, Indonesian Institute of Sciences (LIPI), Serpong, Indonesia.*
[2] *Cancer Chemoprevention Research Center, Faculty of Pharmacy, Universitas Gadjah Mada, Yogyakarta, Indonesia.*

Keywords:
· Brazilin
· Brazilein
· *Caesalpinia sappan, L.*
· Cisplatin
· Synergistic effect
· WiDr cells

Abstract
Purpose: The aim of this study is to observe the synergistic effect of two active compounds of secang, brazilin and brazilein, combined with cisplatin on WiDr colon cancer cells.
Methods: Cytotoxic activities of brazilin (Bi) and brazilein (Be) in single and in combination with cisplatin (Cisp) were examined by MTT assay. Synergistic effect was analyzed by combination index (CI) parameter. Apoptosis and cell cycle profiles were observed by using flow cytometry.
Results: The result of MTT assay showed that IC_{50} value of brazilin and brazilein on WiDr cancer cells were 41 µM and 52 µM respectively. The combination of ½ IC_{50} of Bi-Cisp reduced cells viability up to 64% and showed synergistic effect with CI value less than 1 (CI = 0.8). The combinations of ½ IC_{50} of Be-Cisp also reduced cells viability up to 78% and showed synergistic effect (CI=0.65). Combination of Bi-Cisp and Be-Cisp induced apoptosis higher than the single treatments. Further analysis on the cell cycle progression showed that single treatment of ½ IC_{50} of Be and Bi induced S-phase and G2/M-phase accumulation, while combination of Be-Cisp and Bi-Cisp enhanced S-phase accumulation.
Conclusion: Both combination of Bi-Cisp and Be-Cisp showed synergistic effect on WiDr cells through induction of apoptosis and halted the cell cycle progression, thus, WiDr cells growth were significantly reduced.

Introduction

Some of colorectal cancer (CRC) cases are associated with poor survival because of *p53* mutation.[1] The *p53* gene is a tumor suppressor and the key regulator of DNA damage responses. This gene plays a role on tumor suppression processes including cell cycle arrest and apoptosis.[2] Mutation in *p53* gene leading to the loss of wild-type *p53* activity is frequently detected in many different tumor types.[3] Enhancing of invasiveness, attenuating of apoptosis and increasing of genomic instability are generally occurred after mutation of *p53*.[4] The *p53*-mutant cancer may not be treated with the same agent as *p53* wild type cancer.

Surgery, chemotherapeutic drugs and radiation therapy are some of the cancer therapies that frequently be used to treat colon cancer patient.[5] Cisplatin and its derivatives are the effective DNA-damaging anti-tumor agent for various human cancers, including colon cancer.[6] The p53 protein is stabilized and its level increases in response to various DNA damaging agents, including cisplatin. However, side effects including resistance to cisplatin arise in *p53*-mutant cancer cells.[7] Thus, we need to investigate potential anticancer compounds that work on p53-independent pathway. Currently, combination of chemotherapy regiments based on platinum-derived compounds with other drugs (co-chemotherapeutic agent) constitute the pharmacological therapy of choice for the treatment of colon cancer. The *p53*-mutant colon cancer may need to be treated with combination therapy.

The major compounds of *Caesalpinia sappan* L. (Caesalpiniaceae) i.e. brazilin and brazilein have been reported to have activities as antiinflammation, antioxidant, hepatoprotective and antiviral.[8–11] Brazilin and brazilein induce apoptosis and inhibit cell growth on several cancer cells.[12–14] Brazilein suppresses cancer cells migration and invasion.[15] Thus, brazilin and brazilein have potential to be developed as co-chemotherapeutic agent. Nevertheless, synergistic effect of combination of brazilin and brazilein with cisplatin against *p53*-mutant WiDr cancer cells has never been reported. In this study, we observed the synergistic cytotoxic effect of combination of brazilin and brazilein with cisplatin on WiDr cancer cells.

Materials and Methods
Chemicals
Brazilin and brazilein were isolated from *Caesalpinia sappan*, L. using previously reported method.[9] Cisplatin was purchased from Wako (Japan).

---

*Corresponding author: Edy Meiyanto, Email : edy_meiyanto@ugm.ac.id

Cell culture

WiDr cell line was obtained Faculty of Medicine, Universitas Gadjah Mada, Yogyakarta.

Cytotoxic assay

The 1×104 cells/well were seeded in 96-well plate. Cells were treated with various concentrations of brazilin, brazilein, and cisplatin in single or in combination then incubated in 37°C, 5% CO_2 for 24 h. Cells were then washed with PBS (Sigma), were treated with 100 μL culture medium containing 0.5 mg/mL MTT (Sigma) and incubated in 37°C, 5% CO_2 for 4 h. The reaction was stopped by adding to the cells with SDS reagent (10% sodium dodecyl sulphate (Merck) in HCl 0.01M (Merck)) then was incubated overnight in room temperature. The absorbance was measured with microplate reader (Bio-Rad) at λ 595 nm.

Cell cycle distribution

Propidium iodide (PI) staining kit (Becton Dickinson) was used to analyze DNA content. 5×104 cells/well were seeded in 24-well plate. Cells were treated with various concentrations of samples in single or in combination then incubated in 37°C, 5% CO_2 for 24 h. Cells were harvested and washed in PBS, fixed with 70% ethanol, labeled with PI (2 μg/mL), and incubated in room temperature, protected from light, for 10 min. The DNA content was analyzed using flow cytometry (Becton Dickinson) and followed by flowing software (version 2.5.1) and Excel MS Office 2013.

Apoptosis detection

Apoptotic cells population was determined using PI-Annexin V assay (Annexin V-FITC Apoptosis Detection Kit Roche). 5×10^4 cells/well were seeded in 24-well plate. Cells were treated with various concentrations of samples either single or in combination for 24 h. Cells were harvested, added with 1× binding buffer, labeled with PI-Annexin V, and incubated at room temperature in the dark for 5 min. The cells suspension was analyzed using a flow cytometry (Becton Dickinson) and followed by flowing software (version 2.5.1) and Excel MS Office 2013.

Statistical analysis

Statistical analysis was performed using Student t-test (Microsoft Excel 2013). *P*-values less than 0.05 were considered significant.

Effects of combinations on growth inhibition were analyzed using the Combination index (CI) equation developed by Reynolds and Maurer.[16]

Results and Discussion

Cytotoxic effect of brazilin and brazilein on WiDr cells.

First, we observed the cytotoxic activity to find out the potency of brazilin and brazilein in inhibiting of WiDr cells proliferation. The cytotoxic activity was performed by using MTT assay. The results showed that brazilin and brazilein inhibited WiDr cells growth in a dose-dependent manner with IC_{50} value were 41 μM and 52 μM respectively (Figure 1), while the IC_{50} value of cisplatin was 15 μM (data not shown).

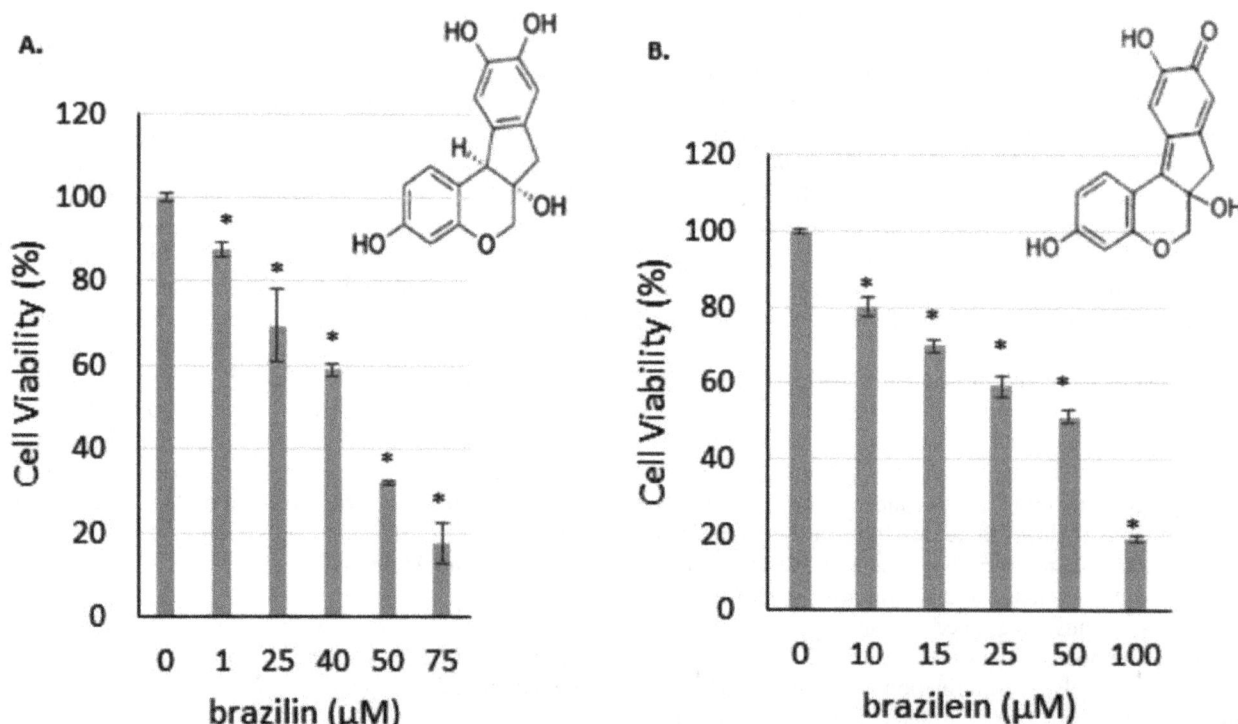

Figure 1. Cytotoxic effect of brazilin and brazilein on WiDr cells. A. brazilin (1-75 μM), B. brazilein (10-100 μM). Cells were treated with various concentrations of samples for 24 h before assessed by MTT assay. Data was collected from three replications (P<0.05).

Synergistic effect of combination of Bi-Cisp and Be-Cisp on WiDr cells growth

Discovery of agents that reduce resistance of chemotherapeutic agent is urgently needed and become one main target of today research. We investigated the effect of brazilin and brazilein in combination with cisplatin, a standard chemotherapeutic agent, on WiDr colon cancer cells. As shown in Figure 2, the combination of 1/10, 1/8, 1/4 and 1/2 IC_{50} of either Bi-Cisp or Be-Cisp showed synergistic effect on inhibition of WiDr cells growth (CI<1). Moreover, the combination of 1/2 IC_{50} of Bi-Cisp inhibited cell viability up to 64%. These data indicate that both compounds are potential to be developed as co-chemotherapeutic agent on colon cancer cells. To understand the mechanism underlies the synergistic effect, we observed the effect of the combinations on cell cycle modulation and on the induction of apoptosis.

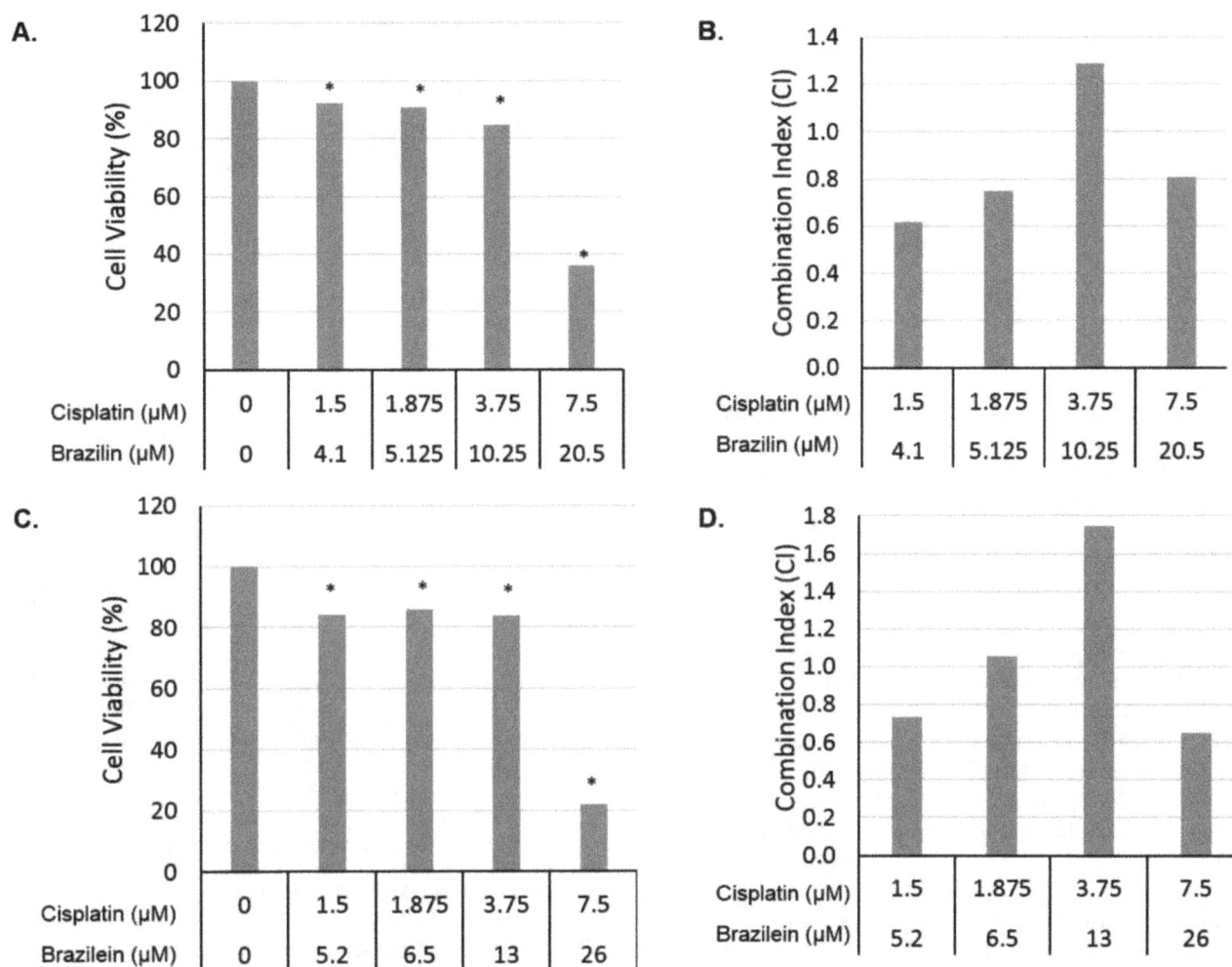

Figure 2. Combination of 1/2 IC_{50} of Bi-Cisp (20.5 µM- 7.5 µM) and Be-Cisp (26 µM- 7.5 µM) synergistically inhibited WiDr cells growth. A. Effect of combination of Bi-Cisp on WiDr cells growth. B. Combination Index (CI) of Bi-Cisp on WiDr cells. C. Combination of Be-Cisp on WiDr cells growth. D. CI of Be-Cisp on WiDr cells. Cells were treated with samples for 24 h before assessed by MTT assay. Data was collected from three replications (P<0.05).

Cell cycle modulation of brazilin and brazilein in combination with cisplatin

We conducted cell cycle analysis to elucidate how brazilin, brazilein and their combination with cisplatin inhibited cells proliferation. The results of cell cycle analysis (Figure 3) showed that single treatment of either brazilin or brazilein caused S-phase and G2/M-phase accumulation. Treatment of 1/2 IC_{50} of brazilein (Figure 3D) induced higher G2/M accumulation compared to 1/2 IC_{50} of brazilin (Figure 3C). On the other hand, single treatment of 1/2 IC_{50} of cisplatin induced S-phase accumulation (Figure 3B). When brazilin or brazilein was combined with cisplatin, the combinations increased cells accumulation in S-phase compared to its single treatment, whereas both combination showed accumulation in G2/M-phase compared to control cells (Figure 3E-G).

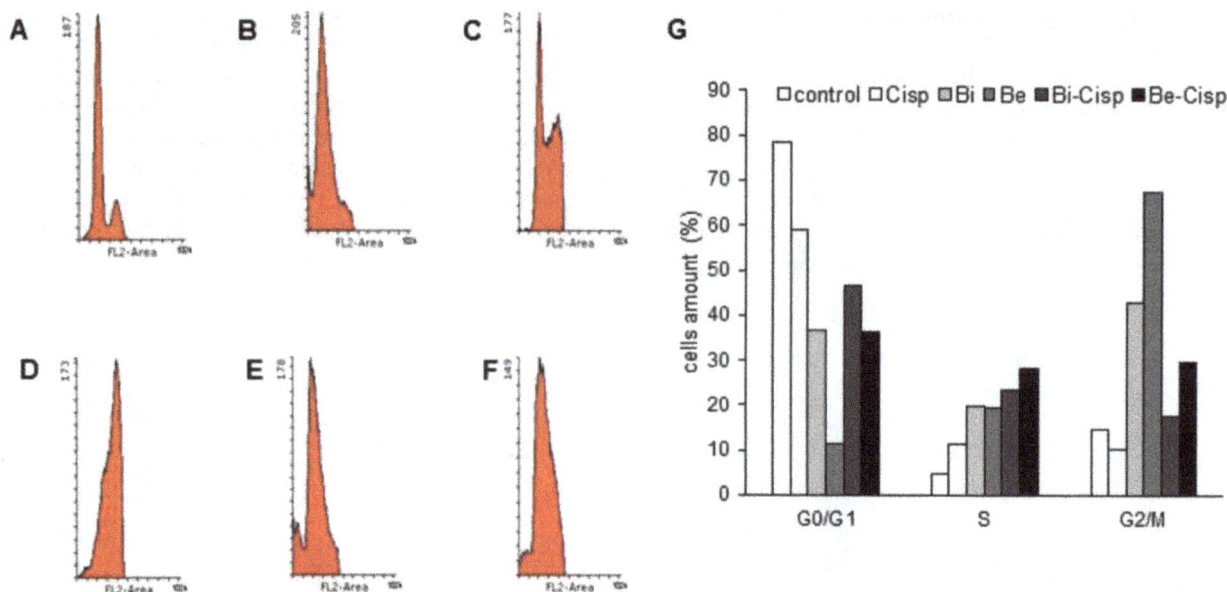

Figure 3. Combination of ½ IC$_{50}$ of Bi-Cisp and Be-Cisp induced S-phase accumulation on WiDr cells. A. Control. B. Cisplatin (7.5 μM). C. Brazilin (20.5 μM). D. Brazilein (26 μM). E. Combination of Bi-Cisp (20.5 μM -7.5 μM). F. Combination of Be-Cisp (26 μM -7.5 μM). G. Cell cycle distribution of ½ IC$_{50}$ of Bi and Be in single and combination with Cisp. Data was collected according to the description in Method.

Apoptosis induction of brazilin and brazilein in combination with cisplatin.

Inhibition of proliferation may be caused by modulation in cell cycle and by the induction of apoptosis. To investigate the effect of brazilin, brazilein and their combination with cisplatin on apoptosis, we did FACS analysis on WiDr cells which were treated with samples and were stained with fluorescein isothiocyanate-conjugated annexin V and fluorescent dye propidium iodide (PI). Single treatment of cisplatin, brazilin and brazilein exhibited 14%, 10% and 12% of total apoptotic cells respectively. Either combination of brazilin-cisplatin or brazilein-cisplatin increased total apoptotic cells up to 22% compared to control or 9% compared to cisplatin alone (Figure 4). Combination of brazilein-cisplatin treatment showed highest accumulation in late apoptotic and necrosis, while combination of brazilin-cisplatin exhibited highest accumulation in early apoptotic cells following 24 hours of incubation. These results suggested that brazilin and brazilein increased the induction of apoptosis of cisplatin on WIDr cells.

Cisplatin is a platinum-based drug that is used for the treatment of a wide-variety of primary human cancers. However, the efficacy of cisplatin is often limited by the rise of drug resistance.[6,7] Brazilin and brazilein are the active compounds from *Caesalpinia sappan* L. The structures of brazilin and brazilein are almost similar, whereas brazilein has C=O group and brazilin does not have C=O group in its structure.[9] In this study, brazilin showed the better cytotoxic effect against WiDr cancer cells than brazilein (Figure 1). Nevertheless, both of compounds performed synergistic effect while were combined with cisplatin.

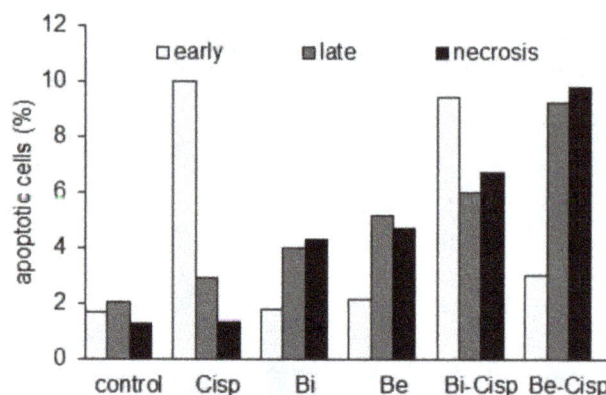

Figure 4. Combination of ½ IC$_{50}$ of Bi-Cisp and Be-Cisp synergistically induced apoptosis on WiDr cells. Cells were treated with Bi, Be and Cisp (20.5 μM, 26 μM, and 7.5 μM respectively) as indicated in the graph for 24 h. Data was collected according to the description in Method.

Cell cycle analysis showed that single treatment of either brazilin or brazilein induced S-phase and G2/M-phase accumulation, while single treatment of cisplatin only accumulated cells in S-phase (Figure 4). Interestingly, when brazilin and brazilein were given as combination with cisplatin, both compounds seemed to work effectively in two fields. Both brazilin and brazilein enhance S-phase accumulation of cell cycle up to 23% and 28% respectively compared to single treatment of cisplatin. The rest of the cells, which were lead to G2/M phase were also blocked by brazilin and brazilein (Figure 4). The mechanism underlies the S-phase and G2/M-phase arrest-induced by brazilin and brazilein needs further investigation. Previous study reported that brazilin induces G2/M arrest through inactivation of histone deacetylase and followed by the activation of CDK inhibitor p27.[14] The G2/M accumulation on brazilein treatment on colon cancer cells may be related with the ability of brazilein to bind with COX2 receptor (data not shown). Brazilein may induce G2/M arrest through inhibition of COX2, which is followed with the activation of p21. The p21 inhibits the CDK1/cyclin B complex and maintains the G2 arrest.[17] Since WiDr cell expresses *p53* mutant, p21 may be induced by p53-independent pathway.[18,19] The S phase arrest-induced by the combination of brazilin-cisplatin and brazilein-cisplatin are possibly due to the action of cisplatin which as reported by Yuan et al,[20] single treatment of cisplatin induces S-phase arrest via activation of CHK1 and CHK2 checkpoint kinase. The proteins induce cell death through DNA damage and cell cycle arrest during S phase. Hence, S-phase arrest induced by cisplatin through CHK1 activation on p53-mutant cells has been reported.[21] Hence, we need to investigate that S-phase arrest induced by both of the combinations underwent apoptosis instead of DNA repair.

Although the total apoptosis event of single treatment of cisplatin, brazilin and brazilein were similar (Figure 2), the three compounds have different pattern. Cisplatin exhibited the highest distribution in early apoptosis. On the other hand, brazilin and brazilein exhibited the highest distribution in late apoptosis. Combination of both brazilin-cisplatin and brazilein-cisplatin enhanced induction of apoptosis compared to cisplatin single treatment. The results support our suggestion that S-phase accumulation induced by the combinations lead to apoptosis instead of DNA repair. Interestingly, even though the total apoptotic events of both of the combinations were similar, combination of brazilin-cisplatin exhibited the highest accumulation in the early apoptotic cells, while combination of brazilein-cisplatin treatment exhibited the highest accumulation in the late apoptotic cells and necrosis. This difference may be due to its different mechanism. Previous study reported that cisplatin induces apoptosis through FAS receptor pathway.[22] FAS/FADD as well as TNF activate procaspase-8 to form caspase-8 and lead to increasing of proapoptotic protein Bax via intrinsic pathway.[23] Caspase-8 also directly activated caspase-3 and 7 and lead to apoptosis via extrinsic pathway.[24] Furthermore, brazilin induces apoptosis by increasing of cleavage caspase 3, cleavage caspase 7 and cleavage PARP,[12] while brazilein directly inhibits anti apoptotic protein surviving.[25] The *p53* is a transcription factor for pro-apoptotic protein, while *NFκB* is a transcription factor for anti-apoptotic protein such as Bcl-2 and surviving.[26] Hsieh reported that brazilein inhibits activation of NFκB.[15] On *p53*-mutated cells with loss most of pro-apoptotic protein expression, inhibition of NFκB activation which down-regulates anti-apoptotic protein and followed by apoptosis induction is an important mechanism to suppress cancer cells growth. Downregulation of of anti-apoptotic protein induces activation of caspase-9 and caspase-3 and followed with apoptosis phenomena.[25,27,28] Those support our finding that the combination of brazilin-cisplatin and brazilein-

cisplatin work synergistically to induce apoptosis on WiDr cells.

Combination of several therapies facilitates the blockade of several survival mechanisms in cancer cells and their microenvironment, achieving a synergistic therapeutic effect.[29] On combination therapy, reducing of concentration without reducing the effect may be feasible. It overcomes side effects of chemotherapeutic agent. Brazilin and brazilein are potential to be developed as a co-chemotherapeutic agent with cisplatin for treating colon cancer cells. However, further investigation need to be done to elucidate the molecular mechanism of brazilin, brazilein and its combination with cisplatin in inducing apoptosis and modulating S-phase and G2/M arrest on WiDr colon cancer cells.

Conclusion
Based on these results, we propose that brazilin and brazilein work synergistically with cisplatin in inhibiting colon cancer WiDr cells growth through a different target in cell cycle modulation and apoptosis induction.

Acknowledgments
This work was supported by the grant of Penelitian Unggulan Perguruan Tinggi (PUPT) 2015 from Indonesian Ministry of Research and Technology and High Education.

Ethical Issues
Not applicable.

Conflict of Interest
The authors declare no conflict of interests.

References
1. Sarasqueta AF, Forte G, Corver WE, de Miranda NF, Ruano D, van Eijk R, et al. Integral analysis of p53 and its value as prognostic factor in sporadic colon cancer. *BMC Cancer* 2013;13:277. doi: 10.1186/1471-2407-13-277
2. Bieging KT, Mello SS, Attardi LD. Unravelling mechanisms of p53-mediated tumour suppression. *Nat Rev Cancer* 2014;14(5):359-70. doi: 10.1038/nrc3711
3. Muller PA, Vousden KH. Mutant p53 in cancer: New functions and therapeutic opportunities. *Cancer Cell* 2014;25(3):304-17. doi: 10.1016/j.ccr.2014.01.021
4. Cooks T, Pateras IS, Tarcic O, Solomon H, Schetter AJ, Wilder S, et al. Mutant p53 prolongs nf-kappab activation and promotes chronic inflammation and inflammation-associated colorectal cancer. *Cancer Cell* 2013;23(5):634-46. doi: 10.1016/j.ccr.2013.03.022
5. Guillou PJ, Quirke P, Thorpe H, Walker J, Jayne DG, Smith AM, et al. Short-term endpoints of conventional versus laparoscopic-assisted surgery in patients with colorectal cancer (mrc clasicc trial): Multicentre, randomised controlled trial. *Lancet* 2005;365(9472):1718-26. doi: 10.1016/S0140-6736(05)66545-2

6. Shen DW, Pouliot LM, Hall MD, Gottesman MM. Cisplatin resistance: A cellular self-defense mechanism resulting from multiple epigenetic and genetic changes. *Pharmacol Rev* 2012;64(3):706-21. doi: 10.1124/pr.111.005637

7. Gadhikar MA, Sciuto MR, Alves MV, Pickering CR, Osman AA, Neskey DM, et al. Chk1/2 inhibition overcomes the cisplatin resistance of head and neck cancer cells secondary to the loss of functional p53. *Mol Cancer Ther* 2013;12(9):1860-73. doi: 10.1158/1535-7163.MCT-13-0157

8. Liu AL, Shu SH, Qin HL, Lee SM, Wang YT, Du GH. In vitro anti-influenza viral activities of constituents from caesalpinia sappan. *Planta Med* 2009;75(4):337-9. doi: 10.1055/s-0028-1112208

9. Nirmal NP, Rajput MS, Prasad RG, Ahmad M. Brazilin from caesalpinia sappan heartwood and its pharmacological activities: A review. *Asian Pac J Trop Med* 2015;8(6):421-30. doi: 10.1016/j.apjtm.2015.05.014

10. Cuong TD, Hung TM, Kim JC, Kim EH, Woo MH, Choi JS, et al. Phenolic compounds from caesalpinia sappan heartwood and their anti-inflammatory activity. *J Nat Prod* 2012;75(12):2069-75. doi: 10.1021/np3003673

11. Liang CH, Chan LP, Chou TH, Chiang FY, Yen CM, Chen PJ, et al. Brazilein from caesalpinia sappan l. Antioxidant inhibits adipocyte differentiation and induces apoptosis through caspase-3 activity and anthelmintic activities against hymenolepis nana and anisakis simplex. *Evid Based Complement Alternat Med* 2013;2013:864892. doi: 10.1155/2013/864892

12. Lee DY, Lee MK, Kim GS, Noh HJ, Lee MH. Brazilin inhibits growth and induces apoptosis in human glioblastoma cells. *Molecules* 2013;18(2):2449-57. doi: 10.3390/molecules18022449

13. Tao LY, Li JY, Zhang JY. Brazilein, a compound isolated from caesalpinia sappan linn., induced growth inhibition in breast cancer cells via involvement of gsk-3beta/beta-catenin/cyclin d1 pathway. *Chem Biol Interact* 2013;206(1):1-5. doi: 10.1016/j.cbi.2013.07.015

14. Kim B, Kim SH, Jeong SJ, Sohn EJ, Jung JH, Lee MH, et al. Brazilin induces apoptosis and g2/m arrest via inactivation of histone deacetylase in multiple myeloma u266 cells. *J Agric Food Chem* 2012;60(39):9882-9. doi: 10.1021/jf302527p

15. Hsieh CY, Tsai PC, Chu CL, Chang FR, Chang LS, Wu YC, et al. Brazilein suppresses migration and invasion of mda-mb-231 breast cancer cells. *Chem Biol Interact* 2013;204(2):105-15. doi: 10.1016/j.cbi.2013.05.005

16. Reynolds CP, Maurer BJ. Evaluating response to antineoplastic drug combinations in tissue culture models. *Methods Mol Med* 2005;110:173-83. doi: 10.1385/1-59259-869-2:173

17. Sobolewski C, Cerella C, Dicato M, Ghibelli L, Diederich M. The role of cyclooxygenase-2 in cell proliferation and cell death in human malignancies. *Int J Cell Biol* 2010;2010:215158. doi: 10.1155/2010/215158

18. Ahmed D, Eide PW, Eilertsen IA, Danielsen SA, Eknaes M, Hektoen M, et al. Epigenetic and genetic features of 24 colon cancer cell lines. *Oncogenesis* 2013;2:e71. doi: 10.1038/oncsis.2013.35

19. Park C, Kim GY, Kim GD, Choi BT, Park YM, Choi YH. Induction of g2/m arrest and inhibition of cyclooxygenase-2 activity by curcumin in human bladder cancer t24 cells. *Oncol Rep* 2006;15(5):1225-31.

20. Yuan Z, Guo W, Yang J, Li L, Wang M, Lei Y, et al. Pnas-4, an early DNA damage response gene, induces s phase arrest and apoptosis by activating checkpoint kinases in lung cancer cells. *J Biol Chem* 2015;290(24):14927-44. doi: 10.1074/jbc.M115.658419

21. Shen H, Perez RE, Davaadelger B, Maki CG. Two 4N Cell-Cycle Arrests Contribute to Cisplatin-Resistance. *PLoS ONE.* 2013;8(4):e59848. doi:10.1371/journal.pone.0059848.

22. Rebillard A, Jouan-Lanhouet S, Jouan E, Legembre P, Pizon M, Sergent O, et al. Cisplatin-induced apoptosis involves a fas-rock-ezrin-dependent actin remodelling in human colon cancer cells. *Eur J Cancer* 2010;46(8):1445-55. doi: 10.1016/j.ejca.2010.01.034

23. Huang K, Zhang J, O'Neill KL, Gurumurthy CB, Quadros RM, Tu Y, et al. Cleavage by caspase 8 and mitochondrial membrane association activate the bh3-only protein bid during trail-induced apoptosis. *J Biol Chem* 2016;291(22):11843-51. doi: 10.1074/jbc.M115.711051

24. Florea AM, Busselberg D. Cisplatin as an anti-tumor drug: Cellular mechanisms of activity, drug resistance and induced side effects. *Cancers (Basel)* 2011;3(1):1351-71. doi: 10.3390/cancers3011351

25. Zhong X, Wu B, Pan YJ, Zheng S. Brazilein inhibits survivin protein and mrna expression and induces apoptosis in hepatocellular carcinoma hepg2 cells. *Neoplasma* 2009;56(5):387-92.

26. Zubair A, Frieri M. Role of nuclear factor-κB in breast and colorectal cancer. *Curr Allergy Asthma Rep* 2013;13(1):44-9. doi:10.1007/s11882-012-0300-5.

27. Miyake N, Chikumi H, Takata M, Nakamoto M, Igishi T, Shimizu E. Rapamycin induces p53-independent apoptosis through the mitochondrial pathway in non-small cell lung cancer cells. *Oncol Rep* 2012;28(3):848-54. doi:10.3892/or.2012.1855

28. Rathore R, McCallum JE, Varghese E, Florea AM, Busselberg D. Overcoming chemotherapy drug resistance by targeting inhibitors of apoptosis proteins (iaps). *Apoptosis* 2017;22(7):898-919. doi: 10.1007/s10495-017-1375-1

29. Eldar-Boock A, Polyak D, Scomparin A, Satchi-Fainaro R. Nano-sized polymers and liposomes designed to deliver combination therapy for cancer. *Curr Opin Biotechnol* 2013;24(4):682-9. doi: 10.1016/j.copbio.2013.04.014

6

Variables Associated with Adherence to Stress Ulcer Prophylaxis in Patients Admitted to the General Hospital Wards

Shadi Farsaei[1]*, Sajad Ghorbani[2], Payman Adibi[3]

[1] Department of Clinical Pharmacy and Pharmacy Practice, Isfahan Pharmaceutical Sciences Research Center, Isfahan University of Medical Sciences, Isfahan, Iran.
[2] Department of Clinical Pharmacy and Pharmacy Practice, Isfahan University of Medical Sciences, Isfahan, Iran.
[3] Department of Gastroenterology, Integrative Functional Gastroenterology Research Center, Isfahan University of Medical Sciences, Isfahan, Iran.

Keywords:
· Adherence
· Academic medical center
· Anti-ulcer agents
· Clinical practice guideline

Abstract

Purpose: The dramatic increase in stress ulcer prophylaxis (SUP) prescribing patterns over the past several years has raised concerns regarding to their appropriate utilization. This prospective study attempted to evaluate the trend of adherence to stress ulcer prophylaxis from admission until discharge in non- Intensive care unit (ICU) setting. Additionally, we attempted to find those variables associated with appropriate SUP administration.

Methods: Data collection was performed prospectively to evaluate 195 randomly selected adult patients who received SUP or had indication for that in non-ICU wards of one of the largest referral center in Iran, during 6 months. Adherence was studied according to widely accepted American Society of Health system Pharmacists (ASHP) guideline. Univariate and multivariate logistic regression was also performed to detect associations related to misuse of SUP.

Results: We recognized total inappropriate use of SUP upon admission, during hospital stay and at discharge were somewhat identical at different time points (61%, 80% and 77.4% respectively). On the other hand, since small number of patients experienced SUP underutilization, unfortunately this was not possible to elucidate factors that may have effect on this flawed behavior. However, increasing age was identified to be significant variable in SUP overutilization.

Conclusion: This prospective study highlighted inappropriate overutilization of SUP within non-critically ill patients and found factors which predicted this behavior. Adherence during hospital stay was also calculated for the first time in this study, which was related to SUP adherence upon hospital admission.

Introduction

Stress ulcer is defined as an acute superficial inflammatory lesions of the gastric mucosa induced by abnormally elevated physiological demand such as sepsis, trauma, burns, and neurologic damage.[1-3] Although several factors encompass the pathogenesis of stress related mucosal damage (SRMD), but the main reason is ischemia and reperfusion of the vulnerable area.[4]

SRMD predominantly created in the acid-producing area of the stomach (upper body and fundus), and rarely lead to hemodynamically significant gastrointestinal (GI) bleeding in non-critically ill patients.[3]

These mucosal lesions was preliminary observed in central mucosal layer of stomach fundus in 7 critical ill patients after death at 1969.[5] However, risk of stress ulcer bleeding was high in 1970 (20-30%), but it declined considerably in 1990 (1.5-14%) due to use of prophylaxis medications.[6] Although, risk of GI bleeding is relatively low in non-critically ill patients (0.41%),

but they also could benefit from stress ulcer prophylaxis (SUP) medications.[7]

High rate of SUP prescriptions in intensive care unit (ICU) and general wards necessitated presence of guideline to prevent irrational use of medications.

Therefore, the American Society of Health system Pharmacists (ASHP) was published a guideline for SUP in critically ill patient and suggested two categorical risk factors for SRMD as minor and major risk factors.[8] This guideline declared a lack of evidence to support the use of SUP in non-critically ill patients with less two minor risk factor for clinically significant bleeding.[9,10] Although mechanical ventilation, coagulopathy and history of GI bleeding during past year are significant and independent risk factors for stress ulcer in these patients.[1,8-11]

Proton pump inhibitors (PPIs) and histamine 2 receptor antagonists (H2 antagonists) are the most prescribed

---
*Corresponding author: Shadi Farsaei, Email: Farsaei@pharm.mui.ac.ir

SUP medications in ICU and general wards of hospital.[3,12]

Previous studies were evaluated the use of SUP in ICU and non-ICU patients because of morbidity and mortality of stress ulcer-related bleeding, the cost of drugs and possible complications associated with SUP administration such as infectious problem and drug-drug interactions related to acid suppression therapy (AST).[13-15] These studies showed high rate (56-75%) of irrational prescribing of SUP in non-ICU patients.[14] Although these studies mostly evaluated SUP administration upon admission and at discharge, but data during stay in hospital have been neglected. Therefore, in this study the prevalence of iatrogenic overutilization or underutilization of SUP upon admission, at discharge and during stay in general wards were also evaluated. Additionally, possible factors associated with misuse of AST were reported.

Materials and Methods
Methods
It was the cross sectional prospective study performed in the general medical, emergency, and surgical wards at one of the largest teaching hospital in Iran, from September 2014 to March 2015. This mentioned hospital affiliated with residency and fellowship program with around 800 beds that provides medical services to patients from different parts of the country. In this research, the appropriateness of SUP administration was evaluated according to ASHP guideline in adult patients admitted to the medical, surgical and emergency wards. Therefore, patients who received AST for treatment purposes such as GI bleeding, gastroesophageal reflux disease (GERD), peptic ulcer disease (PUD), and dyspepsia did not fulfilled criteria to include in our study. Moreover, patients who transferred from the ICU were excluded.

Patients were randomly selected from different general wards based on the proportion number of admitted patients in each ward. For simple randomization, we assigned a consecutive number to each individual, thereafter, SPSS random number generator was used to produce random numbers.

In addition, an attempt was made to prevent treatment bias induced by physician awareness.

Data collection was performed to gather information regarding demographic characteristics of patients, prescriber service of SUP, admission diagnosis (medical, surgical and trauma), nutritional status, time spent from ward admission to start SUP, related laboratory data, past medical history of GI problem, and duration of admission in hospital wards.

Furthermore, patients were assessed daily for associated risk factors of SRMD, administration of SUP medication (type, dose, route and duration of SUP medications), and GI bleeding during stay in hospital wards.

According to ASHP guideline and recent performed studies, patients who had 1 absolute indications or at least 2 of the relative indications were eligible for SUP administration in non-ICU setting (Table 1).[8,12,16,17]

Table 1. Major and minor risk factors for SRMD used in our study according to previous guidelines*

Major risk factor
Coagulopathy defined as a platelet count lower than50000 or INR higher than 1.5 or a PTT higher than 2 times the control value
Respiratory failure requiring mechanical ventilation for longer than 48 hours
History of GI ulceration or GI bleeding during past year

Minor risk factor
Head trauma with GCS ≤ 10 or spinal cord injury
Burn more than 35 percent BSA
Sepsis
Renal insufficiency
Hepatic failure
Heart failure
Renal or hepatic transplantation
Partial hepatectomy
Use of warfarin
Occult GI bleeding for six or more days
History of use of NSAID more than 3 month
Prolonged NPO status lasting more than 5 days with GI pathology or after major surgery
Glucocorticoid therapy (more than 250 mg hydrocortisone or the equivalent)
Use of heparin with therapeutic dose
Multiple trauma with ISS ≥ 16

* Prophylaxis is recommended in patients with one of the major risk factor or at least two minor risk factors
SRMD=Stress related mucosal damage, INR=International normalized ratio, PTT= Partial thromboplastin time, GI=Gastrointestinal, GCS= Glasgow Coma Scale, BSA=Body surface area, NSAID= Nonsteroidal anti-inflammatory drugs, NPO= nil per os (nothing by mouth), ISS=Injury severity score

In our study, SUP administration was assessed upon hospital ward admission, at discharge and during hospital ward stay for both patients who received and did not receive SUP medications.

To evaluate appropriateness of SUP administration during hospital ward stay, we used the below formula to calculate the proportion of days which SUP has or has not been prescribed based on guideline during follow up in our study:

Appropriate percent of SUP prescription = number of days which SUP prescription pattern was in compliance with ASHP guideline / duration of follow up × 100.

According to this formula, appropriateness of SUP administration would be considered if this percent was 80-120%. Meanwhile, percentage more than 120% and less than 80% were defined as overutilization and underutilization, respectively.[18]

Finally, the appropriateness of SUP treatment at hospital discharge was investigated and possible factors related to SUP overutilization were reported. In addition, the cost of non-guideline-based SUP medications' use was calculated by multiplying the total number of inappropriately utilized medications with the cost of each one.

Statistical analysis

Mean and standard error [SE] were used to report quantitative results, and both frequencies and percentages were calculated for qualitative data.

Logistic regression was performed to find the relationship between different variables and SUP overutilization at the beginning and during of hospital stay. Univariate regression analysis was first performed to confirm the importance of these factors and thereafter, multiple logistic regression was conducted to probe the relationship between the previously established risk factors and SUP overutilization. Odds ratio and confidence intervals (95% CI) were considered to report the results of logistic regression model. P-value of 0.05 or less was considered significant.

Results

Of the 204 patients were randomly selected during 6-month period study, 4.4% (9 patients) did not include in our study because they received AST for treatment purposes (7 and 2 patients received AST for dyspepsia and PUD, respectively).

Among 195 patients, 56.4%, 29.8%, and 13.9% were from the medical, surgical and emergency wards respectively, and more than 50% of SUP medications were prescribed by three medical services (internal, surgery and infection) (Table 2).

The pharmacological agents commonly used upon hospital ward admission and at discharge were PPIs and H2 blockers. Accordingly, PPIs and H2 blockers were prescribed for 117 (75.5%) and 38 (24.5%) of 155 patients upon hospital ward stay, respectively. PPIs were the most frequent medications administered for

SUP in patients admitted in gastroenterology, internal, infection and heart wards. Whereas, H2 blockers were the most prescribed AST in neurology, emergency and surgery wards. Moreover, intravenous dosage form of SUP medications were mostly used in gastroenterology, heart, surgery and emergency departments (Figure 1). In addition, PPIs were remained the most prescribed SUP at hospital ward discharge. It should be mentioned that, any combination of PPI and H2 blocker was not administered to the study population.

Table 2. Demographic and baseline characteristics of patients completed the study

Characteristic		Numbers, % or Mean (Std.E)
Age	-	54.2 (1.4)
Gender	Male	119 (61)
	Female	76 (39)
Medical diagnosis	Medical	137 (70.3)
	Surgical	54 (27.7)
	Trauma	4 (2.1)
Nutrition	Oral	163 (83.6)
	NPO	21 (10.8)
	Gavage	7 (3.6)
	TPN	3 (1.5)
	PPN	1 (0.5)
Prescriber service	Internal medicine	49 (28)
	Surgery	27 (15.4)
	Infection	26 (14.9)
	Heart	11 (6.3)
	Neurology	9 (5.1)
	Emergency medicine	9 (5.1)
	Gastroenterology	9 (5.1)
	Orthopedist	6 (3.6)
	Neurologist	6 (3.6)
	Oncology	5 (2.9)
	Others	18 (10.3)

Std.E=standard error, NPO=nil per os (nothing by mouth), TPN=total parenteral nutrition, PPN=partial parenteral nutrition

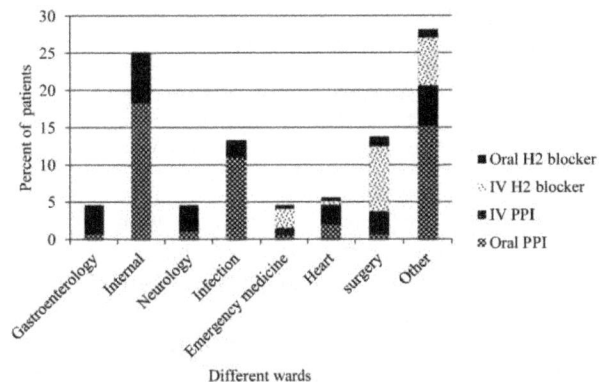

Figure 1. Dosage form of medications administered for stress ulcer prophylaxis based on different wards
IV= Intravenous, PPI= Proton pump inhibitor

The time lasted from hospital ward stay to begin SUP administration was 0.3 ± 0.1 day.

Moreover, duration of patient follow up and taking SUP in the hospital ward were 8.0 ± 0.5 and 7.4 ± 0.5 days, respectively.

Our results revealed inappropriate use of SUP upon admission, during hospital stay and at discharge were 61%, 80% and 77.4%, respectively.

Among included patients, 155 received SUP upon hospital ward admission, 109 (70.33%) patients did not fulfill the criteria to receive SUP. In addition, 10 out of 40 (25%) patients did not receive SUP properly upon admission while they had clear or valid indication.

We also assessed appropriate percent of SUP prescription during hospital ward stay (according to declared formula in method). Therefore, SUP prescriptions were considered over-utilized in 137 of 195 (70.3%) patients in the average of 6.6 ± 0.5 days. However, only in 19 of 195 (9.8%) patients under-utilization were occurred for 3.5 ± 1.3 days. On the other word, SUP was prescribed properly for 28 of 175 (16.0%) patients who received SUP, and 9 of 20 (45.0%) patients who did not receive SUP during hospital ward stay. In general, results revealed SUP was prescribed appropriately for 37 of 195 (19.0%) patients during hospital stay.

At the end, SUP was continued appropriately in 10 of 22 (45.5%) patients at hospital discharge. Moreover, 139 of 173 (80.3%) patients did not receive SUP properly according to guideline (Table 3).

Table 3. Frequency of eligible patients for stress ulcer prophylaxis

Risk factor	Number (% from 195 included patients)	
Major ASHP criteria	Upon ward admission	At hospital discharge
Coagulopathy	29 (16.6)	16 (9.2)
Mechanical ventilation for longer than 48 hours	-	-
History of GI ulceration or GI bleeding during past year	11 (6.3)	11 (6.3)
Patients with at least 1 of the major ASHP criteria *	38 (19.5)	28 (14.3)
Minor ASHP criteria		
Head trauma or spinal cord injury	5 (2.5)	4 (2.1)
Burn more than 35 percent BSA	-	-
Sepsis	3 (1.5)	3 (1.5)
Renal insufficiency	23 (11.8)	18 (9.2)
Hepatic failure	3 (1.5)	3 (1.5)
Heart failure	9 (4.6)	9 (4.6)
Use of warfarin	10 (5.1)	3 (1.5)
History of use of NSAIDs more than 3 month	3 (1.5)	3 (1.5)
Prolonged NPO status lasting more than 5 days with GI pathology or after major surgery	1 (0.5)	5 (2.5)
Glucocorticoid therapy †	16 (8.2)	2 (1.03)
Use of heparin with therapeutic dose	18 (9.8)	7 (3.6)
Patients meeting at least 2 of the minor ASHP criteria *	70 (35.9)	49 (25.1)
Number (%)		
Patients received stress ulcer prophylaxis when it was not indicated	109 (70.3) ‡	12 (54.5) ††
Patients did not receive stress ulcer prophylaxis when it was indicated	10 (25) §	34 (19.6) ‡‡

* This number is less than the sum of total patients meeting ASHP major criteria because some patients had more than 1 criterion
† More than 250 mg hydrocortisone or the equivalent
‡ Among 155 patients who received SUP
§ Among 40 patients who not received SUP
†† Among 22 patients who received SUP
‡‡ Among 173 patients who not received SUP
ASHP= American society of health-system pharmacists, BSA=Body surface area, NSAID= Nonsteroidal anti-inflammatory drugs, NPO= nil per os (nothing by mouth), GI=Gastrointestinal

Consequently, inappropriate administration of SUP upon hospital ward admission, at discharge and during hospital stay were summarized in Figure 2. Non-adherence was higher among those received SUP than who did not receive it in different time of evaluation. However, inappropriate use of SUP increased during hospital stay than upon admission, but it reached the lowest percent at hospital discharge.

The total cost of non-guideline-based SUP medications' use was $3,500 for 204 patients evaluated in our study.

It should be mentioned that intravenous pantoprazole and ranitidine were considered for 70% and 14% of this cost, respectively.

Among 195 patients, only 1 (0.51%) patient experienced GI bleeding during follow up. He admitted to hospital with diagnosis of myocardial infarction and past medical history of GI bleeding. In addition, mortality rate in our study was 11 of 195 (5.64%) patients.

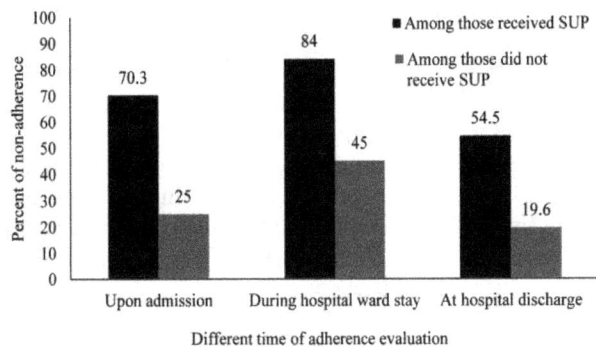

Figure 2. Overview of non-adherence to stress ulcer prophylaxis in general wards
SUP= Stress ulcer prophylaxis

Factors associated with inappropriate SUP administration

All variables were analyzed to evaluate factors affecting adherence to SUP practice. Since small number of patients experienced SUP underutilization during hospital ward stay, unfortunately this was not possible to elucidate factors that may have an effect on this behavior. Therefore, variables that may have dictated overutilization were summarized in Table 4.

According to univariate analysis, a significant increase in the risk of wrong decision to start SUP was observed in female patients ($p = 0.002$). Although it must be noted that the number of minor and major risk factors were not significantly different when variable of gender was studied ($p = 0.81$ and $p = 1.00$ respectively).

Table 4. Variables affecting SUP overuse at admission and during hospital stay

-	Upon hospital admission[μ]					During hospital stay [Ω]				
	Univariate regression		Multivariate regression			Univariate regression		Multivariate regression		
	p-value	OR	p-value	OR	95% CI	p-value	OR	p-value	OR	95% CI
Age	<0.001	1.013	0.024	1.011	1.001-1.020	< 0.001	1.024	0.003	1.018	1.006-1.029
Female gender	0.002	2.471	0.372	1.369	0.687-2.727	< 0.001	3.643	0.911	1.044	0.490-2.223
Duration of hospital stay	0.002	1.053	0.944	1.002	0.959-1.046	< 0.001	1.137	0.170	1.041	0.983-1.103

All p-values calculated by binary logistic regression test
μ: Among patients who received SUP, 46 patients were SUP candidate and in 109 SUP were over-utilized
Ω: Among patients who received SUP, 28 had appropriate adherence and in 137 SUP were over-utilized
OR=odds ratio, CI=confidence interval.

Moreover, older age and longer duration of hospital stay were shown to be a major predictor of SUP overuse ($p = < 0.001$ and $p = 0.002$, respectively). However, only increased age remained statistically significant when multivariate model was developed at hospital admission ($p = 0.024$, OR = 1.011, 95% CI = 1.006-1.029).

It should be mentioned that factors affecting SUP overuse were similar upon hospital admission and during hospital stay in both univariate and multivariate analyses.

Discussion

Although current medical care could decrease the prevalence of stress-related GI bleeding by 17% in recent years, but routine administration of SUP over the years in most non-ICU hospitalized patients has emerged an important challenge in health system.[3,6] This may be related to less defined risk factors which could identify high risk patients who would benefit from SUP use in non-ICU hospitalized patients.[6,19] However, it should be mentioned that these risk factors were well studied and determined in ICU patients.[8,20] Despite this limitation, similar to previous conducted studies, we used the modified version of ASHP risk factors as the guidance to evaluate appropriateness of SUP administration in non-ICU patients.[3]

Our results revealed SUP was prescribed in the majority proportion of included patients upon hospital admission; despite, most of them were considered inappropriate according to guideline. This unsuitable pattern of SUP prescription also remained at discharge. Unfortunately, this dramatic finding is comparable with recent literature review which indicates high percent of patients received SUP improperly upon hospital admission and at discharge (22-93% and 44-88%, respectively).[3,10,12,16,17,21] High prevalence of irrational prescribing in some institutes necessitated clinical pharmacist intervention, which could improve the prescription pattern of SUP administration in certain hospital wards.[22,23]

Different study design (retrospective, cross-sectional and prospective) and institutes where studies were conducted justified this wide range of non-adherence to SUP guideline in previous studies. However, this rate of adherence is relatively higher in ICU patients who have more definitive risk factors to initiate SUP medications.[18] In addition, teaching or nonteaching setting of study could have an effect on inappropriate SUP prescription. Recent studies revealed SUP usage in academic centers were more compliant with the guidelines versus nonacademic hospitals.[17,24,25]

It seems that evaluation of adherence upon admission and at discharge are inadequate to give a complete view of rationale prescribing of SUP medications. Accordingly, we also calculated adherence during hospital stay and unfortunately we found small number of physicians adhered to the SUP guideline during hospitalization which is similar to data related to hospital admission. On the other word, inappropriate beginning of SUP was continued during hospital stay in the same manner. These findings showed first day adherence could be a good predictor of adherence during hospital stay.

We should mention that since we did not find any previous report to calculate this adherence, we theorized that patients who received 80-120% of SUP medications appropriately were adhered to the guideline. Moreover, we did not find the appropriate time needed to pass after risk factors were resolved to stop SUP medications. Therefore, we considered patients ineligible to continue SUP when the appropriate indications were disappeared. However this decision is somewhat more difficult in ICU setting where patients are at increased risk of stress induced ulcers and consequent bleeding.[26]

In addition, we attempted to elucidate some factors that may be associated with adherence to SUP prescriptions. Nonetheless, because of low percentage of underutilized patients, we only could find factors that predicted overutilization.

Although previous conducted studies identified some predictive factors for AST overuse, but data is not enough especially in developing countries and there is controversy among published results.[3,10,21,27-30]

We identified similar risk factors of AST overuse both upon hospital admission and during hospital stay. Increased age, duration of hospital stay, and female gender were suggested to be significant factors that could affect on AST overuse in our results. Nevertheless, only increased age remained significant variable in multivariate analysis among the mentioned factors, while both duration of hospital stay and gender became a trend.

The rational of more AST overuse during longer hospital stay is understandable. Since the sicker patients required longer hospital stay and more medical care, so unconscious physicians may be encouraged to begin SUP to prevent more complication of GI bleeding. It is surprising that, Issa et al[3] also has identified similar factors contributing in SUP overuse. They revealed hospital stay as the only significant factors affecting SUP overuse in multivariate analysis whereas, age and male gender became a trend. However, not only other observational studies did not identify significantly shorter duration of hospital stay in patients who received SUP appropriately, but one of this studies suggested the negative trend between hospital stay and AST overuse.[21,30]

Increased age was another significant factor impacting AST overuse in our study. It is reasonable prediction that unconsciousness physicians considered SUP for advanced age patients predisposing to more medical problems. Other performed studies also confirmed our results.[3,27] A retrospective medical chart review suggested increasing patient age as a clear variable in AST overuse.[31] The results of another retrospective review noted intravenous PPI was overused in inpatients with age ≥ 65 years old.[10]

The reason that female gender was considered as predictive factor for AST overuse in our study is unclear. Furthermore, some previous studies released data showing otherwise, they suggested male gender as associated variable that could significantly predict AST overuse.[21,30] Although other studies found that female gender was independently associated with inappropriate AST prescribing in both primary care and hospitalized patients.[28,29] Review of published studies revealed conflicting results regarding the effect of gender on SUP adherence, but none of them could explain the logic of these inconsistence.

Not surprisingly, overuse of AST is not devoid of side effects. In fact, an increased risk of developing clostridium difficile-associated diarrhea and possibly nosocomial pneumonia may be associated with AST use, which is greater with PPIs.[32,33] However, more evaluation is required to determine this causality.[33] Furthermore, numerous potential interactions such as drug-drug, drug-nutrient and drug-test interactions have been described with variety of mechanism.[34,35]

Therefore, this inappropriate practice of SUP prescribing has substantial burden for both patients and health care providers.

Some limitations of the present prospective study need to be noticed. A relatively small number of studied patients might not be an appropriate sample to completely represent the population of admitted patients in non-ICU wards of this large hospital. Moreover, since mostly residents rather than attending physicians decide to start and continue SUP in academic center, it is difficult to extrapolate the result of one academic center to other hospitals. Not determining the possible complications of SUP administration (e.g., pneumonia or CAD) in the study population can be considered as the other limitation of this study.

However, the prospective design of our study is the strength point of that, because missing data is highly unlikely. Moreover, our results showed variables associated to SUP misuse in one of the largest hospital in a developing country, which give a chance to compare results with other conducted studies. Our results also give wide viewing about SUP adherence upon admission, during hospital stay and upon discharge and could use as a guide for appropriate future practice of physicians. Possible interventions such as application of internal guideline, preparing order template which contains indication of SUP administration, stop orders, automatic switch order from PPI to H2 blocker, education of residents and nursing staff and implementation of clinical pharmacists' activities can be helpful to decrease unnecessary AST use.

Conclusion

We found high inappropriate SUP utilization according to ASHP guideline upon admission, during hospital stay and at discharge (61%, 80% and 77.4%, respectively). This prospective study highlighted unsuitable overutilization of SUP within non-critically ill patients and found factors which predicted this behavior such as older age and longer duration of hospital stay. Adherence during hospital stay was also calculated for the first time in this study and we found it related to SUP adherence upon hospital admission. It is clear that AST overuse may cause significant adverse effects and imposes unnecessary financial burden on both patients and hospital. Therefore, controlled policies require to manage inappropriate SUP administration. Further studies may also need to evaluate variables associated with SUP overuse in the outpatient setting.

Acknowledgments

We would like to thank staff members of Alzahra Hospital for their cooperation (general support). It also should be declared that this study was financially supported by Isfahan University of Medical Sciences.

Ethical Issues

The study protocol was approved by the ethical committee of Isfahan University of Medical Sciences.

Conflict of Interest

The authors have no conflicts of interest to declare.

References

1. Cook DJ, Fuller HD, Guyatt GH, Marshall JC, Leasa D, Hall R, et al. Risk factors for gastrointestinal bleeding in critically ill patients. Canadian critical care trials group. *N Engl J Med* 1994;330(6):377-81. doi: 10.1056/NEJM199402103300601

2. Eisa N, Bazerbachi F, Alraiyes AH, Alraies MC. Q: Do all hospitalized patients need stress ulcer prophylaxis? *Cleve Clin J Med* 2014;81(1):23-5. doi: 10.3949/ccjm.81a.1307

3. Issa IA, Soubra O, Nakkash H, Soubra L. Variables associated with stress ulcer prophylaxis misuse: A retrospective analysis. *Dig Dis Sci* 2012;57(10):2633-41. doi: 10.1007/s10620-012-2104-9

4. Spirt MJ. Stress-related mucosal disease: Risk factors and prophylactic therapy. *Clin Ther* 2004;26(2):197-213.

5. Buendgens L, Koch A, Tacke F. Prevention of stress-related ulcer bleeding at the intensive care unit: Risks and benefits of stress ulcer prophylaxis. *World J Crit Care Med* 2016;5(1):57-64. doi: 10.5492/wjccm.v5.i1.57

6. Grube RR, May DB. Stress ulcer prophylaxis in hospitalized patients not in intensive care units. *Am J Health Syst Pharm* 2007;64(13):1396-400. doi: 10.2146/ajhp060393

7. Qadeer MA, Richter JE, Brotman DJ. Hospital-acquired gastrointestinal bleeding outside the critical care unit: Risk factors, role of acid suppression, and endoscopy findings. *J Hosp Med* 2006;1(1):13-20. doi: 10.1002/jhm.10

8. Ashp therapeutic guidelines on stress ulcer prophylaxis. Ashp commission on therapeutics and approved by the ashp board of directors on november 14, 1998. *Am J Health Syst Pharm* 1999;56(4):347-79.

9. Heidelbaugh JJ, Goldberg KL, Inadomi JM. Overutilization of proton pump inhibitors: A review of cost-effectiveness and risk [corrected]. *Am J Gastroenterol* 2009;104 Suppl 2:S27-32. doi: 10.1038/ajg.2009.49

10. Nasser SC, Nassif JG, Dimassi HI. Clinical and cost impact of intravenous proton pump inhibitor use in non-icu patients. *World J Gastroenterol* 2010;16(8):982-6.

11. Madsen KR, Lorentzen K, Clausen N, Oberg E, Kirkegaard PR, Maymann-Holler N, et al. Guideline for stress ulcer prophylaxis in the intensive care unit. *Dan Med J* 2014;61(3):C4811.

12. Sheikh-Taha M, Alaeddine S, Nassif J. Use of acid suppressive therapy in hospitalized non-critically ill patients. *World J Gastrointest Pharmacol Ther* 2012;3(6):93-6. doi: 10.4292/wjgpt.v3.i6.93

13. Brett S. Science review: The use of proton pump inhibitors for gastric acid suppression in critical illness. *Crit Care* 2005;9(1):45-50. doi: 10.1186/cc2980

14. Mohebbi L, Hesch K. Stress ulcer prophylaxis in the intensive care unit. *Proc (Bayl Univ Med Cent)* 2009;22(4):373-6.

15. Spirt MJ, Stanley S. Update on stress ulcer prophylaxis in critically ill patients. *Crit Care Nurse* 2006;26(1):18-20, 2-8; quiz 9.

16. Bez C, Perrottet N, Zingg T, Leung Ki EL, Demartines N, Pannatier A. Stress ulcer prophylaxis in non-critically ill patients: A prospective evaluation of current practice in a general surgery department. *J Eval Clin Pract* 2013;19(2):374-8. doi: 10.1111/j.1365-2753.2012.01838.x

17. Foroughinia F, Madhooshi M. Attachment to stress ulcer prophylaxis guideline in the neurology wards of two teaching and non-teaching hospitals: A retrospective survey in iran. *J Res Pharm Pract* 2016;5(2):138-41. doi: 10.4103/2279-042X.179582

18. Rafinazari N, Abbasi S, Farsaei S, Mansourian M, Adibi P. Adherence to stress-related mucosal damage prophylaxis guideline in patients admitted to the intensive care unit. *J Res Pharm Pract* 2016;5(3):186-92. doi: 10.4103/2279-042X.185728

19. Janicki T, Stewart S. Stress-ulcer prophylaxis for general medical patients: A review of the evidence. *J Hosp Med* 2007;2(2):86-92. doi: 10.1002/jhm.177

20. Barletta JF, Bruno JJ, Buckley MS, Cook DJ. Stress ulcer prophylaxis. *Crit Care Med* 2016;44(7):1395-405. doi: 10.1097/CCM.0000000000001872

21. Alsultan MS, Mayet AY, Malhani AA, Alshaikh MK. Pattern of intravenous proton pump inhibitors use in icu and non-icu setting: A prospective observational study. *Saudi J Gastroenterol* 2010;16(4):275-9. doi: 10.4103/1319-3767.70614

22. Khalili H, Dashti-Khavidaki S, Hossein Talasaz AH, Tabeefar H, Hendoiee N. Descriptive analysis of a clinical pharmacy intervention to improve the appropriate use of stress ulcer prophylaxis in a hospital infectious disease ward. *J Manag Care Pharm* 2010;16(2):114-21. doi: 10.18553/jmcp.2010.16.2.114

23. Mousavi M, Dashti-Khavidaki S, Khalili H, Farshchi A, Gatmiri M. Impact of clinical pharmacy services on stress ulcer prophylaxis prescribing and related cost in patients with renal insufficiency. *Int J Pharm Pract* 2013;21(4):263-9. doi: 10.1111/ijpp.12005

24. Zeitoun A, Zeineddine M, Dimassi H. Stress ulcer prophylaxis guidelines: Are they being implemented in lebanese health care centers? *World J Gastrointest Pharmacol Ther* 2011;2(4):27-35. doi: 10.4292/wjgpt.v2.i4.27

25. Eid SM, Boueiz A, Paranji S, Mativo C, Landis R, Abougergi MS. Patterns and predictors of proton pump inhibitor overuse among academic and non-academic hospitalists. *Intern Med* 2010;49(23):2561-8.

26. Pines JM, Saltzman JR. Is it time to implement clinical decision rules for upper gi bleeding? Barriers, facilitators, and the need for a collaborative approach. *Gastrointest Endosc* 2016;83(6):1161-3. doi: 10.1016/j.gie.2015.12.016

27. Afif W, Alsulaiman R, Martel M, Barkun AN. Predictors of inappropriate utilization of intravenous proton pump inhibitors. *Aliment Pharmacol Ther* 2007;25(5):609-15. doi: 10.1111/j.1365-2036.2006.03226.x

28. Carey IM, De Wilde S, Harris T, Victor C, Richards N, Hilton SR, et al. What factors predict potentially inappropriate primary care prescribing in older people? Analysis of uk primary care patient record database. *Drugs Aging* 2008;25(8):693-706.

29. Craig DG, Thimappa R, Anand V, Sebastian S. Inappropriate utilization of intravenous proton pump inhibitors in hospital practice--a prospective study of the extent of the problem and predictive factors. *QJM* 2010;103(5):327-35. doi: 10.1093/qjmed/hcq019

30. Mayet AY. Improper use of antisecretory drugs in a tertiary care teaching hospital: An observational study. *Saudi J Gastroenterol* 2007;13(3):124-8.

31. George CJ, Korc B, Ross JS. Appropriate proton pump inhibitor use among older adults: A retrospective chart review. *Am J Geriatr Pharmacother* 2008;6(5):249-54. doi: 10.1016/j.amjopharm.2008.12.001

32. Buendgens L, Bruensing J, Matthes M, Duckers H, Luedde T, Trautwein C, et al. Administration of proton pump inhibitors in critically ill medical patients is associated with increased risk of developing clostridium difficile-associated diarrhea. *J Crit Care* 2014;29(4):696 e11-5. doi: 10.1016/j.jcrc.2014.03.002

33. Alshamsi F, Belley-Cote E, Cook D, Almenawer SA, Alqahtani Z, Perri D, et al. Efficacy and safety of proton pump inhibitors for stress ulcer prophylaxis in critically ill patients: A systematic review and meta-analysis of randomized trials. *Crit Care* 2016;20(1):120. doi: 10.1186/s13054-016-1305-6

34. Juel J, Pareek M, Jensen SE. The clopidogrel-ppi interaction: An updated mini-review. *Curr Vasc Pharmacol* 2014;12(5):751-7.

35. Wedemeyer RS, Blume H. Pharmacokinetic drug interaction profiles of proton pump inhibitors: An update. *Drug Saf* 2014;37(4):201-11. doi: 10.1007/s40264-014-0144-0

7

Cross-Linked Hydrogel for Pharmaceutical Applications

Rabinarayan Parhi

GITAM Institute of Pharmacy, GITAM University, Gandhi Nagar Campus, Rushikonda, Visakhapatnam-530045, Andhra Pradesh, India.

Keywords:
· Hydrogel
· Cross-linking
· Thermoreversible gel
· Polymers

Abstract
Hydrogels are promising biomaterials because of their important qualities such as biocompatibility, biodegradability, hydrophilicity and non-toxicity. These qualities make hydrogels suitable for application in medical and pharmaceutical field. Recently, a tremendous growth of hydrogel application is seen, especially as gel and patch form, in transdermal drug delivery. This review mainly focuses on the types of hydrogels based on cross-linking and; secondly to describe the possible synthesis methods to design hydrogels for different pharmaceutical applications. The synthesis and chemistry of these hydrogels are discussed using specific pharmaceutical examples. The structure and water content in a typical hydrogel have also been discussed.

Introduction

The formulations applied onto the skin surface are broadly classified in to two groups such as topical and transdermal. Topical formulations deliver drug to local area of skin without systemic exposure. On the other hand, transdermal formulations applied to the skin surface for the purpose of delivering and maintaining effective concentration of drug in the systemic circulation.[1] There are three basic types of transdermal formulations such as aerosol sprays, semisolids, and patches. Out of these, semisolid transdermal drug formulations such as creams, ointments, and gels are most commonly used to provide systemic effect by delivering the drug across the skin. Gel, among all, is most preferred because of their excellent appearance, fast drug release, desired consistency, ease of manufacturing and quality assessment, and considerable stability.[2] Most importantly, gels can be modified in order to make it suitable for delivering drug in sustained manner.

An ideal gel should satisfy the following three salient features:[3]

(i) They must have at least two components i.e. the gelling agent and a fluid component.
(ii) Each component should be continuous throughout the system.
(iii) They should exhibit mechanical properties of the solid state.

Gels are transparent or translucent semisolid formulations containing a high ratio of solvent/ gelling agent. In other word, gel can be defined as a semi-solid preparation composed of low concentrations (<15%) of gelator molecules.[4] According to USP, gels are defined as a semisolid, either suspension of small inorganic particles or large organic molecules interpenetrated with liquid.[5] In gel system a liquid phase is constrained within a rigid three dimensional polymeric network thereby exhibiting visco-elastic nature. Gels can be classified into hydrogels and organogels based on the liquid medium entrapped within the polymeric network. Hydrogels are composed of aqueous phase, whereas organogels are composed of aqueous phase along with organic phase.

Hydrogels are hydrophilic, three dimensional cross-linked polymer systems capable of imbibing large amounts of water or biological fluids between their polymeric chains to form aqueous semi-solid/solid gel networks.[6,7] Polymer networks in hydrogel may absorb water from 10–20% (an arbitrary lower limit) up to thousands of times their dry weight.[8,9]

Followings are the main features of hydrogels for which they are widely used in pharmaceutical applications:[10-14]

(i) Both compositionally (such as glycosaminoglycans) and mechanically, hydrogels are similar to the native extracellular matrix, thus can serve as a supporting material for cells during tissue regeneration and carrier in delivering a therapeutic agent.
(ii) It exhibits soft material nature, which encourages uptake of water and thereby forming hydrated yet solid materials, just like cells in the body.
(iii) The elastic property (due to the presence of meshes of the networks) of fully swollen or hydrated hydrogels is found to be minimizing irritation to the surrounding tissues after implantation.

Corresponding author: Rabinarayan Parhi, Email: bhu_rabi@rediffmail.com

(iv) Their hydrophilic and cross-linked property imparts excellent biocompatibility.

(v) Low interfacial tension between the hydrogel surface and body fluid minimizes protein adsorption and cell adhesion, which reduces the chances of a negative immune reaction.

(vi) Mucoadhesive and bioadhesive characteristics of many polymers used in hydrogel preparations (e.g. polyacrylic acid (PAA), polyethylene glycol (PEG), and polyvinyl alcohol (PVA)) enhance drug residence time on the skin/plasma membrane, leading to increase in tissue permeability.

Structure and water content in hydrogel

Presence of water in hydrogels plays an important role in the overall permeation of active ingredients into and out of the gel. Water can be associated to any hydrogel structure in following ways as shown in Figure 1.

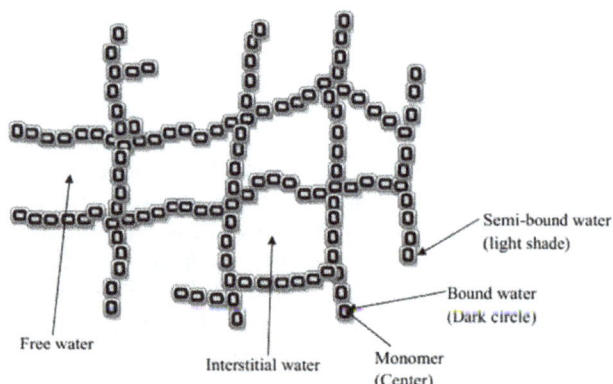

Figure 1. Schematic diagram of molecular structure of hydrogel network with different types of water.

The types of water associated with hydrogel are:
  (i)   Bound water (primary and secondary)
  (ii) Semibound water
  (iii) Interstitial water
  (iv) Free water or bulk water

When a dry hydrogel comes in contact with water, absorption of water into its matrix starts. At first water molecules entering the matrix will directly attach to the hydrophilic groups, forming hydrophilic bound water or primary bound water. The polymeric network swells because of complete hydration of the polar groups that resulted in the exposer of hydrophobic groups. These exposed groups also interact with water molecules, leading to hydrophobically-bound water, or 'secondary bound water'. The combination of primary and secondary bound water is often called the bound water. This water is considered as integral part of hydrogel structure and can only be separated out from the hydrogel under extreme conditions. After the saturation of hydrophilic and hydrophobic groups, the additional water that is absorbed due to the osmotic driving force of the network chains is called free water or bulk water. Between the bound water, present on polymeric monomer surface, and free water, there is a presence of

water layer called semibound water. Interstitial water is present in the interstices of hydrated polymeric network that is trapped physically but not attached to hydrogel network.[7,15]

Classification of hydrogel

Pharmaceutical hydrogels may be classified on the basis of their type of cross-linking or microstructure into following types (Figure 2):

Physical or reversible gel

In the preparation of physical gel, the selection of polymer is crucial and it depends on the two primary criteria; interaction among the chain must be strong enough to form semi-permanent junction in the molecular network and the network should hold large amount of water molecules inside it. The forces involved in the physical gel formation are hydrophobic, electrostatic, and hydrogen bonding between polymer chains.[16,17] Because the network formation by all of these interactions is purely physical, gel formation can be reversed.

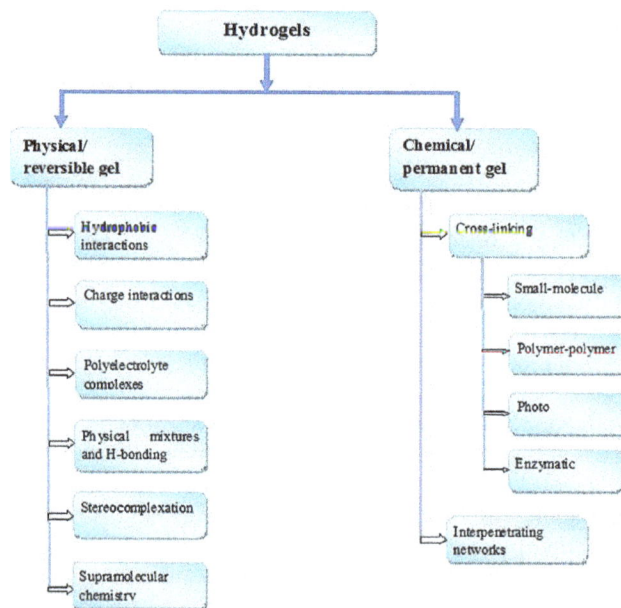

Figure 2. Classification of hydrogels based on cross-linking

Hydrophobic interactions

The mechanism involved in the sol-gel and gel-sol conversion of thermoreversible gel is based on hydrophobic interaction. The polymers showing hydrophobic interaction must be having both hydrophilic and hydrophobic domain, called as amphiphiles. Such amphiphiles are water soluble at low temperature. However, following increased temperature the hydrophobic domains (gelators) aggregate to minimize the hydrophobic surface area contacting the bulk water. This reduces the amount of structured water surrounding the hydrophobic domains and maximizing the solvent entropy. The gelation temperature depends on various parameters such as the concentration of the polymer, the length of the hydrophobic block, and the chemical structure of the polymer.[18]

Poloxamer (PX) is such a polymer which shows thermoreversible property in aqueous solutions. PX consists of hydrophilic poly (ethylene oxide) (PEO) and hydrophobic poly(propylene oxide) (PPO) blocks arranged in a tri-block structure as PEO–PPO–PEO [19]. The gelation of PX depends upon both temperature and concentration and the total gelling process is typically divided into two steps (Figure 3). The first step occurs when the temperature is increased to reach the critical micelle temperature (CMT) and the PX co-polymers aggregate to form spherical micelles. These micelles consist of an outer shell of hydrated swollen PEO chains

with dehydrated PPO blocks as the core. The process develops into the second step when a further increase in the temperature packs the micelles in an orderly manner to form gels.[19] Gelation is also dependent on the concentration of PX molecules in solution. At very low concentrations, PX molecules exist as monomers in solution. Increasing PX concentration up to $10^{-4}\%$ to $10^{-5}\%$ (w/w) leads to a critical micelle concentration (CMC), where spherical micelles started to built up. Further increase in PX concentration leads to a tightly packed system with a gel consistency.[20,21] Between 20-30% (w/v) aqueous solution of PX 407 at cold temperature (4-5°C) forms clear liquid and get transformed to gel at body temperature (37°C).

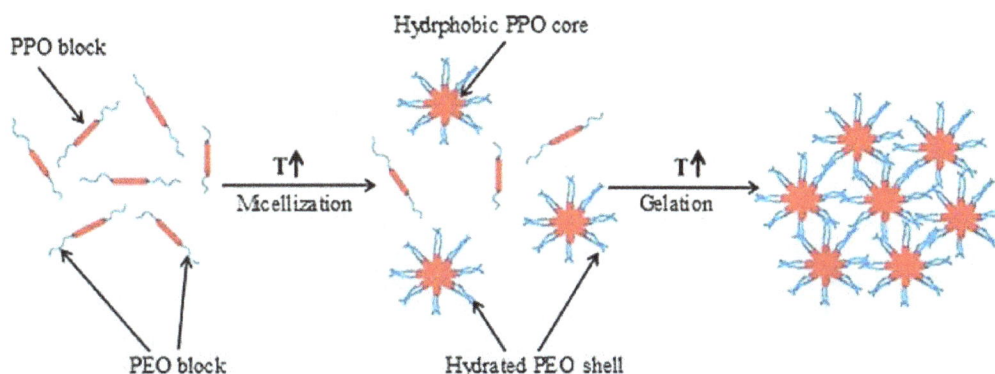

Figure 3. Schematic representation of physical gelation mechanism of PX 407 in water (Modified from reference 20)

Release of the model drug benzoic acid was found to be decreased with the increase in PX 407 concentration. This is probably due to an increase in size and number of micelles leading to decrease in size and number of aqueous channels. Further the modification of benzoic acid to more lipophilic moiety p-hydroxybenzoic acid causes a decrease in its release rate. This could be due to the greater partitioning of lipophilic derivatives into the micellar region within the gel structure.[22] Erukova *et al.* (2000) observed that PX facilitated the permeation of comparatively large molecules, including 2-n-undecylmalonic acid and doxorubicin, across lipid bilayers, whereas the permeation of small solutes (such as ammonium and acetic acid) remained unaffected. They also observed that PX accelerated the translocation of large hydrophobic anions (tetraphenylborate). They attributed the above effect of PX with the content of PEO units i.e. it is enhanced when the portion of PEO block in the copolymer is increased.[23] Gels and niosomal gels of meloxicam were developed using polymers such as PX 407, Chitosan and Carbopol-934. The PX 407 gel or niosomal PX 407 gel showed the superior drug release over the other formulations. Between the two types of gel of PX 407, niosomal gels exhibited superiority over conventional gels for anti-inflammatory test.[24] Thermosensitive gels of drugs such as indomethacin,[25] adriamycin and 5-flurouracil,[26] mitomycin C,[27] and ketoprofen[28] were successfully developed and studied. The gel formed from PX alone (as in case of above) leads to relatively rapid diffusion of drugs out of the

hydrophilic gel matrix by the dilution of water that entered the gel matrix.[29] To circumvent above drawback many researchers have used combination of polymers to reduce the fast entry of water and subsequently diffusion of drug out of gel structure. In addition, it will retain the gel structure for longer period of time and thereby sustain the drug release.

Based on the above fact thermoreversible gels of meloxicam were prepared using PX 407 and PX 188 (20-30% w/w) in combination with different additives such as polyvinylmethylether maleic anhydride copolymer, HPMC, PE-400, DMSO, sodium chloride. Among investigated gel bases, PX 407-HPMC gel was found to be ideal due to its gel strength (1.560±0.0135 N), viscosity (312.3±2.06 cP) and release characteristics.[30] HPMC K100M (2% w/v) and PX 407 (20% w/v) based procaine bioadhesive gels were prepared and the drug release was found to be increased with the increase in drug concentration from 1.5% to 3.5% (w/w) in the gels and the temperature of surrounding solutions from 28°C to 42°C.[31] Pranoprofen release from HPMC and PX 407 based bioadhesive gel was increased with the increase in temperature, which was attributed to increased in activation energy of the drug.[32,33] Similarly, Shin *et al.* (2004) successfully prepared lidocaine HCl gel using HPMC (2% w/v) and PX 407 (20% w/v) for analgesic activity.[34] We have successfully prepared and characterized bioadhesive hydrogels of aceclofenac and metoprolol succinate containing various concentrations of HPMC (0.5-4% w/w) and PX 407 (15-30% w/w).[35,36]

A range of other synthetic amphiphilic thermally gelling polymers have been investigated. Based on the position of hydrophilic and hydrophobic blocks they may be classified in to two categories; symmetric and asymmetric. Symmetric means the presence of hydrophobic block at the center and hydrophilic blocks on either side and vice versa. Examples of this category are PX (discussed in the previous section), PEG- poly (lactide-co-glycolide) (PLGA)-PEG[37] or PLGA-PEG-PLGA[38] etc. Compared to PX systems, PL(G)A-based triblock gelators exhibit better biodegradability, higher gelation temperatures (which is allowing easier handling of injectable preparation), and sustained drug release.[39] Another example of symmetric triblock polymer is Poly (N-isopropylacrylamide) (PNIPAM)-poly (phosphorylcholine)-PNIPAM, which form gels at 6-7 wt % when the temperature exceeded 32°C (is the phase transition temperature of PNIPAM).[40] PNIPAM grafted with other polymers such as hyaluronic acid and chitosan were developed successfully for the sustained release of riboflavin[41] and 5-fluorouracil,[42] respectively. Asymmetric triblock copolymer formed of PEG, PLA, and poly (L-glutamic acid) were also developed and observed that the L-glutamic acid block permits selective modification with specific targeting groups such as the cell-adhesive RGD peptide.[43]

Reverse thermal gelation is also evident from some natural polymers. A biocompatible, parenteral gel composed of chitosan solutions and glycerol-2-phosphate was prepared and the gel was found to be exhibited sol-gel transition at a temperature close to 37°C.[44] Chitosan grafted with PEG (approximately 40 wt %) based thermoreversible gel was prepared and studied for bovine serum albumin (BSA) release. This gel showed an initial burst release for 5 h and afterwards a steady linear release of BSA for a period of approximately 70 h.[45] Liang *et al.* (2004) successfully used thermosensitive methylcellulose to thermally gel aqueous alginate solution blended with various salts such as $CaCl_2$, Na_2HPO_4, and NaCl for the delivery of BSA.[46] Similar thermally triggered transitions have also been exhibited by hydroxypropylcellulose.[47]

Charge interactions

Charge interactions which lead to the formation of hydrogel may occur in two ways; (i) between a polymer and an oppositely charged small molecule as linker, and (ii) between two polymers of opposite charge (Figure 4). This type of cross-linking (or decross-linking) can be triggered by pH changes that ionize or protonate the ionic functional groups. These hydrogels can be tailored to achieve a specific set of thermal, mechanical and degradation profiles. In some cases they can formed in situ, known as in situ gelling hydrogels.[48] A mixture of quaternized chitosan (N-[(2-hydroxy-3-trimethylammonium) propyl] chitosan chloride (HTCC)) and glycerophosphate (GP) forms an ionically cross-linked gel at 37°C which can release doxorubicin hydrochloride as a function of pH.[49] At acidic condition

and physiological condition these hydrogel dissolved and released drug quickly, while it released drug slowly at neutral or basic conditions.

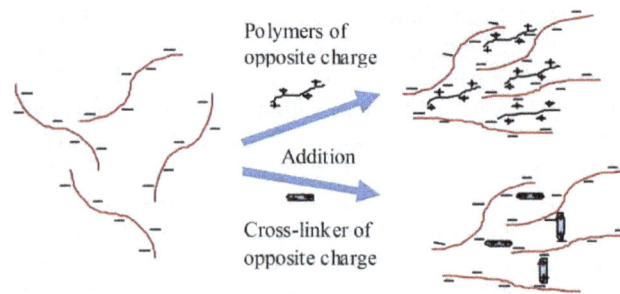

Figure 4. Schematic illustration of mechanism of charge interactions with an oppositely charged polymer and a cross-linker

The charged interactions have been widely investigated for cross-linking in situ gelling hydrogels. The main advantage of this interaction is that biodegradation can occur as ionic species in extracellular fluid which bind competitively with the gel components and as a result decross-linking of network happen. In addition, this approach can also be used to cross-link microparticle or nanoparticle gels to equip it with suitable drug delivery properties. For instance anionic (methacrylic acid (MAA)) and cationic (dimethylaminoethyl methacrylate (DMAEMA)) polymers coated hydroxyethyl methacrylate-derivatized dextran microspheres exhibit spontaneous gelation upon mixing due to ionic complex formation between the oppositely charged microparticles.[50] Another approach, so called ionic-complementarity, uses peptide of alternating positive and negative charge distribution leading to peptide self-assembly. These peptides assume β-sheet secondary structure predominantly, and can form hydrogels. The advantage of this approach is that nanoscopic and/or macroscopic structures with great stability and functionality can be developed by varying peptide concentration, pH, presence of salts, and time.[51]

Polyelectrolyte complexes (PECs)/ Complex coacervate gel

PECs are formed by the electrostatic interactions between two oppositely charged polyelectrolytes in an aqueous solution as shown as in Figure 5. Thus both the polymers must be ionized and have opposite charges. This implies that the reaction can only occur at pH values in the vicinity of the pKa interval of the two polymers.[16] Its distinction from electrostatic interactions is based on the MW of molecules. The PEC is formed between larger molecules with a broad MW range and the association is stronger than other secondary binding interactions like hydrogen bonding (H-bonding) or van der Waals interactions. For example formation of PEC between chitosan, a polycation, with polyanions such as proteins (e.g. collagen, gelatin, albumin), polysaccharides (e.g. alginate, pectin or xanthan) and synthetic polymers (e.g. PAA) were reported.[52]

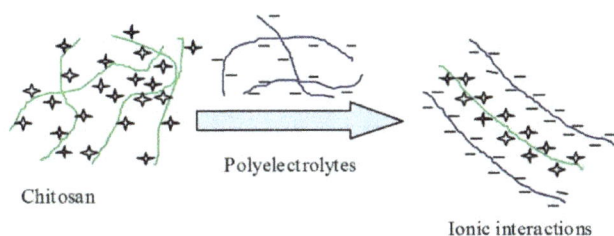

Figure 5. Schematic diagram of PEC mechanism

Chitosan based PEC of metoprolol tartrate were developed in the form of beads and hydrogels by interaction of cationic chitosan with anionic sodium alginate, carboxymethyl cellulose sodium and k-carrageenan using simple ionic gelation technique. Among all the combinations, PEC of chitosan and carboxymethylcellulose sodium exhibited least in vitro drug release and was able to extend the release of metoprolol tartrate up to 12 h.[53] Another chitosan based PEC hydrogel with improved viscoe-lastic behavior was developed using low concentration (0.1 to 0.8%) of chitosan and constant gelatin concentration of 1%.[54] Chang *et al.* (2014) successfully developed PEC of chitosan and poly-(γ-glutamic acid) (γ-PGA) to promote new bone formation in the alveolar socket following tooth extraction.[55] With same composition, a cytocompatible PEC was developed for biological application.[56] A PEC composed of alginate and chitosan was developed and found to be having improved thermal, chemical, and mechanical properties and stability.[57] Sometimes, same polymers having opposite charges, fraction is modified to opposite charge by chemical processes, can also be used to prepare PEC hydrogel. One of such hydrogel was developed with phosphorylated chitosan (a polycation) and chitosan (a polyanion) as an osteoblast carrier. These hydrogels exhibited three-dimensional hierarchically-porous structure and good cyto-biocompatibility for osteoblasts in vitro.[58] Based on above approach, another novel PEC encapsulated dexamethasone hydrogel was prepared using polycationic N-trimethyl chitosan and polyanionic N-carboxymethyl chitosan to target distal intestine.[59] Chitosan, in many drug delivery systems, present as unionized amine form at the neutral/alkaline pH of physiological application sites, while the anionic polyelectrolyte is in the ionized form. In this form to stabilize any PEC is a challenging task, but it can be overcome by using modified chitosan such as quaternized chitosan. This modified chitosan along with PAA were used to prepare PEC hydrogels with improved mechanical properties by in situ polymerization of acrylic acid monomers in the concentrated quaternized chitosan solution.[60]

The advantage of PEC is that it is formed without the use of organic precursors, catalysts, or reactive agents, avoiding the concern about safety in the body. During complexation, polyelectrolytes can either coacervate, or form a more or less compact hydrogel. However, if ionic interactions are too strong, precipitation can occur,[61] which is quite common and hinders the formation of hydrogels. Precipitation can be prevented weakening the electrostatic attraction by the addition of salts, such as NaCl.[16]

Physical mixtures and hydrogen bonding interaction
Hydrogels by H-bonding interactions can be formed by freeze-thaw cycles using PVA alone[62] or in combination with other polymers such as chitosan.[52] In the earlier case crystallization plays a big part in the creation of cross-links between PVA chains during lyophilization. The cross-linking is possible due to the existence of regular pendant hydroxyl groups on PVA that are able to form crystallites by strong inter-chain H-bonding. The crystals formed by this method are generally considered to have a two-molecule monoclinic unit cell, with hydroxyl groups randomly placed on either side of both polymer chains as shown in Figure 6. It has been proposed that in the first freeze-thaw cycle, the initial freezing of water, and associated expansion, leads to increased polymer concentration in the unfrozen phase. Crystallization can then take place within the polymer-rich microphages.[63]

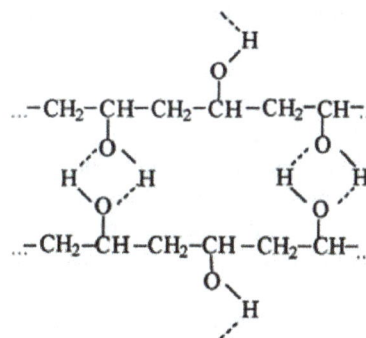

Figure 6. Hydrogen bonding in PVA solutions

Processing parameters such as the concentration, the number of thermal cycles, and the thawing rate affect the mechanical behavior of cryogel. Pazos *et al.* (2009) reported that with increasing number of thermal cycles resulting in the formation of the strongest cryogels because the number of intermolecular hydrogen bonding increases and molecular chains aggregate.[64] They also reported that the increase in thawing rate from 2 (0.333°C/min) to 5 (0.067°C/min) exhibited the same effect on the gel's elastic properties. Meenakshi, and Ahuja, (2015) found that 4 freeze-thaw cycles are optimum for the preparation of composite cryogels of metronidazole with carboxymethyl tamarind kernel polysaccharide and PVA. This cryogel provided 75.77% of drug release over a period of 6h and had better thermal stability.[65]

In case of composite cryogel, mixture of polymers forms junction points in the form of crystallites and inter-polymer interaction after a series of freeze–thaw cycles.[16] These interactions act as cross-linking sites of the hydrogel. Addition of another polymer to PVA negatively affects the formation of PVA crystallites thereby forming hydrogels of less ordered structures. Chitosan-PVA polymer blend is one such example of polymer mixture, where increasing chitosan concentration in the blend reduces the crystallinity of hydrogel.[52] The addition of chitosan decreased maximum strength and thermal stability of PVA cryogel containing minocycline and gentamycin, while it increased the swelling ability, elasticity and porosity of cryogel.[66,67] Contrary to above, Paduraru et al. (2012) reported that strength of the cryogel increased by increasing the microcrystalline cellulose content from 0 to 50 % wt.[68]

H-bonding can also be formed with blend of two or more natural polymers such as hyaluronic acid-methylcellulose, gelatin-agar, and starch-carboxymethyl cellulose. The formation of H-bonding interactions between the polymer chains along with the compatible geometry resulted in the enhanced visco-elastic properties of the hydrogel.[69] The main advantage of above mixture of polymers is the excellent biocompatibility offered by them due to the absence of chemical cross-linkers. However, the problem associated with it is the breaking of H-bonded networks over a few hours in vivo due to influx of water, which restricting their use to short-acting drug release systems.[18]

Stereocomplexation

Stereocomplexation is a synergistic interaction between polymer chains or small molecules of the same chemical composition, occasionally with different chemical composition, but different stereochemistry and stereocomplex formation occur due to the interaction between polymers having different tacticities or configurations.[70] It may be homo-stereocomplexation or hetero-stereocomplexation. In former case the complex formation occurs between same molecules but with different stereochemistry. For example, interaction between polylactide blocks with L- and D-stereochemistry.[70] Another well known example of stereocomplexation is the one between isotactic and syndiotactic poly(methyl methacrylate) (PMMA).[71] Hetero-stereocomplexation occurs between two different molecules with different stereochemistry such as D-PLA and L-configured peptides leuproide, a luteinizing hormone-releasing hormone.[72] Natural polymers such as dextran precursors can be grafted to L-lactide and D-lactide oligomers leading to the spontaneous gelation in water. It provided an excellent biocompatibility and biodegradability.[73]

Like H-bond interactions, stereocomplexation do not need harsh organic solvents and chemical cross-linkers. Main limitation of stereocomplexation is the restricted range of polymer compositions available which can be used i.e. even small changes in the stereochemistry or else changing the composition of matter can significantly weaken or altogether eliminate the stereochemical interaction.

Supramolecular chemistry

Supramolecular chemistry is based on the association of two or more chemical species held together by intermolecular forces. The intermolecular forces includes electrostatic interactions, H-bonding, metal coordination, π- π interaction, Van der Waals forces etc. and the important methods by which supermolecules formed are; molecular self-assembly, folding, host-guest interaction (e.g. inclusion complex), recognization and complexation and mechanical-interlocking.[74]

This approach has wide application such as material technology, catalysis, data storage and processing and in the preparation of medicines. The most common type of cross-linking interaction used to prepare hydrogels is the formation of inclusion complexes. For example, formation of a reversible hydrogel complex between PEO polymers and α-cyclodextrins.[75] Similarly, β-cyclodextrin can be used to gel PPO-grafted dextran into a hydrogel.[76] Self-assembled systems have also been reported that apply both hydrophobic interactions and supermolecular chemistry to facilitate the formation of denser and/or more stable hydrogel networks. A self-assembled system, PEO-poly(R-3-hydroxybutyrate) (PHB)-PEO triblock copolymers, was complexed with α-cyclodextrin to form strong hydrogel networks. The cross-linking was accomplished by (a) the thermal gelation of the hydrophobic PHB segments and (b) the inclusion complexes formed between the PEO segments and cyclodextrin. This system is capable of releasing fluorescein isothiocyanate-dextran for up to one month.[77]

Chemical or permanent gel

Physically cross-linked hydrogels are prepared without the use of cross-linking entities or chemical modification. Despite of the above advantage, it is inflexible towards variables such as gelation time, gel pore size, chemical functionalization, and degradation or dissolution, leading to inconsistent performance in vivo.[52] In contrast, chemically cross-linked hydrogels allows absorption of water and/or bioactive compounds without dissolution and permits drug release by diffusion.[18]

Cross-linking

Chemical cross-linking method uses covalent bonding between polymer chains in order to produce permanent hydrogel. The cross-link formation was carried out by the addition of small cross-linkers molecules, polymer-polymer conjugation, photosensitive agents or by enzyme catalyzed reaction.

Small-molecule cross-linking

Preparation of small-molecule cross linking hydrogels at the minimum requires one polymer and a small molecule as cross-linker in an appropriate solvent. Cross-linkers are molecules with at least two reactive functional groups that allow the formation of bridges between polymeric chains.[78] Small cross-linkers can be of two types; bi-functional molecules or drug molecules. In the former case drug molecule is entrapped within the hydrogel formed due to the interaction between bi-functional molecule and polymer. Moreover, drug molecule having two functional group covalently bonded with polymeric chains to form hydrogel, which avoids the use of cross-linkers. This approach is limited to drug in which two reactive functional groups are available. One such drug molecule is primaquine (a di-amino drug), which has been used to cross-link periodate-oxidized gum arabic into a hydrogel through the rapid formation of Schiff bases between the amine groups and the aldehyde groups present in the drug and polymer, respectively.[79]

The simplest form of the cross-linking takes place between aldehyde and amino groups to form Schiff base. For example, dialdehyde such as glyoxal and particularly glutaraldehyde[46] forms covalent imine bonds with the amino groups of chitosan via Schiff reaction.[80] In other cases, dextran-tyramine[81] and hyaluronic acid-tyramine[82] covalently bonded by using horseradish peroxidase (HRP) and hydrogen peroxide (H_2O_2) as cross-linkers to form hydrogels with improved controllable gelation times ranging from 5 s to 9 min according to the reactant concentrations used. A general disadvantage of each of these small-molecule cross-linking methods is the potential toxicity of residual unreacted cross-linker agents in vivo. For instance, glutaraldehyde and glyoxal are known to be neurotoxic and mutagenic, respectively.[80]

Genipin (a naturally derived chemical from the fruit ofgardenia) widely used as a cross-linking agent alternative to dialdehydes due to its biocompatibility.[83] It was also reported that genipin bind polymers, such as chitosan and gelatin with biological tissues covalently.[84] Furthermore, amino-terminated groups containing molecules such as PEG, N,O-carboxymethyl chitosan,[85] and BSA[86] have been cross-linked to genipin to form hydrogels with flexible dissolution rates from 3 min to more than 100 days. Even though genipin shows good biocompatibility, it is still liable to negatively interact with encapsulated drugs, an unavoidable problem for gelation in the presence of a therapeutic.

This approach used to develop transdermal drug delivery systems for the delivery of oxprenolol HCl,[87] propanolol HCl,[88] 5-fluorouracil,[89] indomethacin from gel beads for the control release.[90]

Polymer-polymer cross-linking or hybrid polymer networks (HPN)
In this type of hydrogel, the cross-linking reaction occurs between a structural unit of a polymeric chain and a structural unit of another polymeric chain of another type. Therefore, polymers must be pre-functionalized with reactive functional groups. Several types of covalent linkages can be made depending on the desired speed of cross-linking, selection of targeted reactive functional groups, and biodegradability of the resulting conjugates.

Widely investigated in situ cross-linking phenomenon is Michael addition between a nucleophile (i.e. an amine or a thiol) and a vinyl group. For example, cross-linking of vinyl sulfone-functionalized dextrans with thiolated PEG. This type of approach provides the flexibility in forming multiple types of bonds, relative biological inertness and finally rapid formation of hydrogel.[91] Another example is the formation of a hydrazone bond between an aldehyde and a hydrazide which facilitates rapid cross-linking of gel precursors.[92] Control release of tissue plasminogen activator and budesonide[93] to the peritoneum was achieved by using hyaluronic acid cross-linking by hydrazone bonds. Similar approaches also been used to design poly (aldehyde guluronate) for the effective delivery of osteoblasts and growth factors.[94]

The major advantages of this approach are the elimination of cross-linker molecules and in situ formation of covalently bonded hydrogels. The main limitation of this approach is the requirement for significant polymeric modification to link functional group to polymeric chain. In addition, the pre-gel polymers are often themselves somewhat cytotoxic, even when prepared from highly biocompatible polymer precursors.

Photo cross-linking
Formation of hydrogels based on photo cross-linking depends on the presence of photo sensitive functional groups. By linking a photo sensitive functional group to a polymer enables it to form cross-linkages upon irradiation with light such as UV light. Chitosan is one such polymer which was studied more compared to other polymers. A photo cross-linked chitosan hydrogel was developed by incorporating azide groups ($-N_3$) to polymeric chain of chitosan. After its exposure to UV light, the azide group is converted to nitrene group (R-N:) which binds free amino groups of chitosan leading to the in situ formation of hydrogel within a minute.[95] Photo cross-linked hydrogel can also be formed between the polymers. One such example is thermo-sensitive chitosan-pluronic hydrogel, where both the polymers were functionalized with photo sensitive acrylate groups ($CH_2=CHCOO-$) by UV irradiation. The resulted cross-linked polymer formed a physical network at temperatures above the lower critical solution temperature (LCST) and the same exhibited the ability to release encapsulated human growth hormone (hGH) in sustained manner.[96] The above combination was also used to deliver plasmid DNA.[97] Another chitosan-PEG-based hydrogel was developed by modifying chitosan with photoreactive azidobenzoic acid and PEG with arginylglycylaspartic acid peptide. Upon UV illumination, a free-radical photo-initiated polymerization took place that led to the formation of hydrogel in situ. Resulted hydrogel helped in targeting the injured myocardium for the delivery of growth factors and cells.[98]

The advantage of this approach is to facilitate easy and speedy formation of hydrogel. It also offers safety and low cost preparation compared to chemical methods, which generally require the addition of different reactive species, initiators, or catalysts. However, this technique requires a photosensitizer and prolonged irradiation, which could also result in local rise of temperature, thereby damaging neighboring cells and tissue.[99]

Enzymatic cross-linking

This is a new approach to form in situ hydrogel using enzyme-catalyzed cross-linking reaction between polymer chains. A number of enzymes including transglutaminases (TG),[100-102] peroxidases,[103,104] tyrosinase,[105] phosphopantetheinyl transferase, lysyl oxidase, plasma amine oxidase, and phosphatases[106] were studied and reported.

TG belong to thiol group of enzymes which catalyze the formation of highly resistant covalent bonds between a free amine group of a protein or peptide-bound lysine and the g-carboxamide group of a protein or peptide-bound glutamine.[106] Yung *et al.* (2007) have successfully developed thermally stable and biocompatible gelatin hydrogels cross-linked by microbial TG (mTG), which is capable of delivering encapsulated regenerative cells (HEK293) in a controlled manner.[100] The same group tested the diffusion of anticancer drug, interleukin-2, from mTG cross-linked gelatin and found that the resulted hydrogels are not only cyto-compatible but also have potential to be used as sustained drug release devices.[101] Between animal derived tissue TG (tTG) and recombinant human TG (hTG) enzymes used for cross-linking of two classes of protein polymers containing either lysine or glutamine under physiological conditions, tTG completed the cross-linking faster (within 2 min) compared to hTG.[102]

HRP and soy bean peroxidase are the most commonly used peroxidase enzymes in the formation of hydrogel. They catalyze the conjugation of phenol and aniline derivatives in the presence of substrate H_2O_2. In this reaction the HRP promptly combines with H_2O_2 and the resulted complex can oxidize hydroxyphenyl groups present in compound such as tyramine and tyrosine.[106] Recently, Kim *et al.* (2011) developed HRP catalyzed injectable tyramine modified hyaluronic acid (HA-Tyr) hydrogels in two steps. In the first step, HA-Tyr conjugate was synthesized by amide bond formation between carboxyl groups of HA and amine groups of tyramine and in the subsequent step HA-Tyr hydrogels were prepared by radical cross-linking reaction using HRP and H_2O_2. This hydrogel was used to deliver dexamethasone intra-articularly for the treatment of rheumatoid arthritis.[103] An enzymatically cross-linked injectable hydrogel was developed from chitosan derivatives, chitosan-glycolic acid, and phloretic acid using HRP and H_2O_2.[104] This hydrogel can be formed (gelation time) from 10 sec to 4 min by using the polymer concentration from 3 to 1% and has potential for cartilage tissue engineering.

Tyrosinases are oxidative enzymes that convert accessible tyrosine residues of proteins (e.g. gelatin) into reactive o-quinone moiety, which can undergo non-enzymatic reactions with available nucleophiles such amino groups of chitosan. Chen *et al.* (2002) developed gelatin gel by two methods namely; (i) cooling the gelatin solution and (ii) tyrosinase-catalyzed hydrogel formation and observed that the second method demonstrated better mechanical properties which can be exploited for medical and industrial applications.[107] Gelatin-chitosan gels were developed using both TG and tyrosinase for comparison and following observations were made; (i) chitosan was not required for transglutaminase-catalyzed gel formation, although gel formation was faster and the resulted gel was stronger in its presence, (ii) TG-catalyzed gelatin-chitosan gels lost the ability to undergo thermally reversible transitions, (iii) tyrosinase-catalyzed gelatin-chitosan gels were considerably weaker than transglutaminase-catalyzed gels, but can be strengthened by cooling below gel-point of gelatin.[105]

Interpenetrating networks (IPNs)

An IPN may be defined as any material that contains two or more polymers in the network form in which one polymer is cross-linked in the presence of other.[108,109] IPNs are considered as "alloys" of cross-linked polymers, which are formed without any covalent bonds between them. These networks cannot be separated unless chemical bonds are broken.[110]

The polymers to be used in the preparation of IPN hydrogel must fulfill following three conditions; at least one polymer must be synthesized and/or cross-linked within the immediate presence of the other, both polymers should have similar kinetics, and there should not be dramatic phase separation between/among the polymers.[111] An IPN is different from other polymer combination because it has no viscoelastic property, and it swells, but does not dissolve in any solvent.[112]

Based on the chemistry of preparation, IPN hydrogels can be classified into following types:[113,114]

(i) Simultaneous IPN: when both the networks are synthesized simultaneously from the precursors at the same time by independent, non-interfering routs.

(ii) Sequential IPN: it is formed by swelling of a single-network hydrogel into a solution containing the mixture of monomer, initiator and activator, with or without a cross-linker.

Sequential IPNs are of two types namely, fully-IPN and semi-IPN based on the presence and absence of cross-linker, respectively.

According to the structure, IPN hydrogels can be classified into three categories:[114]

(i) IPNs: formed by two juxtaposed networks, with many entanglements and physical interactions between them.

(ii) Homo-IPNs: these are developed from the two polymers which are having independent networks, but have same structure.

(iii) Semi- or Pseudo-IPNs: in this type one polymer has a linear instead of a network structure.

There are mainly two classes of polymers which are used to synthesize IPN hydrogels, including natural polymers and their derivatives such as polysaccharides and proteins, and synthetic polymers containing hydrophilic functional groups (e.g. -COOH, -OH, -CONH₂, SO₃H, amines etc).[8]

IPN hydrogels of clarithromycin were synthesized by using three polymers such as chitosan, PAA and poly (vinyl pyrrolidone) (PVP) and two cross-linking agents (e.g. glutaraldehyde and N,N'-methylene-bis-acrylamide). The resulted IPN hydrogels have good mucoadhesion property, which helped the gel to retain in gastric environment of stomach for prolonged period of time. As a result of that IPN hydrogel maintain antibiotic concentration in stomach for prolonged period of time, thereby used as a drug delivery system for treatment of *H. pylori* infection and in management of peptic ulcer.[115] Semi-IPN hydrogels were synthesized by cross-linking chitosan and PVP blend with glutaraldehyde and found that the resulted semi-IPN gels have potential to deliver clarithromycin in the gastric medium.[116] Kulkarni *et al.* (2010) developed IPN hydrogel membranes of prazosin hydrochloride using sodium alginate (SA) and PVA as polymers for transdermal delivery. The stiffness of the film was increased by the addition of cross-linker glutaraldehyde and both the stiffness and in vitro drug release property film depend on the concentrations of

glutaraldehyde in membranes. The prepared IPN membranes extended prazosin hydrochloride release up to 24h, whereas membranes made up off SA and PVA alone showed fast drug release.[117] Microspheres of theophylline were successfully prepared based on IPNs method using chitosan and methylcellulose as polymers and glutaraldehyde as a cross-linker. The encapsulation efficiency was found to be up to 82% and the extended drug release up to 12 h.[118] Likewise, duration of 5-fluorouracil release was significantly sustained for up to 52 h from new thermo-sensitive gels in which a chitosan network is crosslinked with various concentrations of glutaraldehyde that interpenetrates PX gels.[119]

Multicomponent networks as IPNs have better mechanical strength and swelling/deswelling response compared to single-network hydrogels.[120] Furthermore, the cross-linking density, hydrogel porosity, and gel stiffness can be adjusted in IPN-based hydrogels according to the target application. The drawbacks are: (i) it has a problem with encapsulating a wide variety of therapeutic agents, especially sensitive bimolecular, and IPN, particularly sequential type, (ii) preparation requires the use of toxic agents such as initiator, activator and cross-linker in order to initiate or catalyze the polymerization or to catalyze the cross-linking.[121] Difference between physical and chemical hydrogel and types of cross-linked hydrogel along with their polymer system and drug incorporated is presented in Table 1 and Table 2, respectively.

Table 1. Difference between physical and chemical gel.[8]

Physical hydrogel	Chemical hydrogel
Physical hydrogels are formed by molecular entanglements, and/or secondary forces including ionic, H-bonding or hydrophobic forces.	Chemical hydrogels formed by covalent cross-linking.
Above bonds are weak, thus physical hydrogels are considered as reversible gel.	These are termed as permanent or irreversible as covalent bonds are strong.
These are prepared without the use of cross-linking entities or chemical modification.	These are prepared using cross-linking entities or chemical modification.
It is inflexible towards variables such as gelation time, gel pore size, chemical functionalization, and degradation or dissolution, leading to inconsistent performance in vivo.	It is flexible in respect to gelation time, gel pore size, chemical functionalization, and degradation or dissolution.
Physically cross-linked hydrogels are less stable against degradation.	Chemically cross-linked hydrogels are very stable against degradation.
These are homogeneous.	These are non-homogeneous.
Physical hydrogels have hydrophilic and hydrophobic regions present in the polymeric network.	Chemical hydrogels have domains of high cross-link density as compared to conventional hydrogels.
These hydrogels show poor mechanical properties because of the reversible physical interactions.	The mechanical properties of these hydrogels are higher than physically cross-linked hydrogels.
For incorporation of bioactive substances, these gels are of great interest.	These are being used in a number of applications like pharmaceutical, agriculture, food industry, cosmetics, etc.

Table 2. Hydrogel types with their composition and drug incorporated.

Types of hydrogel	Polymer (s)	Drug	References
Hydrophobic interactions	PX 407	Benzoic acid/ p-hydroxybenzoic acid	22
	PX 188, PX 181 and Pluronic P85	2-n-undecylmalonic acid, doxorubicin, ammonium, acetic acid and tetraphenylborate.	23
	PX 407, Chitosan and Carbopol-934	Meloxicam	24
	PX 407	Indomethacin	25
	PX 407	Adriamycin and 5-flurouracil	26
	PX 407	Mitomycin C	27
	HPC and PX 407	Ketoprofen	28
	PX 407 and PX 188, Polyvinylmethylether maleic anhydride copolymer, HPMC, PE-400.	Meloxicam	30
	HPMC K100M and PX 407	Procaine	31
	HPMC and PX 407	Pranoprofen	32, 33
	HPMC and PX 407	Lidocaine HCl	34
	HPMC and PX 407	Aceclofenac and Metoprolol succinate	35, 36
	PNIPAM grafted with hyaluronic acid and chitosan	Riboflavin and 5-fluorouracil	41, 42
	Chitosan grafted with PEG 40	BSA	45
	Alginate solution	BSA	46
Charge interactions	HTCC and GP	Doxorubicin HCl	49
Polyelectrolyte complexes	Chitosan with sodium alginate, carboxymethyl cellulose sodium and k-carrageenan	Metoprolol tartrate	53
	Chitosan and gelatin	----	54
	Chitosan and poly-(γ-glutamic acid) (γ-PGA)	----	55, 56
	Alginate and chitosan	----	57
	Phosphorylated chitosan (a polycation) and chitosan	Osteoblasts	58
	Polycationic N-trimethyl chitosan and polyanionic N-carboxymethyl chitosan	Dexamethasone	59
	Quaternized chitosan and PAA	----	60
Physical mixtures and H-bonding	Carboxymethyl tamarind kernel polysaccharide and PVA	Metronidazole	64
	Chitosan and PVA	Minocycline and Gentamycin	66, 67
	Microcrystalline cellulose and PVA	Vanillin	68
Stereocomplexation	L- and D- PLA	----	70
	Isotactic and syndiotactic PMMA	----	71
	D-PLA and L-leuproide	----	72
	Dextran precursors grafted L-lactide and D-lactide oligomers	----	73
Supramolecular chemistry	PEO polymers and α-cyclodextrins	----	75
	β-cyclodextrin & PPO-grafted dextran	----	76
	PEO-poly(R-3-hydroxybutyrate) (PHB)-PEO triblock copolymers & α-cyclodextrin	----	77
Cross-linking			
(i) Small-molecule cross-linking	Oxidized gum arabic	Primaquine	79
	Genipin	BSA	86
	Chitosan	Oxprenolol HCl	87
		Propanolol HCl	95
		5-Fluorouracil	89
	Chitosan–alginate	Indomethacin	90

Types of hydrogel	Polymer (s)	Drug	References
(ii) Polymer-polymer cross-linking	Hyaluronic acid with amino or aldehyde functionality	Bone morphogenetic protein-2	91
	Cross-linked hyaluronic acid	Tissue plasminogen activator and budesonide	93
	Poly(aldehyde guluronate) and adipic acid dihydrazide	Bone precursor cells and growth factor	94
(iii) Photo cross-linking	Chitosan-pluronic	Human growth hormone (hGH) Plasmid DNA	96 97
	Modified chitosan-PEG	Growth factors and cells	98
(iv) Enzymatic cross-linking	Gelatin cross-linked by mTG	Regenerative cells (HEK293) Interleukin-2	100 101
	Tyramine modified hyaluronic acid by HRP	Dexamethasone	103
Interpenetrating networks	Chitosan, PAA and PVP	Clarithromycin	116
	Chitosan and PVP	Clarithromycin	117
	SA and PVA	Prazosin HCl	118
	Chitosan and methylcellulose	Theophylline	119
	Chitosan and PX	5-fluorouracil	120

Conclusion and future prospective

Over the past 50 years, there has been continuous progress in designing of hydrogels that led to numerous applications such as pharmaceutical, biomedical, agrochemicals, food industry, etc. In pharmaceutical therapeutic delivery, hydrogels are available in various dosage forms such as tablets, capsules, microspheres, transdermal films, wound dressings, etc. These hydrogels are also used to develop catheter, vascular grafts, semiocclusive dressings, mammary implants, transdermal drug delivery systems, scaffold for tissue engineering and medicated patches etc.[6] Despite the wide use, hydrogels suffer significant disadvantages such as low mechanical strength and toughness, difficulties in handling, sterilization, syringability issues. Special structural configurations like slip-link networks, nanocomposite hydrogels, double network hydrogels, multi-functional cross-linked hydrogels, and homogeneous hydrogels can be synthesized to enhance mechanical strength and toughness of resulting hydrogels.[122] These techniques should be followed by a suitable method of polymerization or cross-linking in order to make them desirable for suitable application. Another way to enhance mechanical property along with improved biocompatibility and physical property is to combine both physical and chemical cross-linking in a single hydrogel system.

The syringability issue can be solved to a large extent by designing physical gelators which gel at lower polymer concentrations and at more precise gelation temperatures, like in-situ or thermosensitive gels, would reduce the risk of premature gelation inside the needle upon injection. Similarly, for covalently cross-linked hydrogels, the development of strategies to release cross-linker in a triggered manner inside the body, thereby minimizes the risk of syringe clogging, improve the localization of cross-linker release to minimize in vivo toxicity. This strategy is used to transform hydrogels in to "smart" materials that can respond to changes in their environment. In addition the hydrogel properties can be further modified by incorporation of micro or nano fillers. More recently, hydrogels have been modified into hydrogel microparticles for solubility enhancement purposes.[123,124]

In the present scenario, the focus needs to be shifted towards the development of innovative methods to prepare: (i) hydrophilic polymers of desirable functional groups, (ii) multifunctional/multiarm structures such as grafted or branched co-polymers and star polymers that would offer better properties and suit wider applications in the future.

Acknowledgments

The author thanks management of GITAM University to provide necessary facilities and support.

Ethical Issues

Not applicable.

Conflict of Interest

The author declares no conflicts of interest.

References

1. Delgado-Charro MB, Guy RH. Effective use of transdermal drug delivery in children. *Adv Drug Deliv Rev* 2014;73:63-82. doi: 10.1016/j.addr.2013.11.014
2. Raut S, Bhadoriya SS, Uplanchiwar V, Mishra V, Gahane A, Jain SK. Lecithin organogel: A unique micellar system for the delivery of bioactive agents in the treatment of skin aging. *Acta Pharm Sin B* 2012;2(1):8-15. doi: 10.1016/j.apsb.2011.12.005
3. Gunn C. Disperse systems. In: Carter SJ, editor. *Tutorial Pharmacy*. 6th ed. New Delhi, India: CBS Publishers; 2000. PP. 54-88.
4. Vintiloiu A, Leroux JC. Organogels and their use in drug delivery--A review. *J Control Release*

2008;125(3):179-92.   doi: 10.1016/j.jconrel.2007.09.014

5. Kumar L, Verma R. In vitro evaluation of topical gel prepared using natural polymer. *Int J Drug Deliv* 2010;2(1):58-63.   doi: 10.5138/ijdd.2010.0975.0215.02012

6. Flood P, Page H, Reynaud EG. Using hydrogels in microscopy: A tutorial. *Micron* 2016;84:7-16. doi: 10.1016/j.micron.2016.02.002

7. Singhala R, Gupta K. A Review: Tailor-made hydrogel structures (classifications and synthesis parameters). *Polym Plast Technol Eng* 2016;55(1):54-70.   doi: 10.1080/03602559.2015.1050520

8. Hoffman AS. Hydrogels for biomedical applications. *Adv Drug Deliv Rev* 2002;54(1):3-12. doi: 10.1016/j.addr.2012.09.010

9. Prestwich GD, Marecak DM, Marecek JF, Vercruysse KP, Ziebell MR. Controlled chemical modification of hyaluronic acid: synthesis, applications, and biodegradation of hydrazide derivatives. *J Control Release* 1998;53(1-3):93-103. doi: 10.1016/S0168-3659(97)00242-3

10. Koetting MC, Peters JT, Steichen SD, Peppas NA. Stimulus-responsive hydrogels: Theory, modern advances, and applications. *Mater Sci Eng R Rep* 2015;93:1-49. doi: 10.1016/j.mser.2015.04.001

11. Hennink WE, van Nostrum CF. Novel crosslinking methods to design hydrogels. *Adv Drug Deliv Rev* 2002;54(1):13-36.   doi: 10.1016/S0169-409X(01)00240-X

12. Lee KY, Mooney DJ. Hydrogels for tissue engineering. *Chem Rev* 2001;101(7):1869-79. doi: 10.1021/cr000108x

13. Tessmar JK, Gopferich AM. Matrices and scaffolds for protein delivery in tissue engineering. *Adv Drug Deliv Rev* 2007;59(4-5):274-91.   doi: 10.1016/j.addr.2007.03.020

14. Peppas NA, Bures P, Leobandung W, Ichikawa H. Hydrogels in pharmaceutical formulations. *Eur J Pharm Biopharm* 2000;50(1):27-46.   doi: 10.1016/S0939-6411(00)00090-4

15. Hoffman AS. Hydrogels for biomedical applications. *Adv Drug Deliv Rev* 2012;64:18-23.   doi: 10.1016/j.addr.2012.09.010

16. Berger J, Reist M, Mayer JM, Felt O, Gurny R. Structure and interactions in chitosan hydrogels formed by complexation or aggregation for biomedical applications. *Eur J Pharm Biopharm* 2004;57(1):35-52.

17. Boucard N, Viton C, Domard A. New aspects of the formation of physical hydrogels of chitosan in a hydroalcoholic medium. *Biomacromolecules* 2005;6(6):3227-37. doi: 10.1021/bm050653d

18. Hoare TR, Kohane DS. Hydrogels in drug delivery: Progress and challenges. *Polymer* 2008;49(8):1993-2007. doi: 10.1016/j.polymer.2008.01.027

19. Escobar-Chavez JJ, Lopez-Cervantes M, Naik A, Kalia YN, Quintanar-Guerrero D, Ganem-Quintanar

A. Applications of thermo-reversible pluronic F-127 gels in pharmaceutical formulations. *J Pharm Pharm Sci* 2006;9(3):339-58.

20. Antunes FE, Gentile L, Rossi CO, Tavano L, Ranieri GA. Gels of Pluronic F127 and nonionic surfactants from rheological characterization to controlled drug permeation. *Colloids Surf B Biointerfaces* 2011;87(1):42-8. doi: 10.1016/j.colsurfb.2011.04.033

21. Van Hemelrijck C, Muller-Goymann CC. Rheological characterization and permeation behavior of poloxamer 407-based systems containing 5-aminolevulinic acid for potential application in photodynamic therapy. *Int J Pharm* 2012;437(1-2):120-9. doi: 10.1016/j.ijpharm.2012.07.048

22. Gilbert JC, Hadgraft J, Bye A, Brookes LG. Drug release from Pluronic F-127 gels. *Int J Pharm* 1986;32(2-3):223-8.   doi: 10.1016/0378-5173(86)90182-1

23. Erukova VY, Krylova OO, Antonenko YN, Melik-Nubarov NS. Effect of ethylene oxide and propylene oxide block copolymers on the permeability of bilayer lipid membranes to small solutes including doxorubicin. *Biochim Biophys Acta* 2000;1468(1-2):73-86. doi: 10.1016/S0005-2736(00)00244-3

24. El-Badry M, Fetih G, Fathalla D, Shakeel F. Transdermal delivery of meloxicam using niosomal hydrogels: in vitro and pharmacodynamic evaluation. *Pharm Dev Technol* 2015;20(7):820-6.   doi: 10.3109/10837450.2014.926919

25. Miyazaki S, Tobiyama T, Takada M, Attwood D. Percutaneous Absorption of Indomethacin from Pluronic F-127 Gels in Rats. *J Pharm Pharmacol* 1995;47:455-7.   doi: 10.1111/j.2042-7158.1995.tb05829.x

26. Miyazaki S, Takeuchi S, Yokouchi C, Takada M. Pluronic F-127 gels as a vehicle for Topical administration of Anticancer Agents. *Chem Pharm Bull* 1984;32(10):4205-8. doi: 10.1248/cpb.32.4205

27. Miyazaki S, Ohkawa Y, Takada M, Atwood D. Antitumor effect of PF-127 gel containing mytomicin C on sarcoma-180 ascites tumor in mice. *Chem Pharm Bull* 1986;34:2224-6.

28. El-Kattan AF, Asbill CS, Kim N, Michniak BB. Effect of formulation variables on the percutaneous permeation of ketoprofen from gel formulations. *Drug Deliv* 2000;7(3):147-53.   doi: 10.1080/10717540050120188

29. Chen PC, Kohane DS, Park YJ, Bartlett RH, Langer R, Yang VC. Injectable microparticle-gel system for prolonged and localized lidocaine release. II. In vivo anesthetic effects. *J Biomed Mater Res A* 2004;70(3):459-66. doi: 10.1002/jbm.a.30101

30. Inal O, Yapar EA. Effect of mechanical properties on the release of meloxicam from poloxamer gel bases. *Indian J Pharm Sci* 2013;75(6):700-6.

31. Jin WG, Shin SC. Preparation and evaluation of procaine gels for the enhanced local anesthetic action. *Arch Pharm Res* 2008;31(2):235-41.   doi: 10.1007/s12272-001-1147-9

32. Choi JS, Shin SC. Preparation and evaluation of pranoprofen gel for percutaneous administration. *Drug Dev Ind Pharm* 2007;33(1):19-26. doi: 10.1080/03639040600975071

33. Shin SC, Cho CW. Enhanced transdermal delivery of pranoprofen from the bioadhesive gels. *Arch Pharm Res* 2006;29(10):928-33. doi: 10.1007/bf02973916

34. Shin SC, Cho CW, Yang KH. Development of lidocaine gels for enhanced local anesthetic action. *Int J Pharm* 2004;287(1-2):73-8. doi: 10.1016/j.ijpharm.2004.08.012

35. Singh S, Parhi R, Garg A. Formulation of topical bioadhesive gel of aceclofenac using 3-level factorial design. *Iran J Pharm Res* 2011;10(3):435-45.

36. Parhi R. Development and optimization of pluronic® F127 and HPMC based thermosensitive gel for the skin delivery of metoprolol succinate. *J Drug Deliv Sci Technol* 2016;36:23-33. doi: 10.1016/j.jddst.2016.09.004

37. Singh S, Webster DC, Singh J. Thermosensitive polymers: synthesis, characterization, and delivery of proteins. *Int J Pharm* 2007;341(1-2):68-77. doi: 10.1016/j.ijpharm.2007.03.054

38. Lee WC, Li YC, Chu IM. Amphiphilic poly(D,L-lactic acid)/poly(ethylene glycol)/poly(D,L-lactic acid) nanogels for controlled release of hydrophobic drugs. *Macromol Biosci* 2006;6(10):846-54. doi: 10.1002/mabi.200600101

39. Qiao M, Chen D, Ma X, Liu Y. Injectable biodegradable temperature-responsive PLGA-PEG-PLGA copolymers: synthesis and effect of copolymer composition on the drug release from the copolymer-based hydrogels. *Int J Pharm* 2005;294(1-2):103-12. doi: 10.1016/j.ijpharm.2005.01.017

40. Li C, Tang Y, Armes SP, Morris CJ, Rose SF, Lloyd AW, *et al.* Synthesis and characterization of biocompatible thermo-responsive gelators based on ABA triblock copolymers. *Biomacromolecules* 2005;6(2):994-9. doi: 10.1021/bm049331k

41. Ha DI, Lee SB, Chong MS, Lee YM, Kim SY, Park YH. Preparation of thermo-responsive and injectable hydrogels based on hyaluronic acid and poly(N-isopropylacrylamide) and their drug release behaviors. *Macromol Res* 2006;14(1):87-93. doi: 10.1007/bf03219073

42. Bae JW, Go DH, Park KD, Lee SJ. Thermosensitive chitosan as an injectable carrier for local drug delivery. *Macromol Res* 2006;14(4):461-5. doi: 10.1007/bf03219111

43. Deng C, Tian H, Zhang P, Sun J, Chen X, Jing X. Synthesis and characterization of RGD peptide grafted poly(ethylene glycol)-b-poly(L-lactide)-b-poly(L-glutamic acid) triblock copolymer. *Biomacromolecules* 2006;7(2):590-6. doi: 10.1021/bm050678c

44. Molinaro G, Leroux JC, Damas J, Adam A. Biocompatibility of thermosensitive chitosan-based hydrogels: an in vivo experimental approach to injectable biomaterials. *Biomaterials* 2002;23(13):2717-22. doi: 10.1016/S0142-9612(02)00004-2

45. Bhattarai N, Ramay HR, Gunn J, Matsen FA, Zhang M. PEG-grafted chitosan as an injectable thermosensitive hydrogel for sustained protein release. *J Control Release* 2005;103(3):609-24. doi: 10.1016/j.jconrel.2004.12.019

46. Liang HF, Hong MH, Ho RM, Chung CK, Lin YH, Chen CH, et al. Novel method using a temperature-sensitive polymer (methylcellulose) to thermally gel aqueous alginate as a pH-sensitive hydrogel. *Biomacromolecules* 2004;5(5):1917-25. doi: 10.1021/bm049813w

47. Uraki Y, Imura T, Kishimoto T, Ubukata M. Body temperature-responsive gels derived from hydroxypropylcellulose bearing lignin. *Carbohydr Polym* 2004;58(2):123-30. doi: 10.1016/j.carbpol.2004.05.019

48. Buwalda SJ, Boere KW, Dijkstra PJ, Feijen J, Vermonden T, Hennink WE. Hydrogels in a historical perspective: From simple networks to smart materials. *J Control Release* 2014;190:254-73. doi: 10.1016/j.jconrel.2014.03.052

49. Wu J, Su ZG, Ma GH. A thermo- and pH-sensitive hydrogel composed of quaternized chitosan/glycerophosphate. *Int J Pharm* 2006;315(1-2):1-11. doi: 10.1016/j.ijpharm.2006.01.045

50. Van Tomme SR, Van Steenbergen MJ, De Smedt SC, Van Nostrum CF, Hennink WE. Self-gelling hydrogels based on oppositely charged dextran microspheres. *Biomaterials* 2005;26(14):2129-35. doi: 10.1016/j.biomaterials.2004.05.035

51. Chen P. Self-assembly of ionic-complementary peptides: a physicochemical viewpoint. *Colloids Surf Physicochem Eng Aspects* 2005;261(1-3):3-24. doi: 10.1016/j.colsurfa.2004.12.048

52. Bhattarai N, Gunn J, Zhang M. Chitosan-based hydrogels for controlled, localized drug delivery. *Adv Drug Deliv Rev* 2010;62(1):83-99. doi: 10.1016/j.addr.2009.07.019

53. Saleem MA, Kulkarni R, Patil Noornadim G. Formulation and evaluation of chitosan based polyelectrolyte complex hydrogels for extended release of metoprolol tartrate. *Res J Pharm Technol* 2011;4(12):1844-51.

54. Derkach SR, Voronko NG, Sokolan NI. The rheology of hydrogels based on chitosan-gelatin (bio)polyelectrolyte complexes. *J Dispersion Sci Technol* 2017;38(10):1427-34. doi: 10.1080/01932691.2016.1250218

55. Chang HH, Wang YL, Chiang YC, Chen YL, Chuang YH, Tsai SJ, et al. A novel chitosan-γpga polyelectrolyte complex hydrogel promotes early new bone formation in the alveolar socket following tooth extraction. *PLoS One* 2014;9(3):e92362. doi: 10.1371/journal.pone.0092362

56. Kang HS, Park SH, Lee YG, Son TI. Polyelectrolyte complex hydrogel composed of chitosan and poly(γ-glutamic acid) for biological application: preparation,

physical properties, and cytocompatibility. *J Appl Polym Sci* 2007;103(1):386-94. doi: 10.1002/app.24623

57. Kulig D, Zimoch-Korzycka A, Jarmoluk A, Marycz K. Study on alginate-chitosan complex formed with different polymers ratio. *Polymers* 2016;8(5):167. doi: 10.3390/polym8050167

58. Li QL, Chen ZQ, Darvell BW, Liu LK, Jiang HB, Zen Q, et al. Chitosan-phosphorylated chitosan polyelectrolyte complex hydrogel as an osteoblast carrier. *J Biomed Mater Res B Appl Biomater* 2007;82(2):481-6. doi: 10.1002/jbm.b.30753

59. Zaino C, Zambito Y, Mollica G, Geppi M, Serafini MF, Carelli V, et al. A novel polyelectrolyte complex (PEC) hydrogel for controlled drug delivery to the distal intestine. *Open Drug Deliv J* 2007;1:68-75. doi: 10.2174/1874126600701010068

60. You J, Xie S, Cao J, Ge H, Xu M, Zhang L, et al. Quaternized chitosan/poly(acrylic acid) polyelectrolyte complex hydrogels with tough, self-recovery, and tunable mechanical properties. *Macromolecules* 2016;49(3):1049-59. doi: 10.1021/acs.macromol.5b02231

61. Yao KD, Tu H, Cheng F, Zhang JW, Liu J. pH-sensitivity of the swelling of a chitosan-pectin polyelectrolyte complex. *Angew Makromol Chem* 1997;245(1):63-72. doi: 10.1002/apmc.1997.052450106

62. Ricciardi R, Gaillet C, Ducouret G, Lafuma F, Laupretre F. Investigation of the relationships between the chain organization and rheological properties of atactic poly(vinyl alcohol) hydrogels. *Polymer* 2003;44(11):3375-80. doi: 10.1016/S0032-3861(03)00246-5

63. McGuinness GB, Vrana NE, Liu Y. Polyvinyl alcohol-based cryogels: tissue engineering and regenerative medicine. In: Mishra M, editor. *Encyclopedia of Biomedical Polymers and Polymeric Biomaterials*. CRC Press; 2015. PP. 6743-6753.

64. Pazos V, Mongrain R, Tardif JC. Polyvinyl alcohol cryogel: Optimizing the parameters of cryogenic treatment using hyperelastic models. *J Mech Behav Biomed Mater* 2009;2(5):542-9. doi: 10.1016/j.jmbbm.2009.01.003

65. Meenakshi, Ahuja M. Metronidazole loaded carboxymethyl tamarind kernel polysaccharide-polyvinyl alcohol cryogels: Preparation and characterization. *Int J Biol Macromol* 2015;72:931-8. doi: 10.1016/j.ijbiomac.2014.09.040

66. Sung JH, Hwang MR, Kim JO, Lee JH, Kim YI, Kim JH, et al. Gel characterisation and in vivo evaluation of minocycline-loaded wound dressing with enhanced wound healing using polyvinyl alcohol and chitosan. *Int J Pharm* 2010;392(1-2):232-40. doi: 10.1016/j.ijpharm.2010.03.024

67. Hwang MR, Kim JO, Lee JH, Kim YI, Kim JH, Chang SW, et al. Gentamicin-loaded wound dressing with polyvinyl alcohol/dextran hydrogel: Gel characterization and in vivo healing evaluation. *AAPS PharmSciTech* 2010;11(3):1092-103. doi: 10.1208/s12249-010-9474-0

68. Paduraru OM, Ciolacu D, Darie RN, Vasile C. Synthesis and characterization of polyvinyl alcohol/cellulose cryogels and their testing as carriers for a bioactive component. *Mater Sci Eng C* 2012;32(8):2508-15. doi: 10.1016/j.msec.2012.07.033

69. Lapasin R, Pricl S. Rheology of industrial polysaccharides: theory and application. Cornwall, UK: Blackie Academic and Professional; 1995.

70. Tsuji H. Poly(lactide) Stereocomplexes: Formation, Structure, Properties, Degradation, and Applications. *Macromol Biosci* 2005;5(7):569-97. doi: 10.1002/mabi.200500062

71. Fox TG, Garrett BS, Goode WE, Gratch S, Kincaid JF, Spell A, et al. Crystalline polymers of methyl methacrylate. *J Am Chem Soc* 1958;80(7):1768-9. doi: 10.1021/ja01540a068

72. Slager J, Glandnikoff M, Domb AJ. Stereocomplexes, based on biodegradable polymers and bioactive macromolecules. *Macromol Symp* 2001;175(1):105-15.

73. Bos GW, Jacobs JJ, Koten JW, Van Tomme S, Veldhuis T, van Nostrum CF, *et al.* In situ crosslinked biodegradable hydrogels loaded with IL-2 are effective tools for local IL-2 therapy. *Eur J Pharm Sci* 2004;21(4):561-7. doi: 10.1016/j.ejps.2003.12.007

74. Oshovsky GV, Reinhoudt DN, Verboom W. Supramolecular Chemistry in Water. *Angew Chem Int Ed Engl* 2007;46(14):2366-93. doi: 10.1002/anie.200602815

75. Huh KM, Ooya T, Lee WK, Sasaki S, Kwon IC, Jeong SY, *et al.* Supramolecular-structured hydrogels showing a reversible phase transition by inclusion complexation between poly(ethylene glycol) grafted dextran and α-cyclodextrin. *Macromolecules* 2001;34(25):8657-62. doi: 10.1021/ma0106649

76. Choi HS, Kontani K, Huh KM, Sasaki S, Ooya T, Lee WK, et al. Rapid induction of thermoreversible hydrogel formation based on poly(propylene glycol)-grafted dextran inclusion complexes. *Macromol Biosci* 2002;2(6):298-303.

77. Li J, Li X, Ni X, Wang X, Li H, Leong KW. Self-assembled supramolecular hydrogels formed by biodegradable PEO-PHB-PEO triblock copolymers and alpha-cyclodextrin for controlled drug delivery. *Biomaterials* 2006;27(22):4132-40. doi: 10.1016/j.biomaterials.2006.03.025

78. Berger J, Reist M, Mayer JM, Felt O, Peppas NA, Gurny R. Structure and interactions in covalently and ionically crosslinked chitosan hydrogels for biomedical applications. *Eur J Pharm Biopharm* 2004;57(1):19-34. doi: 10.1016/S0939-6411(03)00161-9

79. Nishi KK, Jayakrishnan A. Self-gelling primaquine-gum arabic conjugate: an injectable controlled

delivery system for primaquine. *Biomacromolecules* 2007;8(1):84-90. doi: 10.1021/bm060612x

80. Shim WS, Kim JH, Kim K, Kim YS, Park RW, Kim IS, et al. pH- and temperature-sensitive, injectable, biodegradable block copolymer hydrogels as carriers for paclitaxel. *Int J Pharm* 2007;331(1):11-8. doi: 10.1016/j.ijpharm.2006.09.027

81. Jin R, Hiemstra C, Zhong Z, Feijen J. Enzyme-mediated fast in situ formation of hydrogels from dextran-tyramine conjugates. *Biomaterials* 2007;28(18):2791-800. doi: 10.1016/j.biomaterials.2007.02.032

82. Kurisawa M, Chung JE, Yang YY, Gao SJ, Uyama H. Injectable biodegradable hydrogels composed of hyaluronic acid-tyramine conjugates for drug delivery and tissue engineering. *Chem Commun* 2005;(34):4312-4. doi: 10.1039/b506989k

83. Jin J, Song M, Hourston DJ. Novel chitosan-based films cross-linked by genipin with improved physical properties. *Biomacromolecules* 2004;5(1):162-8. doi: 10.1021/bm034286m

84. Sung HW, Liang IL, Chen CN, Huang RN, Liang HF. Stability of a biological tissue fixed with a naturally occurring crosslinking agent (genipin). *J Biomed Mater Res* 2001;55(4):538-46.

85. Chen SC, Wu YC, Mi FL, Lin YH, Yu LC, Sung HW. A novel pH-sensitive hydrogel composed of N,O-carboxymethyl chitosan and alginate cross-linked by genipin for protein drug delivery. *J Control Release* 2004;96(2):285-300. doi: 10.1016/j.jconrel.2004.02.002

86. Butler MF, Ng YF, Pudney PDA. Mechanism and kinetics of the crosslinking reaction between biopolymers containing primary amine groups and genipin. *J Polym Sci A Polym Chem* 2003;41(24):3941-53. doi: 10.1002/pola.10960

87. Bolgul Y, Hekimoglu S, Sahinerdemli I, Kas HS. Evaluation of oxprenolol hydrochloride permeation through isolated human skin and pharmacodynamic effect in rats. *STP Pharm Sci* 1998;8(3):197-201.

88. Thacharodi D, Rao KP. Development and in vitro evaluation of chitosan-based transdermal drug delivery systems for the controlled delivery of propranolol hydrochloride. *Biomaterials* 1995;16(2):145-8. doi: 10.1016/0142-9612(95)98278-M

89. Denkbas EB, Seyyal M, Piskin E. Implantable 5-fluorouracil loaded chitosan scaffolds prepared by wet spinning. *J Memb Sci* 2000;172(1-2):33-8. doi: 10.1016/S0376-7388(00)00314-8

90. Mi FL, Sung HW, Shyu SS. Drug release from chitosan-alginate complex beads reinforced by a naturally occurring cross-linking agent. *Carbohydr Polym* 2002;48(1):61-72. doi: 10.1016/S0144-8617(01)00212-0

91. Hiemstra C, van der Aa LJ, Zhong ZY, Dijkstra PJ, Feijen J. Novel in situ forming, degradable dextran hydrogels by michael addition chemistry: Synthesis, rheology, and degradation. *Macromolecules* 2007;40(4):1165-73. doi: 10.1021/ma062468d

92. Bulpitt P, Aeschlimann D. New strategy for chemical modification of hyaluronic acid: preparation of functionalized derivatives and their use in the formation of novel biocompatible hydrogels. *J Biomed Mater Res* 1999;47(2):152-69.

93. Ito T, Yeo Y, Highley CB, Bellas E, Benitez CA, Kohane DS. The prevention of peritoneal adhesions by in situ cross-linking hydrogels of hyaluronic acid and cellulose derivatives. *Biomaterials* 2007;28(6):975-83. doi: 10.1016/j.biomaterials.2006.10.021

94. Lee KY, Alsberg E, Mooney DJ. Degradable and injectable poly(aldehyde guluronate) hydrogels for bone tissue engineering. *J Biomed Mater Res* 2001;56(2):228-33.

95. Ono K, Saito Y, Yura H, Ishikawa K, Kurita A, Akaike T, et al. Photocrosslinkable chitosan as a biological adhesive. *J Biomed Mater Res* 2000;49(2):289-95.

96. Yoo HS. Photo-cross-linkable and thermo-responsive hydrogels containing chitosan and pluronic for sustained release of human growth hormone (hGH). *J Biomater Sci Polym Ed* 2007;18(11):1429-41. doi: 10.1163/156856207782246803

97. Lee JI, Kim HS, Yoo HS. DNA nanogels composed of chitosan and Pluronic with thermo-sensitive and photo-crosslinking properties. *Int J Pharm* 2009;373(1-2):93-9. doi: 10.1016/j.ijpharm.2009.01.016

98. Yeo Y, Geng W, Ito T, Kohane DS, Burdick JA, Radisic M. Photocrosslinkable hydrogel for myocyte cell culture and injection. *J Biomed Mater Res B Appl Biomater* 2007;81(2):312-22. doi: 10.1002/jbm.b.30667

99. Lukaszczyk J, Smiga M, Jaszcz K, Adler HJ, Jahne E, Kaczmarek M. Evaluation of oligo(ethylene glycol) dimethacrylates effects on the properties of new biodegradable bone cement compositions. *Macromol Biosci* 2005;5(1):64-9. doi: 10.1002/mabi.200400135

100. Yung CW, Wu LQ, Tullman JA, Payne GF, Bentley WE, Barbari TA. Transglutaminase crosslinked gelatin as a tissue engineering scaffold. *J Biomed Mater Res A* 2007;83(4):1039-46. doi: 10.1002/jbm.a.31431

101. Yung CW, Bentley WE, Barbari TA. Diffusion of interleukin-2 from cells overlaid with cytocompatible enzyme-crosslinked gelatin hydrogels. *J Biomed Mater Res A* 2010;95(1):25-32. doi: 10.1002/jbm.a.32740

102. Davis NE, Ding S, Forster RE, Pinkas DM, Barron AE. Modular enzymatically crosslinked protein polymer hydrogels for in situ gelation. *Biomaterials* 2010;31(28):7288-97. doi: 10.1016/j.biomaterials.2010.06.003

103. Kim KS, Park SJ, Yang JA, Jeon JH, Bhang SH, Kim BS, et al. Injectable hyaluronic acid-tyramine hydrogels for the treatment of rheumatoid arthritis.

Acta   Biomater   2011;7(2):666-74.   doi: 10.1016/j.actbio.2010.09.030

104. Jin R, Moreira Teixeira LS, Dijkstra PJ, Karperien M, van Blitterswijk CA, Zhong ZY, et al. Injectable chitosan-based hydrogels for cartilage tissue engineering. *Biomaterials* 2009;30(13):2544-51. doi: 10.1016/j.biomaterials.2009.01.020

105. Chen T, Embree HD, Brown EM, Taylor MM, Payne GF. Enzyme-catalyzed gel formation of gelatin and chitosan: potential for in situ applications. *Biomaterials* 2003;24(17):2831-41. doi: 10.1016/S0142-9612(03)00096-6

106. Teixeira LS, Feijen J, van Blitterswijk CA, Dijkstra PJ, Karperien M. Enzyme-catalyzed crosslinkable hydrogels: Emerging strategies for tissue engineering. *Biomaterials* 2012;33(5):1281-90. doi: 10.1016/j.biomaterials.2011.10.067

107. Chen T, Embree HD, Wu LQ, Payne GF. In vitro protein-polysaccharide conjugation: tyrosinase-catalyzed conjugation of gelatin and chitosan. *Biopolymers* 2002;64(6):292-302. doi: 10.1002/bip.10196

108. Singh P, Kumar SK, Keerthi TS, Mani TT, Getyala A. Interpenetrating polymer network (IPN) microparticles and advancement in novel drug delivery system: a review. *Pharm Sci Monitor* 2012;3(1):1826-37.

109. Rokhade AP, Patil SA, Aminabhavi TM. Synthesis and characterization of semi-interpenetrating polymer network microspheres of acrylamide grafted dextran and chitosan for controlled release of acyclovir. *Carbohydr Polym* 2007;67(4):605-13. doi: 10.1016/j.carbpol.2006.07.001

110. Myung D, Waters D, Wiseman M, Duhamel PE, Noolandi J, Ta CN, et al. Progress in the development of interpenetrating polymer network hydrogels. *Polym Adv Technol* 2008;19(6):647-57. doi: 10.1002/pat.1134

111. Margaret MT, Brahmaiah B, Krishna PV, Revathi B, Nama S. Interpenetrating polymer network (IPN) microparticles an advancement in novel drug delivery system: a review. *Int J Pharm Res Bio Sci* 2013;2(3):215-24.

112. Kudela V. Hydrogels. In: Kroschwitz JI, editor. *Encyclopedia of polymer science and engineering.* New York: Wiley; 1987. PP. 783-807.

113. Qadri MF, Malviya R, Sharma PK. Biomedical applications of interpenetrating polymer network system. *Open Pharm Sci J* 2015;2:21-30. doi: 10.2174/1874844901502010021

114. Dragan ES. Design and applications of interpenetrating polymer network hydrogels. A review. *Chem Eng J* 2014;243:572-90. doi: 10.1016/j.cej.2014.01.065

115. Kumar GA, Wadood SA, Datta MS, Ramchand D. Interpenetrating polymeric network hydrogel for stomach-specific drug delivery of clarithromycin: Preparation and evaluation. *Asian J Pharm* 2010;4(4):179-84. doi: 10.4103/0973-8398.76738

116. Vaghani SS, Patel MM. pH-sensitive hydrogels based on semi-interpenetrating network (semi-IPN) of chitosan and polyvinyl pyrrolidone for clarithromycin release. *Drug Dev Ind Pharm* 2011;37(10):1160-9. doi: 10.3109/03639045.2011.563422

117. Kulkarni RV, Sreedhar V, Mutalik S, Setty CM, Sa B. Interpenetrating network hydrogel membranes of sodium alginate and poly(vinyl alcohol) for controlled release of prazosin hydrochloride through skin. *Int J Biol Macromol* 2010;47(4):520-7. doi: 10.1016/j.ijbiomac.2010.07.009

118. Rokhade AP, Shelke NB, Patil SA, Aminabhavi TM. Novel interpenetrating polymer network microspheres of chitosan and methylcellulose for controlled release of theophylline. *Carbohydr Polym* 2007;69(4):678-87. doi: 10.1016/j.carbpol.2007.02.008

119. Chung TW, Lin SY, Liu DZ, Tyan YC, Yang JS. Sustained release of 5-FU from Poloxamer gels interpenetrated by crosslinking chitosan network. *Int J Pharm* 2009;382(1-2):39-44. doi: 10.1016/j.ijpharm.2009.07.035

120. Zhang Y, Liu J, Huang L, Wang Z, Wang L. Design and performance of a sericin-alginate interpenetrating network hydrogel for cell and drug delivery. *Sci Rep* 2015;5:12374. doi: 10.1038/srep12374

121. Ahmed EM. Hydrogel: Preparation, characterization, and applications: A review. *J Adv Res* 2015;6(2):105-21. doi: 10.1016/j.jare.2013.07.006

122. Naficy S, Kawakami S, Sadegholvaad S, Wakisaka M, Spinks GM. Mechanical properties of interpenetrating polymer network hydrogels based on hybrid ionically and covalently crosslinked networks. *J Appl Polym Sci* 2013;130(4):2504-13. doi: 10.1002/app.39417

123. Mahmood A, Ahmad M, Sarfraz RM, Minhas MU. β-CD based hydrogel microparticulate system to improve the solubility of acyclovir: Optimization through in-vitro, in-vivo and toxicological evaluation. *J Drug Deliv Sci Technol* 2016;36:75-88. doi: 10.1016/j.jddst.2016.09.005

124. Mahmood A, Ahmad M, Sarfraz RM, Minhas MU. Development of Acyclovir Loaded β-Cyclodextring-Poly Methacrylic Acid Hydrogel Microparticles: An In Vitro Characterization. *Adv Polym Technol* 2016:21711. doi: 10.1002/adv.21711

8

Formulation of Menthol-Loaded Nanostructured Lipid Carriers to Enhance Its Antimicrobial Activity for Food Preservation

Parizad Piran[1], Hossein Samadi Kafil[2,3], Saeed Ghanbarzadeh[4], Rezvan Safdari[3], Hamed Hamishehkar[3]*

[1] Biotechnology Research Center, Tabriz University of Medical Sciences, Tabriz, Iran.

[2] Infectious and Tropical Diseases Research Center, Tabriz University of Medical Sciences, Tabriz, Iran.

[3] Drug Applied Research Center, Tabriz University of Medical Sciences, Tabriz, Iran.

[4] Zanjan Pharmaceutical Nanotechnology Research Center, and Department of Pharmaceutics, Faculty of Pharmacy, Zanjan University of Medical Sciences, Zanjan, Iran.

Keywords:
· Menthol
· Nanostructure lipid carriers
· NLC
· Antimicrobial activity
· Food preservative

Abstract

Purpose: Due to the antimicrobial property, menthol have significant potential for food preservation and foodstuff shelf life improvement. Nevertheless, menthol instability, insolubility, and rapid crystallization in aqueous media make it unsuitable for used in food products. This work was aimed to prepare menthol-loaded nanostructured lipid carriers (NLCs) to enhance its antimicrobial activity.

Methods: Morphology, particle size and size distribution, encapsulation efficiency percent (EE%), and physical stability of the optimized formulation, prepared by hot melt homogenization method, were characterized by scanning electron microscopy, particle size analyzing, gas chromatography, and X-ray diffraction (XRD) methods. Minimum inhibitory concentration and minimum bactericidal concentration of menthol-loaded NLCs were evaluated and compared with conventional menthol emulsion against various Gram-positive (*Staphylococcus aureus*, *Bacillus cereus*) and Gram-negative bacteria (*Escherichia coli*), as well as one fungus (*Candida albicans*).

Results: Menthol-loaded NLCs were spherically shaped nanosized (115.6 nm) particles with narrow size distribution (PDI = 0.2), suitable menthol EE% (98.73%), and appropriate physical stability after 90 days of storage period. XRD results indicated that menthol was in the amorphous form in the nanoparticles matrix. Antibacterial assay results revealed that the menthol-loaded NLCs exhibited significantly higher *in vitro* antimicrobial property than conventional menthol emulsion. The results also indicated that menthol-loaded NLCs had better effect on fungi than bacteria, and furthermore, antibacterial efficiency on Gram-positive bacteria was higher than Gram-negative bacteria.

Conclusion: In conclusion, NLCs could be a promising carrier for improvement of antimicrobial activity and preservation efficacy of essential oils in foodstuffs.

Introduction

Increased concern of consumers on the various side effects of synthetic preservatives and development of antibiotic resistant strains have attracted great attention to the use of natural compounds with antimicrobial activity in food and pharmaceutical industries.[1] Essential oils are volatile, natural, aromatic oily liquids that can be obtained from several parts of the plants such as leaves and flowers. Due to the aromatic property of essential oils, they have been widely used in cosmetic industries for the production of soaps, perfumes, and toiletries.[2] The large bioactivity of essential oils has been confirmed by several studies, including antibacterial, antiviral, anti-inflammatory, antifungal, antimutagenic, anticarcinogenic, and antioxidant activities. This group of oils may provide the natural antimicrobials that food industry requires leading to reduced need for synthetic preservative excipients.[3,4] The main constituents of essential oils have unsaturated carbon chains, which is well-known that are susceptibility to oxidation mediated by light or heat. The high volatility of essential oils also limits their free use without a vehicle. Furthermore, the low aqueous solubility limits the possible application of essential oils in aqueous based foodstuffs such as beverages. All of these factors limit the application of essential oils as candidates for preserving food solutions.[5] Menthol is a monocyclic monoterpene alcohol naturally obtained from peppermint or other mint oils. It is widely used as a flavoring agent for toothpaste, hygiene products, chewing gum, etc. Menthol is generally available in the form of crystals or granules with a melting point at 41-43 °C. Although, previous researches have shown that menthol has antibacterial and antifungal activity, its high volatility, instability, insolubility, and rapid crystallization in aqueous mediums are the crucial problems concerning its applications and shelf life.[6] The

---

*Corresponding author: Hamed Hamishehkar, Email: hamishehkarh@tbzmed.ac.ir

microencapsulation method is an appropriate technique to solve above mentioned problems. In this perspective, encapsulation procedures provide an effective protection of naturally compounds against chemical reactions and undesirable interactions with other components in food. Furthermore, it improves solubility, diminish migration, and preserve the bioactive compounds stability during food processing and storage.[7] In food engineering, protection of bioactive compounds such as vitamins, antioxidants, proteins, and lipids could be achieved using nano encapsulation technique to produce functional foods with enhanced functionality and stability.[8] As lipid based nanoparticles are composed by lipids, they have the ability of interaction with several bacterial and fungal cell types.[9,10] Therefore, in the present study menthol-loaded nanostructured lipid carriers (NLCs) were prepared to improve the solubility, stability, and antimicrobial efficacy of menthol for potential application as preservative in food industry.

Materials and Methods
Materials
Menthol, Tween® 80, Mueller Hinton Agar, Mueller Hinton Broth and Nutrient dextrose agar were supplied from Merck Chemicals Co. (Germany). Poloxamer® 407 was obtained from Sigma-Aldrich Company (USA). Glyceryl Palmtostearate (Precirol ATO-5®) was kindly donated from Gattefossé Company (France). Miglyol® 812 was prepared from Sasol Company (Germany). All other used chemicals and reagents were of analytical grade.

Preparation of menthol-loaded NLCs and emulsion
Menthol-loaded NLCs were prepared by hot melt homogenization method as described previously.[11] Briefly, 200 mg menthol was dissolved in 200 mg Miglyol® and added to 1.8 g melted Precirol® at about 70 °C. Subsequently, Poloxamer® (1.5 g) was dissolved in water and added drop-wise into the oil phase under stirring at 20000 rpm by a homogenizer (DIAX 900, Heidolph, Germany). Finally, after 15 min, keeping the temperature at 70 °C and the same stirring rate allowed the hot formulation to cool down at room temperature. NLC structures are usually composed of solid lipid (e.g. Precirol®) and liquid lipid (e.g. Miglyol®). To have an equivalent comparison between NLC and emulsion in their antimicrobial activity evaluation, a similar liquid lipid was chosen for the preparation of NLC and emulsion. Emulsion was also prepared by gradual water addition into the mixture of menthol (200 mg), Miglyol® (2 g), and Tween® 80 (200 mg) under stirring with homogenizer (5000 rpm). Each formulation was prepared and characterized in triplicate.

Characterization of menthol-loaded NLCs
Particle size distribution of prepared NLCs was analyzed using dynamic light scattering system (DLS) and reported as intensity-weighted average (z average) and polydispersity index (PDI). Zeta potential of prepared nanoparticles was also analyzed by the same system

(Nano ZS, Malvern, UK). The morphology of prepared nanoparticles was obtained using scanning electron microscope (SEM) (LEO 1430VP, UK & Germany) operating at 15 kV. The specimens were mounted on a metal stub with double-sided adhesive tape and coated under vacuum with gold (100-150 A°) in an argon atmosphere prior to observation using a direct current sputtering technique (DST3, Nanostructured Coating Co., Tehran, Iran. In order to assess the effect of nanoparticles' preparation process on crystallographic patterns of menthol and lipids, XRD analysis was performed using an X-ray diffractometer (D-5000, Siemen, Germany, 2° to 40°) at a scan rate of 0.05 °/s to assess the crystalline structures of menthol, Precirol®, and Poloxamer® and optimized NLCs formulation.

Determination of encapsulation efficiency (EE%) and loading capacity (LC%)
The EE% and LE% values were expressed as the percentage of encapsulated menthol to the added menthol or to the used lipid, respectively. EE% was determined by the first separation of the un-entrapped menthol by centrifugation method using Amicon® Ultra-15 with MWCO of 100 kDa (Millipore, Germany) tube. The formulation was added to the upper chamber of the Amicon® tube, and then the tube was centrifuged (Sigma 3K30, Germany) at 5000 rpm for 5 minutes. The clear solution in the bottom of Amicon® tube was used for the determination of unloaded menthol. The EE% and LC% of menthol-loaded NLCs formulations were calculated according to the following equations:

$$EE(\%) = \frac{W_{(Initial\ Menthol)} - W_{(Free\ Menthol)}}{W_{(Initial\ Menthol)}} \times 100 \qquad (1)$$

$$LC(\%) = \frac{W_{(Entrapped\ Menthol)}}{W_{(Total\ lipid)}} \times 100 \qquad (2)$$

where, in equation (1), $W_{(Initial\ Menthol)}$ is the amount of initial menthol used, and $W_{(Free\ Menthol)}$ is the amount of free menthol detected in the lower chamber of Amicon® tube after centrifugation of the NLCs formulation (extracted by ether in triplicate). Accordingly, in equation (2), $W_{(Entrapped\ Menthol)}$ is the amount of loaded menthol, and $W_{(Total\ lipid)}$ is the amount of used lipid in the preparation process. The rinsed formulation was used for the further experiments.

Physical stability
Samples (15 mL) of each formulation were stored in plastic tubes in the dark place at room temperature (25 ± 1 °C), and the physical stability of the menthol-loaded NLCs was evaluated in terms of the mean particle size of NLCs after 90 days.

Gas chromatography
The concentration of menthol was determined using gas chromatography method (Fisons 8160, Milan, Italy, equipped with a flame ionization detector). The DB5 capillary column (30 m in length, 0.25 mm diameter, and 0.25 μm film thickness) was used to separate and

quantify the sample compounds. The carrier gas (Helium 99.999%) flow rate was 2.0 mL/min. The temperatures were as follows: injector = 250 °C, detector = 250 °C, column = 50-250 °C (4 °C/min) and injected volume = 1 μL. Data were collected and processed by a computer equipped with Chromcard software (Fisons, Milan, Italy). The reference standard of the menthol was accurately weighed and dissolved in diethyl ether to produce the stock standard solution and was subsequently diluted to a series of appropriate concentration for construction of calibration curves and determination of the limit of quantification (LOQ). The internal standard solution was added in each concentration solution. Calibration curves were constructed with six different concentrations by plotting the peak area ration of analyte to internal standard versus analyte concentration. Calibration curves showed good linearity (0.9966) over a relatively wide concentration range 3.0-7.5 mg/100 mL, and LOQ was calculated as 0.134 mg/mL.

Microbial strains
The antimicrobial activity of the menthol essential oil formulations was tested against four food-related microorganisms including one Gram-negative bacterium (*Escherichia coli* ATCC 25922), two Gram-positive bacteria (*Staphylococcus aureus* ATCC 25923 and *Bacillus cereus* ATCC 11778), and fungi (*Candida albicans* ATCC 10231). All the microorganisms were provided by the microbiological laboratory, Drug Applied Research Center, Tabriz University of Medical Science, Tabriz, Iran. After activating, the cultures of bacteria were maintained in their appropriate agar media at 4 °C and used as stock cultures. A single colony from the stock plate was transferred into Mueller Hinton Broth and incubated over night at 37 °C. After incubation, the cells were harvested by centrifugation at 3000 rpm for 15 min, washed twice, and re-suspended in saline solution to provide an optical density equal to 0.5 McFarland standard turbidity (equivalent to 10^7 colony forming units (CFU) /mL of bacterial and 10^8 CFU/mL of fungi).

Determination of minimum inhibitory concentration (MIC) and minimum bactericidal concentration (MBC) of menthol
The MIC values were assessed using the broth microdilution method by sterile 96-well microtitre plates.[12] Bacterial strains were cultured overnight at 37 °C in Muller Hinton Broth. Two fold serial dilutions of the menthol-loaded NLCs with medium were prepared in concentration of 4000 to 7.81 μg/mL for assessment of MIC for *E. coli*, *S. aureus*, and *B. Cereus*. 180 μL of prepared diluted solutions was transferred into 96-well microtitre plates, and then 20 μl of standardized microorganism suspensions was added and incubated at 37 °C for 24 h. After incubation time, turbidity of tubes was evaluated to determine bacterial growth, and last dilution with no turbidity (lack of growth) was considered as MIC. There were different control groups:

a) media, b) media + menthol free NLC and emulsion, c) media + menthol-loaded NLC and emulsion (without addition of bacteria), d) media + menthol free NLC and emulsion with addition of bacteria, and e) media + bacteria. Turbidity of wells was measured spectrophotometrically (Ultrospec 2000, Pharmacia Biotech, UK) at the wave length of 620 nm. Subsequently, to determine the MBC, samples (5 μL) from tubes in which no growth was observed were cultured in plate (containing Mueller Hinton agar medium) and incubated for 24 h at 37 °C. To determine the MIC value for *C. albicans*, 16 dilution series from 2496 to 4.87 μg/mL of menthol were prepared, and 50 μL of fungi suspension was added and incubated at 37 °C for 24 h, and the MIC value was determined as the lowest concentration of essential oil inhibiting visible growth of fungi on the agar plate when there was visible growth on the control plates.[13] Each experiment was performed in triplicate. All procedures were performed under sterile conditions. In each test, microorganism strain in Muller Hinton broth (with blank NLCs or emulsion) and Muller Hinton Broth alone were used as positive and negative growth controls, respectively.

Statistical analysis
All experiments were repeated in triplicate, and the data were expressed as a mean value ± standard deviation (SD). Statistical analysis was performed using one-way analysis of variance (ANOVA) with multiple comparisons between deposition data using a Tukey honest significant difference (HSD) test using SPSS software (version 13.0, Chicago, IL, USA). A P-value <0.05 was considered statistically significant.

Results and Discussion
Preparation, characterization and stability of menthol formulations
Particle size and size distribution are the key parameters of colloidal systems and have significant effects on the final nanoparticles' behavior including dissolution, bioavailability, content uniformity, and stability. Dynamic light scattering (DLS) is widely used to determine the size and size distribution of small particles suspended in liquid medium.[14] A PDI value of 0.1 to 0.25 indicates a narrow size distribution whereas a PDI value greater than 0.5 indicates a broad distribution.[15] Particle size and PDI value of prepared emulsions were 1489 nm and 0.556, respectively. The particle size and size distribution of prepared menthol-loaded NLCs were analyzed, and the size distribution profile of optimal formulation is represented in Figure 1a. The particle size and PDI were in the ranges of 115.6–155.8 nm and 0.243–0.445, respectively. The low PDI value indicates the narrow size distribution of prepared NLCs formulation.[14] Optimum formulation had z-average value of 115.6 nm and PDI value of 0.243. Lower particle size of nanoparticles resulted in higher clearness of the prepared nano suspension considered as a critical advantage for the drinking stuffs such as beverages. On

the other hand, one of the strategies to address stability issues is the particle size; lower particles reduce the sedimentation rate, and therefore, the particles can stay suspended longer in nano suspension formulations. Furthermore, a narrow particle size distribution can minimize the saturation solubility difference and drug concentration gradients within the medium and thus inhibit the occurrence of Ostwald ripening.[16] SEM images of nanoparticles showed spherical particles which verified the size analysis data of NLCs (Figure 1b). Particle size of menthol-loaded NLCs was found to be affected by the type of surfactant, lipid to surfactant ratio, solid lipid to liquid lipid ratio, and formulation parameters such as temperature and homogenizer speed (data are not shown). Using nanoparticles, the particle size remained as the most important parameter, as many of the chemical and physical properties, such as surface-to-volume ratio inversely proportional to the diameter of the nanoparticles, are strongly dependent on the

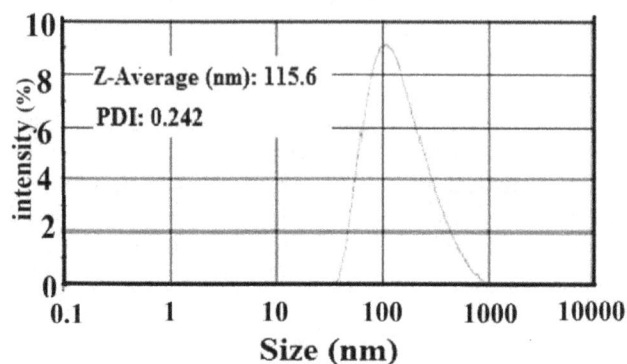

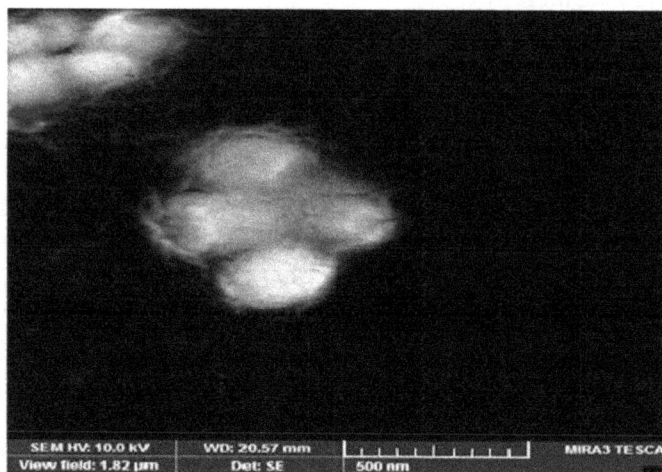

nanoparticle diameter. Smaller nanoparticles resulted in larger surface area, and therefore, more loading sites were available for applications.[17,18] Proper concentration of surfactants is also of great impact on the quality of NLCs dispersions. High concentration of emulsifier reduces the surface tension and facilitates the particle partition during homogenization process. In this study, menthol-loaded NLC resulted in the particle size of 136.8 ± 19.1 nm and PDI of 0.23. The PDI value less than 0.3 is considered uniform and narrow size distribution which guarantees reproducible drug delivery.[15] The results also indicated that particle size and size distribution of produced nanoparticles were relatively stable during 90 days of storage period (141.8 ± 21.4 and 0.35, respectively), which is a critical advantage for a nanoparticular formulation and guarantees the stability of nanoparticles in distribution mediums such as drinking stuffs.

Figure 1. Particle size distribution profile and scanning electron microscopy (SEM) image of optimum nanostructured lipid carriers (NLCs) formulation.

EE% of optimized NLCs formulation was found 98.73% $\pm$ 0.5 with LC% of 9.8% $\pm$ 0.05. High EE% was predictable due to the high lipophilicity of menthol and high concentration of Poloxamer® as surfactant in the NLCs formulation. Furthermore, polymorphic and crystallization form of Precirol® in NLCs formulation is another reason for higher EE% value of NLCs.[19] EE and LC percentage values for emulsion system were achieved 91.4% and 9.1 %, respectively. Representative chromatograms of menthol standard solution and menthol-loaded NLCs formulation after injection into GC column are shown in Figure 2. The peak of menthol was appeared at 10.39 min.

XRD analysis

The physical state of the nanoparticles was analyzed by X-ray diffraction method (Figure 3). The diffraction pattern of menthol exhibits several sharp peaks, indicating the crystalline nature of menthol. The characteristic main peak for menthol was absent in the XRD pattern of NLCs formulation, suggesting the

change from menthol crystallinity status to amorphous status. Diffraction pattern of Precirol® and Poloxamer® in NLCs was much weaker than that of bulk lipid. It indicates that Precirol® in menthol-loaded NLCs was partially recrystallized and formed the less-ordered crystals.

Determination of the MIC and MBC values of menthol formulations

Plant's essential oils and extracts have been used for many thousands of years in food preservation, pharmaceuticals, alternative medicine, and natural therapies. It is necessary to scientifically investigate those plants used in traditional medicine to improve the quality of healthcare.[19] In the present study, the absorbance of microtiter plate before and after the incubation of bacteria, with different concentrations of menthol-loaded NLCs and emulsion, was assessed spectrophotometrically. After incubation and increasing the number of bacteria it is possible to find out the MIC values of menthol-loaded NLCs and emulsion. As shown in Table 1, the growth of Bacillus cereus, Staphylococcus aureus, and Escherichia coli was inhibited at concentration of 125, 250, and 500 µg/mL of menthol in the case of NLCs formulation, respectively. However, the corresponding MIC values for menthol emulsion were 1000, 1000, and 2000 µg/mL, indicating that loading of menthol in NLCs formulation could decrease the amount of necessary menthol for preserving foodstuffs from microorganism growth and spoilage in comparison with emulsion formulation. Addition of low amount of menthol not only is economical, but also may prevent the change in taste and color of the foodstuffs.

Table 1. Minimum inhibitory concentration (MIC) and minimum bactericidal concentration (MBC) of Menthol-loaded NLCs and emulsion.

Microorganism	MIC (µg/mL)		MBC (µg/mL)	
	Emulsion	NLCs	Emulsion	NLCs
Staphylococcus aureus	1000	125	4000	500
Bacillus cereus	2000	250	4000	1000
Escherichia coli	2000	500	>4000	>4000
Candida albicans	156	78	468	117

MIC and MBC values of menthol-loaded NLCs and menthol emulsion formulations against different microorganism are shown in Table 1. Usually the MIC values are considered as different if there is more than one dilution difference between the MIC values. The results showed that in case of the all tested microorganisms when menthol-loaded NLCs were used, the MIC mean values were significantly lower than the when menthol emulsion were used. This suggested the transport mechanisms through the cell membrane of the microorganisms and as a result increasing the antibacterial and antifungal efficiency. On the other hand, menthol-loaded NLCs and emulsion showed lower MIC values, and as a result, higher antibacterial impact on *B. cereus* in comparison with other microorganisms. Correspondingly, both NLCs and emulsion formulations exhibited the highest MIC values in the case of *E. coli*, suggesting that menthol possesses higher antibacterial efficiency against the Gram-positive bacteria (Figure 4). Antimicrobial effect of menthol may be due to the alteration of plasma membrane permeability and leakage of intracellular materials.[20,21] However, considering the relation of physicochemical characteristics of the drugs (such as lipophilicity and water solubility), this mechanism appears to be dependent on the lipid composition and net surface charge of the bacterial membranes. Furthermore, the essential oil might cross the cell membranes, penetrate the interior of the cell, and interact with intracellular sites critical for antibacterial activity. The outer layer of the Gram-negative outer membrane is composed primarily of lipopolysaccharide molecules and forms hydrophilic permeability barrier providing protection against the effects of highly hydrophobic materials. This may explain the low sensitivity of Escherichia coli to the cytotoxic effect of the lipophilic monoterpenes such as menthol.[22,23] NLC formulations also showed promising antifungal activity against candida (Table 1). The successful antifungal activity of NLC loaded with miconazole,[24] ketoconazole,[25] nystatin,[26] and fluconazole[27] were also reported indicating the encouraging approach of NLC against candid a. Although several studies showed that menthol and peppermint oil have shown antibacterial activity, the exact mechanism of action is not clearly explained. In a recent study, diamond nanoparticles were used to load menthol against biofilm formation.[28] The growth of *S. aureus* and *E. coli* made biofilms were inhibited more than 10 folds. The toxic effects on the membrane are often used to reveal the antimicrobial activity of the oil.

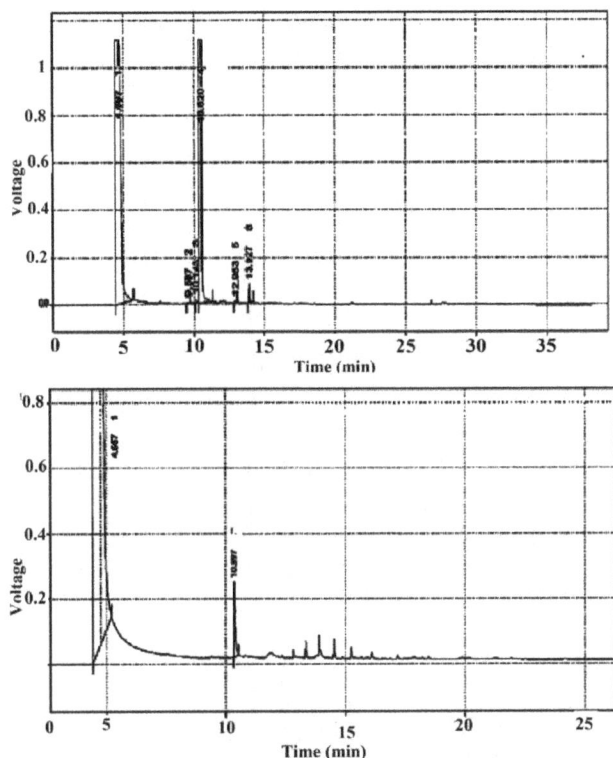

Figure 2. Representative chromatograms of Menthol in Menthol standard solution and Menthol-loaded nanostructured lipid carriers (NLCs).

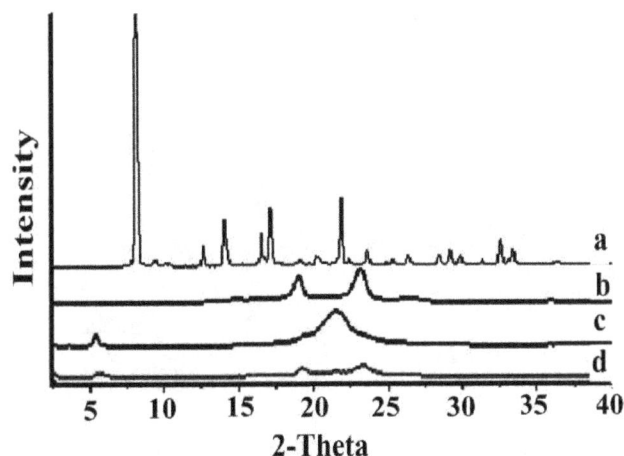

Figure 3. X-Ray diffraction patterns of Menthol, Precirol®, Poloxamer® and nanostructured lipid carriers (NLCs) formulation.

Trombetta et al. (2005) who explored the mechanism of action of three monoterpenes, speculated that the antimicrobial effect of monoterpenes such as (+)-menthol, thymol and linalyl acetate, is partially due to the disruption of the lipid fraction of the plasma membrane, causing in changed permeability and leakage of intracellular materials.[28,29] Emulsions are homogeneous thermodynamically stable transparent dispersions of two immiscible liquids stabilized by an interfacial film of surfactants. However, one major drawback of emulsions is that formation requires high surfactant concentration, which causes toxicity when used in pharmaceutical applications. On the other hand, NLCs could be prepared by a simple and industrially scaling up homogenization method. It has been demonstrated that NLCs increase the retention of a drug in the particle, hence, enhancing the release time and reducing the amount of drug required for the therapeutic action. This proficiency could be employed in controlling essential oils release to improve efficacy and reduce the amount and toxicity of used essential oils. Besides, controlling the release of drug molecule, nanocarriers also protect essential oils against possible thermal or photo degradation, oxidation, or evaporation which guarantees increased stability, flavor, and function, consequently prolonging the final product shelf life. Considering these features, these systems can actually represent an interesting approach for overcoming essential oils restrictions. Nanocarriers could also protect essential oils against possible thermal- or photo-degradation, oxidation or evaporation, assure increased stability, flavor, and function, and consequently extend the final product shelf life.[30]

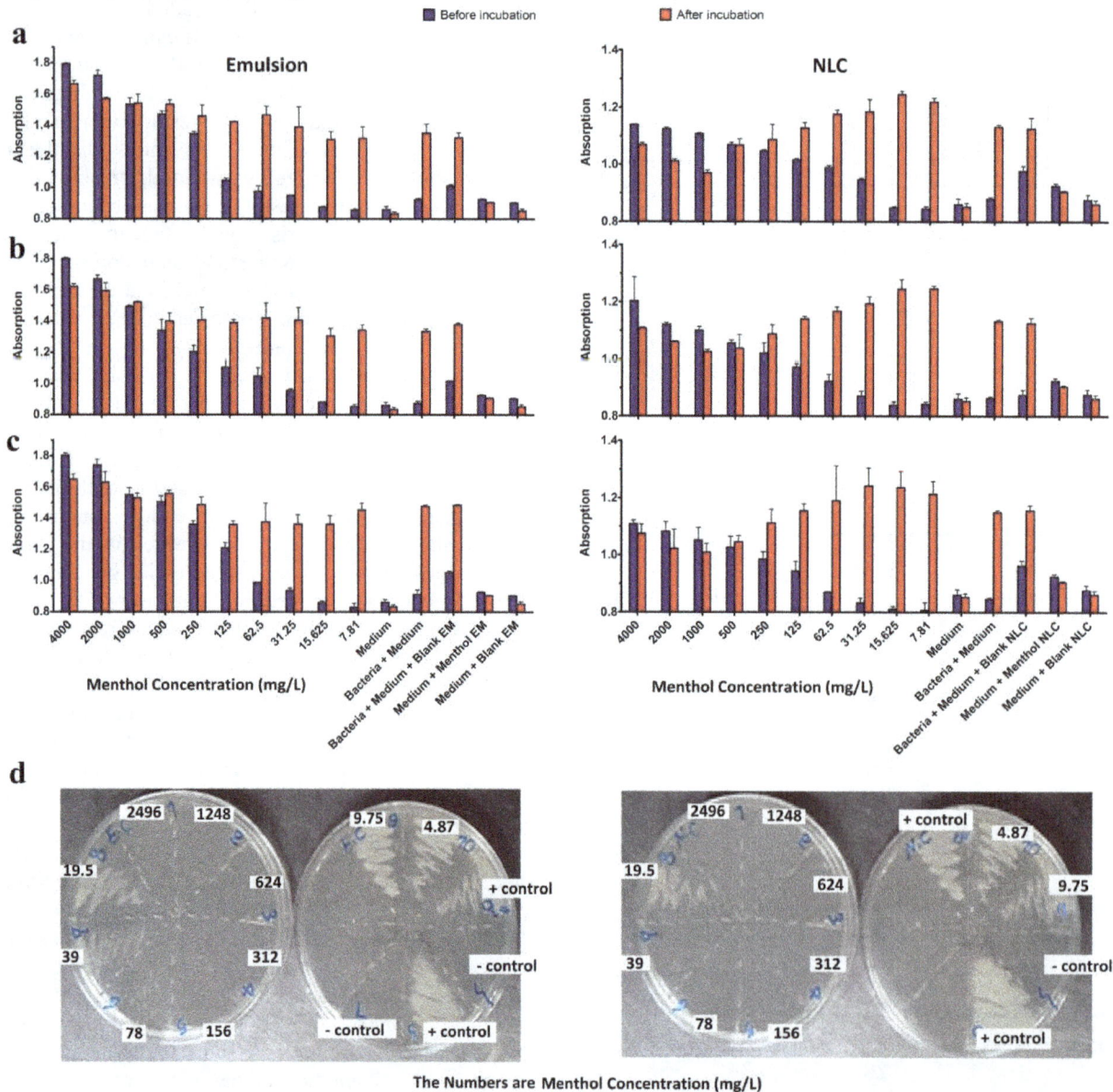

Figure 4. Minimum inhibition concentration (MIC) of conventional emulsion (left) and nanostructured lipid carriers (NLCs) (right) of Menthol against a) *Bacillus cereus,* b) *Escherichia coli,* c) *Bacillus cereus and* d) *Candida albicans*

Conclusion

Menthol was successfully loaded into NLCs in the amorphous structure in the ratio of 1:10 Menthol:lipid by dissolving in the oil phase. Menthol-loaded NLCs were around 100 nm with narrow size distribution (PDI 0.2). The antimicrobial efficiency of the encapsulated menthol was tested on four different microorganisms, demonstrating that MIC and MBC values in the case of NLCs were lower than the menthol emulsion. It can be concluded that essential oils could be used as antibacterial supplement and food preserving agents; however, further investigations are required on the potential antibacterial applicability of this nanostructure in other applications such as topical and oral uses especially against the drug-resistant microorganisms.

Acknowledgments

This paper was financially supported by Tabriz University of Medical Sciences.

Ethical Issues

Not applicable.

Conflict of Interest

The authors declare no conflict of interests.

References

1. Aneja KR, Sharma C, Joshi R. Antimicrobial activity of terminalia arjuna wight & arn.: An ethnomedicinal plant against pathogens causing ear infection. *Braz J Otorhinolaryngol* 2012;78(1):68-74.
2. Edris AE. Pharmaceutical and therapeutic potentials of essential oils and their individual volatile constituents: A review. *Phytother Res* 2007;21(4):308-23. doi: 10.1002/ptr.2072
3. Reichling J, Schnitzler P, Suschke U, Saller R. Essential oils of aromatic plants with antibacterial, antifungal, antiviral, and cytotoxic properties--an overview. *Forsch Komplementmed* 2009;16(2):79-90. doi: 10.1159/000207196
4. Nerio LS, Olivero-Verbel J, Stashenko E. Repellent activity of essential oils: A review. *Bioresour Technol* 2010;101(1):372-8. doi: 10.1016/j.biortech.2009.07.048
5. Gutierrez J, Barry-Ryan C, Bourke P. The antimicrobial efficacy of plant essential oil combinations and interactions with food ingredients. *Int J Food Microbiol* 2008;124(1):91-7. doi: 10.1016/j.ijfoodmicro.2008.02.028
6. Sokovic MD, Vukojevic J, Marin PD, Brkic DD, Vajs V, van Griensven LJ. Chemical composition of essential oils of thymus and mentha species and their antifungal activities. *Molecules* 2009;14(1):238-49. doi: 10.3390/molecules14010238
7. Carneiro HCF, Tonon RV, Grosso CRF, Hubinger MD. Encapsulation efficiency and oxidative stability of flaxseed oil microencapsulated by spray drying using different combinations of wall materials. *J Food Eng* 2013;115(4):443-51. doi: 10.1016/j.jfoodeng.2012.03.033
8. Augustin MA, Hemar Y. Nano- and micro-structured assemblies for encapsulation of food ingredients. *Chem Soc Rev* 2009;38(4):902-12. doi: 10.1039/b801739p
9. Lin C-H, Chen C-H, Lin Z-C, Fang J-Y. Recent advances in oral delivery of drugs and bioactive natural products using solid lipid nanoparticles as the carriers. *J Food Drug Anal* 2017;25(2):219-34. doi: 10.1016/j.jfda.2017.02.001
10. Singh P, Kim YJ, Zhang D, Yang DC. Biological synthesis of nanoparticles from plants and microorganisms. *Trends Biotechnol* 2016;34(7):588-99. doi: 10.1016/j.tibtech.2016.02.006
11. Hamishehkar H, Shokri J, Fallahi S, Jahangiri A, Ghanbarzadeh S, Kouhsoltani M. Histopathological evaluation of caffeine-loaded solid lipid nanoparticles in efficient treatment of cellulite. *Drug Dev Ind Pharm* 2015;41(10):1640-6. doi: 10.3109/03639045.2014.980426
12. Wiegand I, Hilpert K, Hancock RE. Agar and broth dilution methods to determine the minimal inhibitory concentration (mic) of antimicrobial substances. *Nat Protoc* 2008;3(2):163-75. doi: 10.1038/nprot.2007.521
13. Samber N, Khan A, Varma A, Manzoor N. Synergistic anti-candidal activity and mode of action of mentha piperita essential oil and its major components. *Pharm Biol* 2015;53(10):1496-504. doi: 10.3109/13880209.2014.989623
14. Brar SK, Verma M. Measurement of nanoparticles by light-scattering techniques. *TrAC Trend Anal Chem* 2011;30(1):4-17. doi: 10.1016/j.trac.2010.08.008
15. Wu L, Zhang J, Watanabe W. Physical and chemical stability of drug nanoparticles. *Adv Drug Deliv Rev* 2011;63(6):456-69. doi: 10.1016/j.addr.2011.02.001
16. Qian C, McClements DJ. Formation of nanoemulsions stabilized by model food-grade emulsifiers using high-pressure homogenization: Factors affecting particle size. *Food Hydrocolloid* 2011;25(5):1000-8. doi: 10.1016/j.foodhyd.2010.09.017
17. He C, Hu Y, Yin L, Tang C, Yin C. Effects of particle size and surface charge on cellular uptake and biodistribution of polymeric nanoparticles. *Biomaterials* 2010;31(13):3657-66. doi: 10.1016/j.biomaterials.2010.01.065
18. Jiang J, Oberdörster G, Biswas P. Characterization of size, surface charge, and agglomeration state of nanoparticle dispersions for toxicological studies. *J Nanopart Res* 2009;11(1):77-89. doi: 10.1007/s11051-008-9446-4
19. Holley RA, Patel D. Improvement in shelf-life and safety of perishable foods by plant essential oils and smoke antimicrobials. *Food Microbiol* 2005;22(4):273-92. doi: 10.1016/j.fm.2004.08.006
20. Patel T, Ishiuji Y, Yosipovitch G. Menthol: A refreshing look at this ancient compound. *J Am Acad*

Dermatol 2007;57(5):873-8. doi: 10.1016/j.jaad.2007.04.008

21. Kamatou GP, Vermaak I, Viljoen AM, Lawrence BM. Menthol: A simple monoterpene with remarkable biological properties. *Phytochemistry* 2013;96:15-25. doi: 10.1016/j.phytochem.2013.08.005

22. Al-Bayati FA. Isolation and identification of antimicrobial compound from mentha longifolia l. Leaves grown wild in iraq. *Ann Clin Microbiol Antimicrob* 2009;8:20. doi: 10.1186/1476-0711-8-20

23. Hanamanthagouda MS, Kakkalameli SB, Naik PM, Nagella P, Seetharamareddy HR, Murthy HN. Essential oils of lavandula bipinnata and their antimicrobial activities. *Food Chem* 2010;118(3):836-9. doi: 10.1016/j.foodchem.2009.05.032

24. Mendes AI, Silva AC, Catita JA, Cerqueira F, Gabriel C, Lopes CM. Miconazole-loaded nanostructured lipid carriers (nlc) for local delivery to the oral mucosa: Improving antifungal activity. *Colloids Surf B Biointerfaces* 2013;111:755-63. doi: 10.1016/j.colsurfb.2013.05.041

25. Souto EB, Muller RH. The use of sln and nlc as topical particulate carriers for imidazole antifungal agents. *Pharmazie* 2006;61(5):431-7.

26. Pinto Reis C, Vasques Roque L, Baptista M, Rijo P. Innovative formulation of nystatin particulate systems in toothpaste for candidiasis treatment. *Pharm Dev Technol* 2016;21(3):282-7. doi: 10.3109/10837450.2014.999783

27. Gupta M, Vyas SP. Development, characterization and in vivo assessment of effective lipidic nanoparticles for dermal delivery of fluconazole against cutaneous candidiasis. *Chem Phys Lipids* 2012;165(4):454-61. doi: 10.1016/j.chemphyslip.2012.01.006

28. Turcheniuk V, Raks V, Issa R, Cooper IR, Cragg PJ, Jijie R, et al. Antimicrobial activity of menthol modified nanodiamond particles. *Diam Relat Mater* 2015;57:2-8. doi: 10.1016/j.diamond.2014.12.002

29. Phunpee S, Saesoo S, Sramala I, Jarussophon S, Sajomsang W, Puttipipatkhachorn S, et al. A comparison of eugenol and menthol on encapsulation characteristics with water-soluble quaternized beta-cyclodextrin grafted chitosan. *Int J Biol Macromol* 2016;84:472-80. doi: 10.1016/j.ijbiomac.2015.11.006

30. Bilia AR, Guccione C, Isacchi B, Righeschi C, Firenzuoli F, Bergonzi MC. Essential oils loaded in nanosystems: A developing strategy for a successful therapeutic approach. *Evid Based Compl Alt Med* 2014;2014:14. doi: 10.1155/2014/651593

9

Caffeine Neuroprotective Mechanism Against β-Amyloid Neurotoxicity in SHSY5Y Cell Line: Involvement of Adenosine, Ryanodine, and N-Methyl-D-Aspartate Receptors

Mojtaba Keshavarz*, Majid Reza Farrokhi, Atena Amiri

Shiraz Neuroscience Research Center, Shiraz University of Medical Sciences, Shiraz, Iran.

Keywords:
· Caffeine
· N-methyl-D-Aspartate
· Adenosine
· Dantrolene
· β-amyloid

Abstract

Purpose: Some reports have shown neuroprotective effects of caffeine in several neurodegenerative disorders. However, its mechanism of action is not completely clear. Therefore, the aim of this study was to explore the interference of ryanodine, N-methyl-D-aspartate (NMDA) and adenosine modulators with the neuroprotective effects of caffeine against β-amyloid (Aβ) neurotoxicity in the SHSY5Y cells.

Methods: The SHSY5Y cells were treated with Aβ23-35 (20µM) and/or caffeine (0.6 and 1mM), or both for 24 hours. Adenosine (20, 40, 60, 80, 100µM), NMDA (20, 50, 70, 90µM), dantrolene (2, 4, 6, 8, 10µM) were also added to the medium and incubated for 24 hours. The cell viability was measured via the MTT (3-[4,5-dimethylthiazol-2-yl]-2,5-diphenyl tetrazolium bromide) method. The data were analyzed using one-way ANOVA followed by Bonferroni test.

Results: Caffeine at all the used concentrations (0.6, 0.8, 0.9, 1, and 3mM) significantly protected neuronal cells against Aβ neurotoxicity. Adenosine at the concentrations of 20, 40, 80 and 100µM diminished the neuroprotective effects of caffeine (0.6 and 1mM) against Aβ neurotoxicity. NMDA at the concentrations of 20, 50, 70 and 90µM blocked caffeine (0.6 and 1mM) neuroprotective effects. Dantrolene at the concentration of 2, 4, 6, 8 and 10µM diminished the neuroprotective effects of caffeine (0.6mM) and at the concentrations of 2 and 10µM impede caffeine (1mM) neuroprotection against Aβ neurotoxicity.

Conclusion: Caffeine produced neuroprotective effect against Aβ neurotoxicity. Blockade of adenosine and NMDA receptors, as well as the activation of ryanodine receptors, may contribute to the neuroprotective effects of caffeine.

Introduction

Extracellular aggregation of β-amyloid peptides (Aβ) and hyperphosphorylated tau protein (neurofibrillary tangles) may be the most important causes of neural degeneration in Alzheimer's disease (AD).[1] Moreover, accumulating data have implied that deregulated calcium signaling may have an important contribution to the neural cell death in AD.[2] Interestingly, altered intracellular calcium homeostasis emerges earlier than neuropathological abnormalities observed in AD.[3]

Calcium is an important signal transduction molecule[4] which is involved in a wide range of neural functions like cell growth, differentiation, metabolism, exocytosis, and apoptosis.[4] Several neuronal systems, including N-methyl-D-Aspartate (NMDA), adenosine and ryanodine receptors maintain the intracellular concentration of calcium within a narrow normal range.[5-7] On the other hand, ryanodine, NMDA and adenosine receptors have possible roles in the pathophysiology and treatment of AD.[8-10] Thus, these receptors may be the targets of neuroprotective agents in AD.

Caffeine is the most popular psychoactive drug around the world[11] with important modulatory effects on intracellular calcium in the central nervous system (CNS).[5,12] Caffeine effects may be related to the non-specific modulation of several systems in the CNS. At the normal daily consumption (2.4 to 4.0 mg/kg or 2 to 4 cups of coffee per person),[11] the primary target of caffeine is the non-selective antagonism of adenosine receptors.[13] Ryanodine receptors are the other physiological targets of caffeine in the CNS which mediates caffeine-induced intracellular calcium release.[14] In contrast, caffeine effects on the NMDA receptors are not fully elucidated.

Recent evidence has shown that caffeine exerts profound effects on motor, behavior, information processing, and cognitive performance.[15] It has been also demonstrated that caffeine can produce neuroprotective effects in different neurodegenerative diseases.[16] In-vivo and in-vitro studies have also shown that caffeine or coffee has protective effects against AD.[17] However, the exact mechanism of

---
*Corresponding author: Mojtaba Keshavarz, Email: mkeshavar@sums.ac.ir

neuroprotective effects of caffeine in AD is not completely clear. Therefore, the aim of this study was to explore the interference of ryanodine, NMDA and adenosine modulators with the neuroprotective effects of caffeine against Aβ neurotoxicity in the SHSY5Y cell line.

Materials and Methods
Materials
Human SHSY5Y cells were purchased from Pasteur Institute (Tehran, Iran). Cell culture materials including DMEM/F12, FBS (fetal bovine serum), and Penicillin-Streptomycin were obtained from Gibco® life technologies™ (New York, USA). Aβ25-35, caffeine, dantrolene sodium salt, NMDA, and adenosine were purchased from Sigma-Aldrich (St. Louis, USA).

Neuronal Cell Culture
The human SHSY5Y cells were grown in DMEM/F12 (1:1) media supplemented with 10 % fetal bovine serum, 100U/ml penicillin, and 100μg/ml streptomycin. The cells were seeded at a density of 10^5cells/well in the 96-well plates for the MTT (3-[4,5-dimethylthiazol-2-yl]-2,5-diphenyl tetrazolium bromide) experiments. The plates were maintained at 37°C in 95 % humidified atmosphere (air) with 5 % CO_2. After 24 hr of incubation, the cells were treated with Aβ and/or other agents.

Aβ25–35 Preparation
Aβ25–35 was dissolved in sterile distilled water at a concentration of 2μg/μl and kept at −70 °C until use. For the aggregation process, Aβ25–35 was incubated at 37 °C for 4 days before the administration in the cell culture.

Treatment
Caffeine, dantrolene (a ryanodine receptor antagonist), adenosine and NMDA were dissolved in PBS (Phosphate Buffered Solutions). The effective concentration of Aβ25-35 and caffeine was obtained through dose response experiments and MTT assay. On the day of treatment, the serum-free medium was treated with Aβ23-35 (20μM, selected according to pilot studies) and/or caffeine (0.6 and 1mM, selected according to pilot studies), or both for 24 hours. Adenosine (20, 40, 60, 80, 100μM), NMDA (20, 50, 70, 90μM), dantrolene (2, 4, 6, 8, 10μM) were also added to the medium and incubated for 24 hours.

Cell Viability Assay
Twenty-four hours after treatments, 5 mg/ml MTT reagent was added to the cell culture media. Four hours later, the media was gently removed and the precipitations in each well were dissolved in 100 μl of DMSO. We measured the absorbance at 570 nm using a microplate reader (Synergy HT, Biotek®) as an index of neuronal viability.

Statistical analysis
The variables were analyzed using one-way ANOVA followed by Bonferroni test. The significance level was considered as <0.05. All analyses were performed suing SPSS software version 23.

Results and Discussion
Aβ at a concentration of 20μM decreased about 71% in the neural viability in the SY-SY5Y cell lines compared with the control group. Moreover, our analysis showed that different concentrations of caffeine significantly protected neuronal cells against Aβ neurotoxicity ($F_{(df)}$= 16.81(6), p= 0.000). We chose two concentration of caffeine (0.6 and 1 mM) to evaluate the interaction of adenosine, NMDA, and dantrolene with caffeine neuroprotective effects.

Adenosine at the concentrations of 20, 40, 60, 80 and 100μM diminished the neuroprotective effects of caffeine (0.6mM) against Aβ neurotoxicity ($F_{(9)}$= 21.35, p=0.000) (Figure 1). Moreover, adenosine at the concentrations of 20, 40, 80 and 100μM blocked caffeine (1mM) neuroprotective effects against Aβ neurotoxicity ($F_{(9)}$= 8.77, p=0.000) (Figure 2). There was a significant difference between different concentrations of adenosine (without caffeine) against Aβ neurotoxicity ($F_{(3)}$=4.902, p=0.019). The pairwise comparison showed that adenosine only at a concentration of 80μM reduced Aβ neurotoxicity compared with the Aβ-treated group (p=0.036).

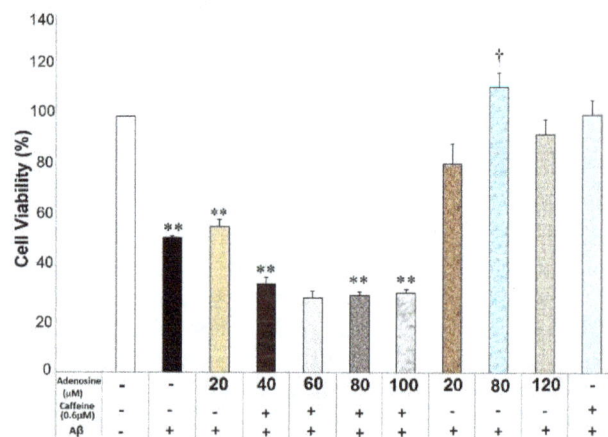

Figure 1. Adenosine affected caffeine (0.6mM) neuroprotective effects against Aβ neurotoxicity in the SHSY5Y neuroblastoma cells. Data are the mean + standard error of four experiments and were analyzed using one-way ANOVA followed by Bonferroni test. ** shows the significance at 0.001 compared with the β-amyloid (Aβ) + caffeine (0.6mM)-treated group, and † significance at 0.05 compared with the Aβ-treated group. Cell viability was assessed via MTT (3-[4,5-dimethylthiazol-2-yl]-2,5-diphenyl tetrazolium bromide) test.

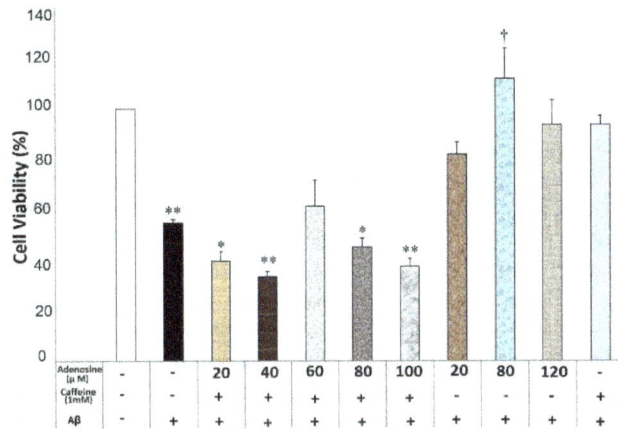

Figure 2. Adenosine affected caffeine (1mM) neuroprotective effects against Aβ neurotoxicity in the SHSY5Y neuroblastoma cells. Data are the mean + standard error of four experiments and were analyzed using one-way ANOVA followed by Bonferroni test. * and ** shows the significance at 0.05 and 0.001 compared with the β-amyloid (Aβ) + caffeine (1mM)-treated group, respectively, and † significance at 0.05 compared with the Aβ-treated group. Cell viability was assessed via MTT (3-[4,5-dimethylthiazol-2-yl]-2,5-diphenyl tetrazolium bromide) test.

Dantrolene at the concentration of 2, 4, 6, 8 and 10μM diminished the neuroprotective effects of caffeine (0.6mM) against Aβ neurotoxicity ($F(7)= 43.75$, $p=0.000$) (Figure 3). Furthermore, dantrolene at the concentrations of 2 and 10μM impeded the caffeine (1mM) neuroprotection against Aβ neurotoxicity ($F(7)=16.26$, $p=0.000$)(Figure 4). In contrast, dantrolene at the concentrations of 4, 6 and 8μM had no effect on the caffeine (1mM) neuroprotection (Figure 4). There was a significant difference between the different concentration of dantrolene (without caffeine use) against Aβ neurotoxicity ($F(4)=8.81$, $p=0.001$), though the pairwise comparison showed no significant difference between each concentration of dantrolene and the Aβ-treated group ($p>0.05$).

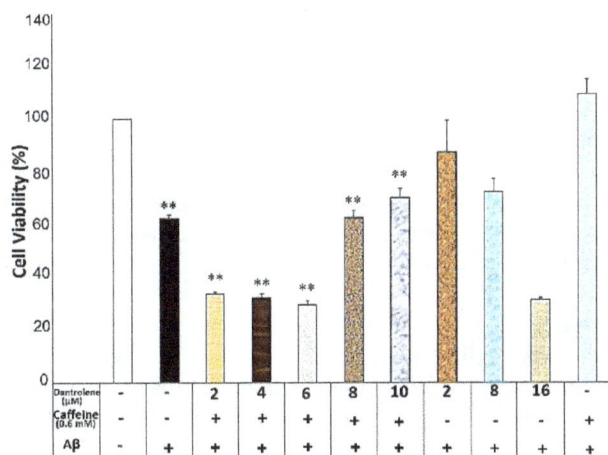

Figure 3. Dantrolene affected caffeine (0.6mM) neuroprotective effects against Aβ neurotoxicity in the SHSY5Y neuroblastoma cells. Data are the mean + standard error of four experiments and were analyzed using one-way ANOVA followed by Bonferroni test. ** shows the significance at 0.001 compared with the β-amyloid (Aβ) + caffeine (0.6mM)-treated group. Cell viability was assessed via MTT (3-[4,5-dimethylthiazol-2-yl]-2,5-diphenyl tetrazolium bromide) test.

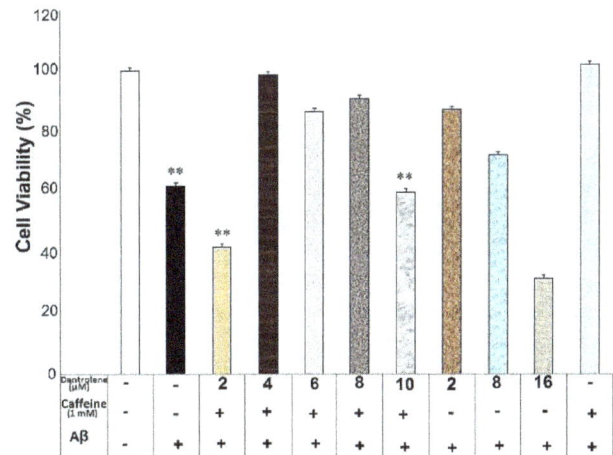

Figure 4. Dantrolene affected caffeine (1mM) neuroprotective effects against Aβ neurotoxicity in the SHSY5Y neuroblastoma cells. Data are the mean + standard error of four experiments and were analyzed using one-way ANOVA followed by Bonferroni test. ** shows the significance at 0.001 compared with the β-amyloid (Aβ) + caffeine (1mM)-treated group. Cell viability was assessed via MTT (3-[4,5-dimethylthiazol-2-yl]-2,5-diphenyl tetrazolium bromide) test.

NMDA at the concentrations of 20, 50, 70 and 90 μM inhibited caffeine (0.6 and 1mM) neuroprotective effects against Aβ neurotoxicity ($F(6)=23.29$, $p=0.000$ and $F(6)= 42.95$, $p=0.000$, respectively) (Figure 5 and 6). There was a significant difference regarding neuronal death between different concentrations of NMDA alone groups, Aβ-treated group and the vehicle treated group ($F(3)= 0.657$, $p=0.594$). Each concentration of NMDA (20, 80 and 120μM) significantly reduced neuronal viability compared with the vehicle-treated group ($p<0.05$) (Figure 5). However, there was no significant difference between NMDA alone groups and Aβ-treated group ($p>0.05$) (Figure 5).

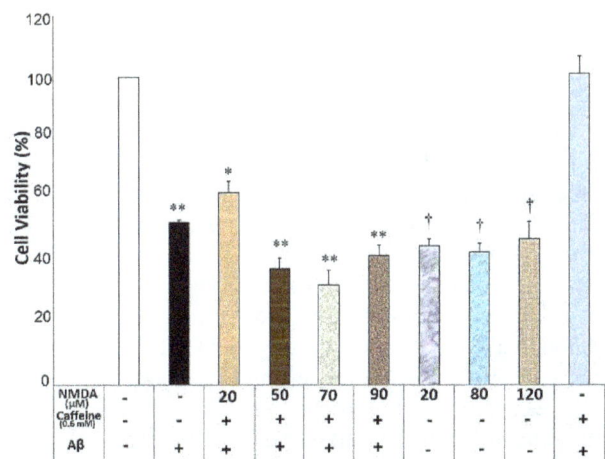

Figure 5. N-Methyl-D-Aspartate (NMDA) affected caffeine (0.6mM) neuroprotective effects against Aβ neurotoxicity in the SHSY5Y neuroblastoma cells. Data are the mean + standard error of four experiments and were analyzed using one-way ANOVA followed by Bonferroni test. * and ** shows the significance at 0.05 and 0.001 compared with the β-amyloid (Aβ) + caffeine (0.6mM)-treated group, respectively, and † is significance at 0.001 compared with the vehicle-treated group. Cell viability was assessed via MTT (3-[4,5-dimethylthiazol-2-yl]-2,5-diphenyl tetrazolium bromide) test.

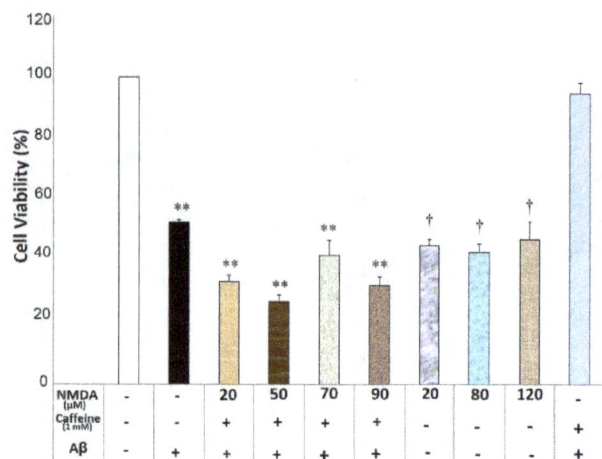

Figure 6. N-Methyl-D-Aspartate (NMDA) affected caffeine (1mM) neuroprotective effects against Aβ neurotoxicity in the SHSY5Y neuroblastoma cells. Data are the mean + standard error of four experiments and were analyzed using one-way ANOVA followed by Bonferroni test. ** shows the significance at 0.001 compared with the β-amyloid (Aβ) + caffeine (1mM)-treated group, and † is significance at 0.001 compared with the vehicle-treated group. Cell viability was assessed via MTT (3-[4,5-dimethylthiazol-2-yl]-2,5-diphenyl tetrazolium bromide) test.

Accumulating evidence confirms the idea that Aβ species have a prominent role in the pathophysiology of AD by inducing neurodegeneration and cognitive dysfunction.[18] Thus, confronting Aβ–induced neural damage may be a hopeful strategy for curing this disorder or preventing disease progression.[18] Our study, in line with previous ones, confirmed neuroprotective effects of caffeine against Aβ neurotoxicity in a neuronal cell line. In agreement, Dall'Igna et al showed that caffeine reduced Aβ neurotoxicity in the rat cerebellar neuronal culture[19] and reversed Aβ-induced cognitive deficit in an animal model of AD.[20] Epidemiologic studies have also revealed that the incidence of AD inversely correlated to the caffeine consumption.[17,21] In contrast, some reports have shown that acute administration of caffeine may worsen neurological condition.[22] Inconsistencies about neuroprotective effects of caffeine may mainly be related to the methodological differences in the studies.

Adenosine is an endogenous neuromodulator that influences many functions in the CNS.[23] Adenosine fulfills homeostatic and neuromodulatory roles in the CNS by controlling neurotransmission and neuronal excitability.[24] Although adenosine has four receptors (A_1R, $A_{2A}R$, $A_{2B}R$, and A_3R), most of its functions might be related to A_1 and A_{2A} receptors.[24] Adenosine and its receptors have important roles in the pathogenesis of neurodegenerative disorders like AD, though the exact function of this neuromodulator should be elucidated.[5] It has been suggested that caffeine neuroprotective effects may be related to the inhibition of adenosine receptors.[20] Our study showed that adenosine impeded neuroprotective effects of caffeine against Aβ neurotoxicity. Thus, the results of our study imply that the blockade of adenosine receptors may be responsible, at least partly, for the neuroprotective effects of caffeine in the cellular model of

AD. In this regard, it has been shown that blockade of A_1 and A_{2A} receptors produces neuroprotective effects.[19,20,22] Our study showed that dantrolene, a ryanodine receptor antagonist,[25] reduced neuroprotective effects of caffeine against Aβ neurotoxicity. Dantrolene modulates intracellular calcium by stabilizing and inhibiting RyR.[25] It can be implicated that caffeine neuroprotective effect may contribute, at least in part, to the RyR-mediated calcium release from the endoplasmic reticulum. There are considerable controversies about the intracellular calcium and RyR roles in the pathogenesis of AD. In agreement with our results, systemic administration of dantrolene has increased amyloid plaque formation and deteriorated hippocampal neuronal damage in a transgenic model of AD.[26] Accordingly, it has been proposed that increased RyR activity may attempt to maintain intracellular calcium homeostasis in the early stages of AD.[27] In line with this, it has been shown that inability of neurons to up-regulate RyR3 made them more vulnerable to the insults like Aβ exposure, excitotoxicity, and oxidative stress.[28] Thus, RyR hyperactivity in AD may be protective and/or a part of a mechanism to compensate calcium deregulation in AD.[27] In contrast, short-term treatment with dantrolene has stabilized intracellular calcium, decreased amyloid load, and reversed cognitive decline and memory impairments in various AD mouse models.[29,30]

NMDA receptors are glutamate receptors with high permeability to calcium[6] that have critical roles in synaptic plasticity, long-term potentiation and learning and memory.[31] In contrast, hyperactivation of these receptors may lead to disrupting calcium homeostasis, neuronal damage, and excitotoxicity.[32] Accumulating evidence has been shown that NMDA receptor-mediated excitotoxicity may be involved in the Aβ neurotoxicity.[33] Our study showed that NMDA reduced caffeine neuroprotective effects against Aβ neurotoxicity. Thus, it can be implicated that caffeine neuroprotective effects may in part be related to the NMDA blockade. To best of our knowledge, there is very limited information in the literature about caffeine interaction with NMDA receptors. However, caffeine may mimic NMDA antagonist effects in some brain regions[34] and its interaction with NMDA receptors may exert beneficial effects in neurodegenerative disorders.[35] Thus, it is possible to assume that direct or indirect blockade of NMDA receptors may contribute to the caffeine neuroprotective effects.

Limitations
The main limitation of this study may be the administration of non-specific modulators of adenosine and RyR. Thus, using specific modulators of these receptors may help to further clarify exact mechanism of action of caffeine in managing neurodegenerative disorders.

Conclusion
Caffeine produced neuroprotective effect against Aβ neurotoxicity in SHSY5Y cell line. The exact

mechanism of caffeine neuroprotective effects is not completely clear. However, blockade of adenosine and NMDA receptors, as well as activation of RyR receptors, may contribute to the neuroprotective effects of caffeine. However, future studies with more selective and specific modulators of adenosine and RyR may confirm the results of this study. Moreover, we cannot rule out other mechanisms that may be involved in the neuroprotective effects of caffeine against Aβ neurotoxicity.

Acknowledgments
We like to appreciate deputy for research of Shiraz University of Medical Sciences for financial support of this project.

Ethical Issues
Not applicable

Conflict of Interest
Non-declared

References
1. Selkoe DJ, Hardy J. The amyloid hypothesis of alzheimer's disease at 25 years. *EMBO Mol Med* 2016;8(6):595-608. doi: 10.15252/emmm.201606210
2. Popugaeva E, Pchitskaya E, Bezprozvanny I. Dysregulation of neuronal calcium homeostasis in alzheimer's disease - a therapeutic opportunity? *Biochem Biophys Res Commun* 2017;483(4):998-1004. doi: 10.1016/j.bbrc.2016.09.053
3. Chui DH, Tanahashi H, Ozawa K, Ikeda S, Checler F, Ueda O, et al. Transgenic mice with alzheimer presenilin 1 mutations show accelerated neurodegeneration without amyloid plaque formation. *Nat Med* 1999;5(5):560-4. doi: 10.1038/8438
4. Berridge MJ, Bootman MD, Lipp P. Calcium--a life and death signal. *Nature* 1998;395(6703):645-8. doi: 10.1038/27094
5. Gomes CV, Kaster MP, Tome AR, Agostinho PM, Cunha RA. Adenosine receptors and brain diseases: Neuroprotection and neurodegeneration. *Biochim Biophys Acta* 2011;1808(5):1380-99. doi: 10.1016/j.bbamem.2010.12.001
6. Rozov A, Burnashev N. Fast interaction between ampa and nmda receptors by intracellular calcium. *Cell Calcium* 2016;60(6):407-14. doi: 10.1016/j.ceca.2016.09.005
7. Yamazawa T, Murayama T, Oyamada H, Suzuki J, Kurebayashi N, Kanemaru K, et al. Correlation of molecular dynamics analysis and calcium signaling in mutant ryanodine receptors. *Biophys J* 2016;110(3):263a. doi: 10.1016/j.bpj.2015.11.1437
8. Danysz W, Parsons CG. Alzheimer's disease, beta-amyloid, glutamate, nmda receptors and memantine--searching for the connections. *Br J Pharmacol* 2012;167(2):324-52. doi: 10.1111/j.1476-5381.2012.02057.x
9. Lacampagne A, Liu X, Reiken S, Bussiere R, Meli AC, Lauritzen I, et al. Post-translational remodeling of ryanodine receptor induces calcium leak leading to alzheimer's disease-like pathologies and cognitive deficits. *Acta Neuropathol* 2017. doi: 10.1007/s00401-017-1733-7
10. Woods LT, Ajit D, Camden JM, Erb L, Weisman GA. Purinergic receptors as potential therapeutic targets in alzheimer's disease. *Neuropharmacology* 2016;104:169-79. doi: 10.1016/j.neuropharm.2015.10.031
11. Fredholm BB, Battig K, Holmen J, Nehlig A, Zvartau EE. Actions of caffeine in the brain with special reference to factors that contribute to its widespread use. *Pharmacol Rev* 1999;51(1):83-133.
12. McPherson PS, Kim YK, Valdivia H, Knudson CM, Takekura H, Franzini-Armstrong C, et al. The brain ryanodine receptor: A caffeine-sensitive calcium release channel. *Neuron* 1991;7(1):17-25.
13. Clark I, Landolt HP. Coffee, caffeine, and sleep: A systematic review of epidemiological studies and randomized controlled trials. *Sleep Med Rev* 2017;31:70-8. doi: 10.1016/j.smrv.2016.01.006
14. Liu J, Supnet C, Sun S, Zhang H, Good L, Popugaeva E, et al. The role of ryanodine receptor type 3 in a mouse model of alzheimer disease. *Channels (Austin, Tex)* 2014;8(3):230-42.
15. Rosso A, Mossey J, Lippa CF. Caffeine: Neuroprotective functions in cognition and alzheimer's disease. *Am J Alzheimers Dis Other Demen* 2008;23(5):417-22. doi: 10.1177/1533317508320083
16. Kolahdouzan M, Hamadeh MJ. The neuroprotective effects of caffeine in neurodegenerative diseases. *CNS Neurosci Ther* 2017;23(4):272-90. doi: 10.1111/cns.12684
17. Perez A, Li T, Hernandez S, Zhang R, Cao C. The rationale of using coffee and melatonin as an alternative treatment for alzheimer's disease. *J Alzheimers Dis Parkinsonism* 2016;6:205. doi: 10.4172/2161-0460.1000205
18. Ahmad A, Ali T, Park HY, Badshah H, Rehman SU, Kim MO. Neuroprotective effect of fisetin against amyloid-beta-induced cognitive/synaptic dysfunction, neuroinflammation, and neurodegeneration in adult mice. *Mol Neurobiol* 2017;54(3):2269-85. doi: 10.1007/s12035-016-9795-4
19. Dall'Igna OP, Porciuncula LO, Souza DO, Cunha RA, Lara DR. Neuroprotection by caffeine and adenosine a2a receptor blockade of beta-amyloid neurotoxicity. *Br J Pharmacol* 2003;138(7):1207-9. doi: 10.1038/sj.bjp.0705185
20. Dall'Igna OP, Fett P, Gomes MW, Souza DO, Cunha RA, Lara DR. Caffeine and adenosine a(2a) receptor antagonists prevent beta-amyloid (25-35)-induced cognitive deficits in mice. *Exp Neurol* 2007;203(1):241-5. doi: 10.1016/j.expneurol.2006.08.008

21. Maia L, de Mendonca A. Does caffeine intake protect from alzheimer's disease? *Eur J Neurol* 2002;9(4):377-82.

22. de Mendonça A, Sebastião AM, Ribeiro JA. Adenosine: Does it have a neuroprotective role after all? *Brain Res Rev* 2000;33(2):258-74. doi: 10.1016/S0165-0173(00)00033-3

23. Martins IJ. Sirtuin 1 and adenosine in brain disorder therapy. *J Clin Epigenet* 2017;3(1). doi: 10.21767/2472-1158.100045

24. Fredholm BB, Chen JF, Cunha RA, Svenningsson P, Vaugeois JM. Adenosine and brain function. *Int Rev Neurobiol* 2005;63:191-270. doi: 10.1016/s0074-7742(05)63007-3

25. Del Prete D, Checler F, Chami M. Ryanodine receptors: Physiological function and deregulation in alzheimer disease. *Mol Neurodegener* 2014;9:21. doi: 10.1186/1750-1326-9-21

26. Zhang H, Sun S, Herreman A, De Strooper B, Bezprozvanny I. Role of presenilins in neuronal calcium homeostasis. *J Neurosci* 2010;30(25):8566-80. doi: 10.1523/jneurosci.1554-10.2010

27. Supnet C, Bezprozvanny I. The dysregulation of intracellular calcium in alzheimer disease. *Cell Calcium* 2010;47(2):183-9. doi: 10.1016/j.ceca.2009.12.014

28. Allan Butterfield D. Amyloid β-peptide (1-42)-induced oxidative stress and neurotoxicity: Implications for neurodegeneration in alzheimer's disease brain. A review. *Free Radic Res* 2002;36(12):1307-13. doi: DOI:10.1080/1071576021000049890

29. Oules B, Del Prete D, Greco B, Zhang X, Lauritzen I, Sevalle J, et al. Ryanodine receptor blockade reduces amyloid-beta load and memory impairments in tg2576 mouse model of alzheimer disease. *J Neurosci* 2012;32(34):11820-34. doi: 10.1523/jneurosci.0875-12.2012

30. Peng J, Liang G, Inan S, Wu Z, Joseph DJ, Meng Q, et al. Dantrolene ameliorates cognitive decline and neuropathology in alzheimer triple transgenic mice. *Neurosci Lett* 2012;516(2):274-9. doi: 10.1016/j.neulet.2012.04.008

31. Morris RG, Anderson E, Lynch GS, Baudry M. Selective impairment of learning and blockade of long-term potentiation by an n-methyl-d-aspartate receptor antagonist, ap5. *Nature* 1986;319(6056):774-6. doi: 10.1038/319774a0

32. Weilinger NL, Lohman AW, Rakai BD, Ma EM, Bialecki J, Maslieieva V, et al. Metabotropic nmda receptor signaling couples src family kinases to pannexin-1 during excitotoxicity. *Nat Neurosci* 2016;19(3):432-42. doi: 10.1038/nn.4236

33. Wang R, Reddy PH. Role of glutamate and nmda receptors in alzheimer's disease. *J Alzheimers Dis* 2017;57(4):1041-8. doi: 10.3233/jad-160763

34. Dall'Igna OP, Da Silva AL, Dietrich MO, Hoffmann A, de Oliveira RV, Souza DO, et al. Chronic treatment with caffeine blunts the hyperlocomotor but not cognitive effects of the n-methyl-d-aspartate receptor antagonist mk-801 in mice. *Psychopharmacology (Berl)* 2003;166(3):258-63. doi: 10.1007/s00213-002-1362-1

35. Brothers HM, Marchalant Y, Wenk GL. Caffeine attenuates lipopolysaccharide-induced neuroinflammation. *Neurosci Lett* 2010;480(2):97-100. doi: 10.1016/j.neulet.2010.06.013

10

The Effect of Dried *Glycyrrhiza Glabra L*. Extract on Obesity Management with Regard to PPAR-γ2 (Pro12Ala) Gene Polymorphism in Obese Subjects Following an Energy Restricted Diet

Nazli Namazi[1,2], Mohammad Alizadeh[2], Elham Mirtaheri[2], Safar Farajnia[3]*

[1]*Diabetes Research Center, Endocrinology and Metabolism Clinical Sciences Institute, Tehran University of Medical Sciences, Tehran, Iran.*
[2]*Nutrition Research Center, Faculty of Nutrition, Tabriz University of Medical Sciences, Tabriz, Iran.*
[3]*Drug Applied Research Center, Tabriz University of Medical Sciences, Tabriz, Iran.*

Keywords:
· Licorice
· Hypocaloric diet
· Nutrigenetics
· PPAR-γ2

Abstract
Purpose: Obesity is a multi-factorial health problem which results from the interaction of environmental and genetic factors. The aim of the present study was to determine the effects of dried licorice extract with a calorie restricted diet on anthropometric indices and insulin resistance with nutrigenetic approach.
Methods: For this pilot, double-blind, placebo-controlled randomized clinical trial, 72 eligible subjects were randomly allocated to Licorice or placebo group. They received a low-calorie diet either with a 1.5 g/day of Licorice extract or placebo for 8 weeks.
Results: There were no significant differences in anthropometric indices and dietary intake in genotype subgroups at the baseline. Findings indicated that supplementation with Licorice extract did not change anthropometric indices and biochemical parameters significantly compared to a hypocaloric diet alone. However, from the nutrigenetic point of view, significant changes in anthropometric indices and QUICKI were observed in the Pro12Pro genotypes compared to the Pro12Ala at the end of the study ($p<0.05$ in all variables). Moreover, no interactive effect of the Licorice supplement and Pro12Ala genotype was found.
Conclusion: In obese subjects, the Pro/Pro polymorphism of the PPAR-γ2 gene seems to induce favourable effects on obesity management. Further studies are needed to clarify whether PPAR-γ2 gene polymorphisms or other obesity genes can affect responses to obesity treatment.

Introduction

Glycyrrhiza glabra L. (Fabaceae) generally which known as Licorice is a medicinal herb that widely grows in Mediterranean region and the south-west Asia. It contains various components with pharmacological properties including glabridin, glycyrrhizin, beta-Glycyhrritinic acid, flavonoids, sterols, amino acids, chalcones, isoflavones and triterpenoidsaponins.[1,2] Licorice root frequently used in traditional medicine particularly for gastric and duodenal ulcers, helicobacter pylori effects and allergenic reactions. Previous studies have reported antioxidant, anti-mutagenic, anti-inflammatory, anti-viral, anti-bacterial and anti-asthmatic properties for licorice and its components.[1,3] Additionally in the resent years, the anti-obesity effects of Licorice and its effective ingredients have been reported.[4-9]
Obesity is a chronic metabolic disorder which defines as excessive or abnormal fat accumulation.[10] Obesity is one of the greatest health threats and it can result in a number of chronic diseases including cardiovascular

diseases, diabetes, dyslipidemia and some cancers.[10] Due to a dramatic increase in obesity prevalence, researchers attempt to find effective medications or supplements for obesity management.[4] Previous studies have demonstrated several side effects for anti-obesity biochemical medications.[11] Therefore, tendency to using complementary therapies such as medicinal herbs is increasing.[11] It has been suggested that Licorice can affect obesity and its complications including insulin resistance and lipid profile through various mechanisms.[12-14] However, there are limited clinical trials with contrary results for anti-obesity properties of Licorice.[4,15-17]
Obesity is a multi-factorial health problem which results from the interaction among metabolic, physiological, social, behavioural, and genetic factors.[10] Proliferator-activated receptor gamma-2 (PPAR-γ2) has been considered as a candidate gene for obesity phenotype and its complications.[18] PPAR-γ gene, a type II nuclear receptor located on

---
*Corresponding author: Safar Farajnia, Email: farajnias@tbzmed.ac.ir

chromosome 3p-25 in humans. The PPAR-γ2 isoform is expressed exclusively in adipose tissue, and it plays a main role in adipogenic differentiation, lipogenesis, energy homeostasis and insulin sensitivity.[19,20] Pro12Ala (rs1801282) is one of known single nucleotide polymorphisms (SNPs) of PPAR-γ2 gene. Following a missense mutation (CCA→ GCA), Proline is substituted to Alanine at codon 12 exon B and it can affect transcriptional activity of PPAR-γ2 gene.[21] Some previous studies have indicated effective roles for Pro12Ala genotype in response to dietary interventions for obesity management.[22,23]

Since PPAR- γ2 gene polymorphism (Pro12Ala) is a common obesity candidate gene and its prevalence has been determined in Iranian population,[24] we considered it for the present study. To the best of our knowledge, the effects of supplementation with licorice extract for obesity management have been evaluated in limited clinical trials. Moreover, it seems the effect of Licorice with respect to genetic differences and gene-diet interactions has not been evaluated so far. Therefore, the aim of the present study was to determine the effects of dried licorice extract with a calorie restricted diet on anthropometric indices and insulin resistance with nutrigenetic view point, considering the polymorphism of PPAR- γ2 (Pro12Ala) gene.

Materials and Methods
Subjects
The present study was a part of a study on obesity gene polymorphisms with 216 sample size. The intervention section was conducted on 72 volunteer obese subjects in Tabriz, Iran. Iranian subjects aged 20–50 years old with a body mass index (BMI) equal or more than 30.0 kg/m^2 were recruited at Sheykhoraees Clinic from March to September 2012. The exclusion criteria were as follows: cardiovascular diseases, liver, thyroid and kidney disorders, diabetes, smoking, taking any anti-obesity medications, vitamin-mineral supplements, antioxidant medications and herbal drugs throughout 3 months ago, menopause, pregnancy and lactation.

At the beginning of the trial, all eligible volunteers signed a written consent form.

Study design
This study was a pilot, double-blind, placebo-controlled randomized clinical trial. Based on the findings of a previous study on frequency of the PPAR-γ2 (Pro12Ala) gene polymorphism in Iranian obese subjects (30.8%),[24] we recruited 216 obese subjects who referred to the obesity clinic and basically screened them for presence of Pro12Ala polymorphism. For getting additional information on the intervention, a 2:1 allocation rate was used.[25] Finally, 72 subjects were selected based on this SNP, 24 Ala carriers (Pro/Ala genotype) and 48 non-Ala carriers (Pro/Pro).

The participants were randomly allocated to two groups using a block randomization procedure (random number table; block size=2). After matching the subjects based on sex, age and BMI, they were allocated into each arm of the trial. To maintain blinding, randomization and allocation was conducted by a subject with no involvement in the trial. In addition, the researchers and participants remained blind throughout randomization and allocation until data analysis. Both groups received a balanced calorie-restricted diet. A dietician designed an individualized diet that was explained in details in our previous study.[12] Intervention and placebo group took 1.5 gr/day (three 500 mg capsules; one capsule 30 min before each main meal) of dried licorice extract and placebo (corn starch; three 500 mg capsules) for 8 weeks, respectively.

Both supplement and placebo were provided for the participants in similar opaque pockets. The colour and appearance of the capsules were the same in both groups. The subjects received the pockets during the first interview and every 20 days. After randomization, the supplements were distributed among the volunteers based on the allocation code (A or B). To determine compliance with the supplements, the participants were asked to return the pockets (empty or full) in each visit. Therefore, compliance could be estimated by counting the remaining capsules. The participants were warned to be excluded if they had taken less than 90% of the supplements through the intervention. Moreover, the participants were advised to continue their usual physical activities and to contact the researcher for any side effects related to taking the supplements. At baseline, demographic characteristics including age, family history of obesity, disease history, and medications was collected.

Licorice extract characteristics
The licorice extract was prepared by Darook pharmaceutical company (Esfahan, Iran). The dried hydroalcoholic extract of licorice root (ethanol 70: water 30% v/v) contained lowered Glycyrrhizin (<0.01%). The yield of extraction was 10% (10gr extract/100 gr powdered licorice root).

Data collection
Dietary intake, anthropometric indices and physical activity assessments
Dietary intake and anthropometric indices were measured at baseline and at the end of the study. Dietary intake was evaluated using a three-day (two weekdays and one weekend) 24-h food recall. Necessary information about how to estimate and record daily food intake were presented. It was analyzed using the Nutritionist IV software (First Databank Inc., Hearst Corp., San Bruno, CA) modified for Iranian foods for total energy and macronutrients. Weight, height, waist circumference

and hip circumference were measured using standard methods as have been explained elsewhere.[12] Body mass index (BMI) was calculated by dividing weight in kilogram by height in meters squared. Physical activity level was evaluated using International physical activity questionnaire (IPAQ)[26] and then participants were categorized into moderate or sedentary physical activity groups.

Biochemical measurements

At baseline and at the end of the intervention, after 12-14h fasting, 10 mL blood samples were collected from each participant between 8:00 and 9:30 a.m. FBS levels was analyzed on the day of sampling and the remaining serum was stored at -80°C until assay time. FBS concentration was measured by the enzymatic method using an Abbot Model Aclyon 300, USA autoanalyzer with a kit from Pars-Azmon (Tehran, Iran). Insulin concentration was measured using the ELISA method with commercial kit (Monobind, Denmark). The quantitative insulin sensitivity check index (QUICKI) was calculated according to the following formula: QUICKI = [1/ (log (Insulin) + log(FBS)].

Genetic Assessments

Venous blood samples (3mL) were collected and transferred into a Vacutainer tube containing EDTA. DNA was extracted from peripheral blood, on the basis of the Cinagen Kit dNp protocol (DNG plus DNA Extraction Kit, Sinagene Company, Tehran, Iran). To determine the SNPs, polymerase chain reaction (PCR), followed by restriction fragment length polymorphism (RFLP) assays was used. The sequences of PCR primers for Pro12Ala PPARγ2 variant (rs1801282) were as follows:

Forward primer: 5'-TCTGGGAGATTCTCCTATTGGC-3'
Reverse primer: 5'-CTGGAAGACAAACTACAAGAG-3'

PCR premix consisted of PCR buffer 10 mM, dNTP 0.2 mM, Mgcl 1.5 mM, each primer (0.8 pM/μl) with 1 U Tag polymerase. Cycling was performed in a thermal cycler as: 95 °C for 4 min, 94 °C for 1 min, 58 °C for 1min, Go to 2 for 38 cycles, 72 °C for 5 min. Then, the PCR product was digested with HhaI restriction enzyme for 1.5 h at 37 °C using 2 μl Buffer tango (10×) and HhaI 0.5μl (Fermentas, Lithuania). The digested products were analyzed by electrophoresis in a 2.5% agarose gel stained with ethidium bromide that was exposed under UV to visualize the fragments. Genotyping was repeated in all Pro12Ala heterozygotes and randomly selected Pro12 homozygotes; their reproducibility was 100%.

Statistical analysis

The Kolmogorov-Smirnov test was used for evaluating the normality of the data distribution. The results are reported as mean±SD and Median (25th, 75th) for data with normal and non-normal distribution, respectively. For comparison data and detection the differences among the study groups, one-way ANOVA (all the variables except insulin) and Kruskal-Wallis H (for insulin) test was used at the beginning and at the end of the trial. The effect of supplement, Pro12Ala gene polymorphism and gene-supplement interactions on changes of anthropometric indices and biochemical parameters was examined using two-way ANOVA test. Statistical analyses of all data were performed using SPSS version 13.0 (SPSS, Chicago, IL, USA), and $p < 0.05$ was considered statistically significant.

Results

A total of 216 obese subjects were screened for the PPARγ (Pro12Ala) gene polymorphism. The prevalence rates were 74.1% (n=160) for Pro/Pro and 25.9% (n=56) for Pro/Ala. Moreover, no participants had the Ala/Ala genotype. Throughout the trial, three subjects in the Licorice group were excluded, because of gastric complications (n=2) and not adhering to the study procedure (n=1). In the placebo group, two subjects were also excluded due to not adhering to the study procedure and gastrointestinal disorder (Figure1). Finally 67 subjects completed the study. The capsule counts indicated that all the participants who completed the study had high compliance (>90%) with the supplementation.

The baseline characteristics of participants based on the Pro12Ala polymorphism are indicated in Table 1. No significant differences were observed in the study population at baseline. As shown in Table 2, there were no significant differences in dietary intakes of the comparable groups at the beginning of the trial. At the end of the study, only differences in energy intake among the study groups stratified by the Pro12Ala polymorphism were significant (p<0.01) (Table 2). Reduction in the energy intake of subjects with Pro/Pro genotype who received licorice supplement was significantly more than the Pro/Ala group (-48.0% vs. -33.4%). Table 3 illustrates the effects of supplement, Pro/Ala polymorphism and the gene-supplement interactions on subgroups of PPAR-γ2 gene in the licorice and placebo group. Findings indicated that supplementation with Licorice extract did not change anthropometric indices and biochemical parameters significantly compared to a hypocaloric diet alone. But dependent on the PPAR-γ2 polymorphism, significant changes in body weight, BMI, WC, WHR and QUICKI were observed at the end of the study. Moreover, no interactive effect of licorice supplementation and PPAR-γ (Pro12Ala) was found on anthropometric indices, serum levels of FBS, insulin, and QUICKI (Table 3).

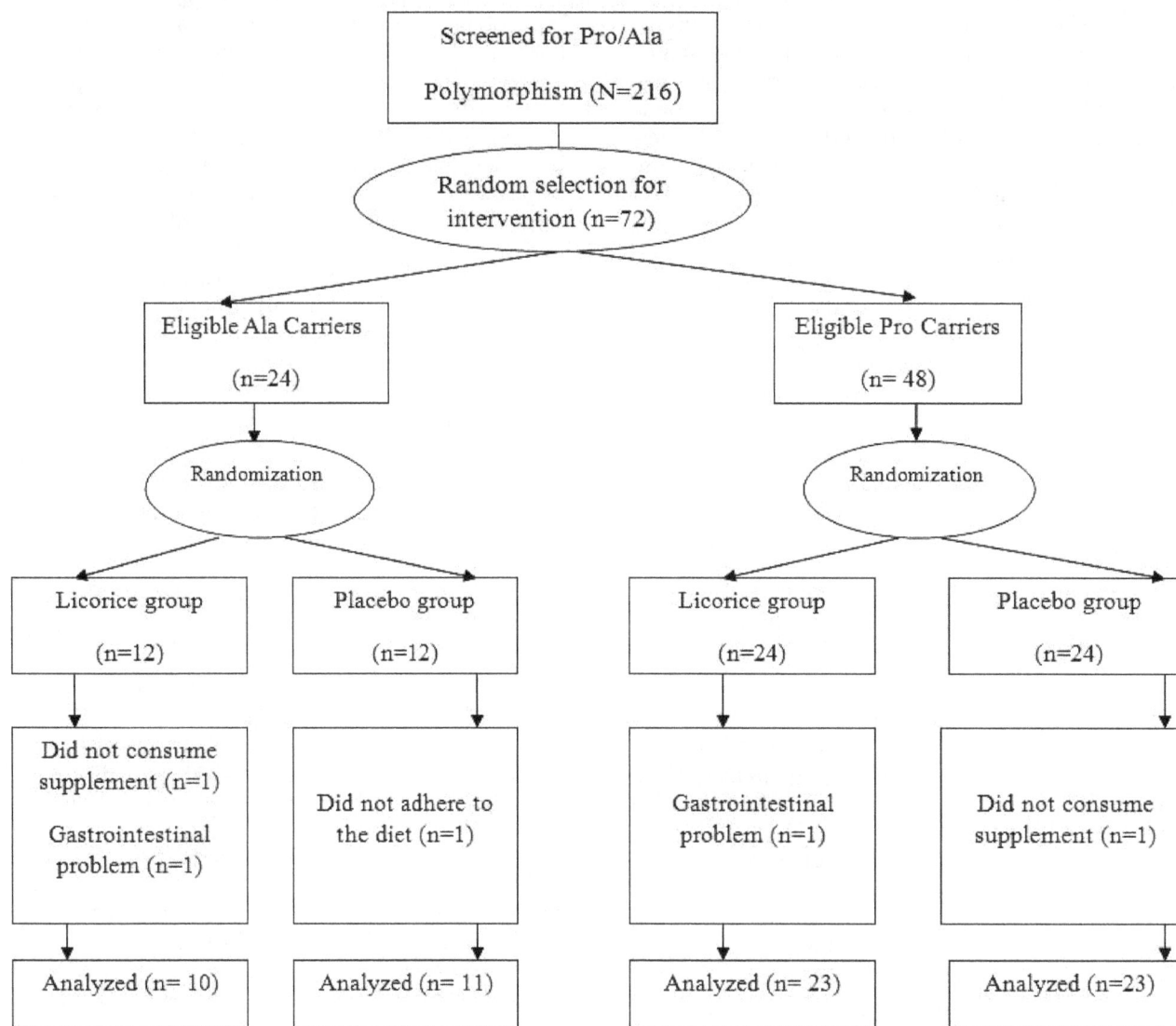

Figure 1. Summary of the randomization, allocation and follow-up of participants in the study groups

Table 1. Anthropometric indices and biochemical parameters of the participants in the Licorice and placebo group based on Pro12Ala genotype at the baseline

-	Licorice Group (n=33)		Placebo Group (n=34)		P-value†
Variables	Pro/Pro	Pro/Ala	Pro/Pro	Pro/Ala	-
Age (years)	37.4 ±14.7*	36.0±8.7	41.8±13.8	42.7±9.1	0.9
Weight (kg)	89.8±18.4	86.3±11.3	83.2±9.8	79.9±5.9	0.3
BMI(kg/m^2)	34.3±5.2	32.9±2.0	33.4±3.3	33.3±2.3	0.4
Waist Circumference (cm)	109.2±14.0	101.2±10.2	110.3±11.0	106.1±9.0	0.09
Hip Circumference (cm)	117.1±10.5	114.4±7.0	112.3±9.3	113.2±6.9	0.6
FBS(mg/dL)	100±8.6	97.2±7.6	97.0±8.6	94.5±6.5	0.2
Insulin	9.0(5.3,13.2)‡	10.5 (7,14.5)	8.5(4.2,10.0)	9.0(4.7,16.6)	0.2**
QUICKI	0.34±0.03	0.34±0.02	0.35±0.02	0.35±0.04	0.8

BMI: Body mass index; FBS: Fasting blood sugar; QUICKI: Quantitative insulin sensitivity check index
*Mean±SD
‡ Median (25th, 75th)
†One-way ANOVA; Comparison of between-group differences at the baseline
** Kruskal-Wallis H

Table 2. Comparison of dietary intake based on the PPAR-γ2 genotype in the Licorice and placebo groups at the baseline and after the intervention

Variables	At the baseline				P-value†	At the end				P-value†
	Licorice		Placebo			Licorice		Placebo		
	Pro/Pro	Pro/Ala	Pro/Pro	Pro/Ala		Pro/Pro	Pro/Ala	Pro/Pro	Pro/Ala	
Energy (kcal/day)	2498±414*	2476±538	2326±382	2436±266	0.7	1297±227	1648±239	1339±230	1480±247	<0.01
Carbohydrate (g/day)	301.2±78.9	314.5±73.5	312.0±59.8	345.4±63.7	0.2	174.1±45.4	208.3±59.1	196.4±47.6	228.6±46.5	0.7
Protein (g/day)	84.9±33.7	109.5±43.6	97.8±20.2	94.9±19.9	0.2	41.9±11.6	39.3±14.6	43.4±7.1	42.2±12.2	0.4
Total fat (g/day)	105.3±45.1	86.6±31.4	89.8±29.8	93.3±37.7	0.9	41.3±15.0	48.0±23.2	42.2±13.2	44.1±14.3	0.3
SFA (g/day)	14.3±7.9	15.0±7.2	13.5±4.7	13.7±4.3	0.8	9.1±3.1	9.3±4.8	4.9±1.2	11.7±5.4	0.3
MUFA (g/day)	15.9±4.4	18.3±5.3	14.3±4.2	15.6±5.9	0.4	6.6±3.7	11.2±3.8	12.2±2.6	13.5±3.8	0.5
PUFA (g/day)	15.4±3.2	16.9±5.4	16.5±2.6	17.4±6.3	0.5	17.1±8.4	19.4±6.4	14.6±5.5	12.2±8.4	0.8
Dietary Fiber (g/day)	10.7±3.9	8.7±3.0	8.7±3.2	9.9±4.6	0.6	12.3±2.7	9.7±3.2	10.5±4.5	11.9±4.1	0.7

SFA: Saturated fatty acid; MUFA: Mono unsaturated fatty acid; PUFA: Poly unsaturated fatty acid
*Mean±SD
†One-way ANOVA: Comparison of between-group differences; **p<0.05 considered significant**

Tabe 3. The effects of supplementation and genotype and their interaction on anthropometric indices and biochemical parameters in each genotype in Licorice and placebo group

Variables	At the baseline				At the end				P-value†		
	Licorice		Placebo		Licorice		Placebo		suppl‡	Geno-type††	Intera-ction**
	Pro/Pro	Pro/Ala	Pro/Pro	Pro/Ala	Pro/Pro	Pro/Ala	Pro/Pro	Pro/Ala			
Weight (kg)	89.8±18.4	86.3±11.3	83.2±9.8	79.9±5.9	82.7±12.5	84.6±10.7	79.9±8.8	78.9±6.7	0.2	**0.03**	0.4
BMI (kg/m²)	34.3±5.2	32.9±2.0	33.4±3.3	33.3±2.3	31.8±4.1	32.2±2.0	32.1±2.6	32.9±2.6	0.2	**0.03**	0.4
WC (cm)	109.2±14.0	101.2±10.2	110.3±11.0	106.1±9.0	102.5±12.1	99.0±8.5	101.5±10.1	104.2±10.5	0.5	**<0.01**	0.5
WHR	0.93±0.08	0.86±0.10	0.98±0.09	0.94±0.09	0.91±0.08	0.85±0.11	0.92±0.11	0.93±0.10	0.5	**0.04**	0.4
FBS (mg/dL)	100±8.6	97.2±7.6	97.0±8.6	94.5±6.5	102.2±6.7	96.8±7.3	96.4±8.1	96.4±5.5	0.8	0.8	0.1
Insulin	9.0 (5.3,13.2)‡	10.5 (7,14.5)	8.5 (4.2,10.0)	9.0 (4.7,16.6)	6.8 (4.6,10.8)	8.1 (5.6,10.5)	4.0 (2.5,7.8)	6.7 (2.7,10.4)	0.7	0.2	0.08
QUICKI	0.34±0.03	0.34±0.02	0.35±0.02	0.35±0.04	0.35±0.04	0.35±0.02	0.38±0.04	0.34±0.02	0.9	**0.04**	0.1

BMI: Body mass index; WC: Waist circumference; WHR: Waist to hip ratio; FBS: Fasting blood sugar; QUICKI: Quantitative insulin sensitivity check index
*Mean±SD; † Two-way ANOVA: Comparison of changes in variables at the end of the study; ‡ The effect of Licorice supplement on outcome variable; †† The effect of PPARγ (Pro12Ala) on outcome variable;** The gene-supplement interaction on outcome variable
p<0.05 considered significant

Discussion

Our findings indicated that independent of the licorice supplementation, body weight, BMI, WC and WHR decreased and QUICKI increased in obese subjects with regard to the Pro12Ala polymorphism of PPAR-γ2 gene. In subjects with Pro/Pro genotype, more changes were observed at the end of the study. Furthermore, no interactions between gene and interventions were found.

There are limited clinical trials on anti-obesity effects of supplementation with Licorice or its active components. Tominaga et al. found that 300 and 1800 mg/day supplementation with Kaneka Glavonoid rich oil [TM] (LFO) suppressed weight gain in overweight subjects after 3 months. In another study by Tominaga et al., 300 mg/day LFO decreased WC and visceral fat after 3 months.[4] According to Armanina et al. study, 3.5 g/day Licorice root did not change BMI in normal weight

subjects after 8 weeks. They suggested that positive effects of licorice may be due to its strong taste that can decrease food intake and appetite.[17] Possible anti-obesity mechanisms for licorice are as follows: 1) regulation of lipid metabolism and lipolysis through effects on gene expression in fatty acid synthesis pathways and increase of fatty acid oxidation[5,2]) activation of PPAR-γ gene[5,3]) reduction in appetite due to strong taste [17] and 4) reduction in fat intestinal absorption.[6]

However, two clinical trials have not shown the anti-obesity effects of licorice. Bell et al. reported that Glavonoid[TM] (Licorice Flavenoid Oil (LFO)) did not reduce body weight and WC in overweight and grade I-II obese subjects after 8 weeks.[16] Hajiaghamohammadi et al. also reported that 2 g/day aqueous licorice extract did not reduce BMI in patients with non-alcoholic fatty liver disease after 8 weeks.[15] Discrepancy in findings might be related to differences in individual's characteristics, study design, dosage and type of licorice supplement, disease background, dietary intake, physical activity level, duration of the intervention and genotypes.

In our study, we compared the efficacy of licorice supplement in combination with a low-calorie diet vs. a low-calorie diet alone with regard to the Pro12Ala polymorphism. It seems that no clinical trial has evaluated the licorice-gene interactions in obesity management. But in some previous studies, the effects of weight-loss diet on subjects with respect to the Pro/Ala genotype were evaluated. In line with our study, Vogel et al., indicated that following a 6-wk very low calorie diet (VLCD), weight reduction in overweight/ obese subjects with Pro12Pro genotype was more than Pro12Ala genotype.[27] But Delahanty et al., demonstrated that independent of intervention (metformin intake and lifestyle changes), weight reduction in pre-diabetic obese subjects with Pro/Ala genotype was more than homozygote subjects after 6 months.[22] Based on Goyenechea et al's study, the Pro12Ala genotype was also more frequently reported in Spanish subjects with successful weight maintenance after 10 weeks of dietary intervention.[28] Curti et al., showed that lifestyle modifications decreased body weight in subjects with high risk of cardiovascular diseases independent of the PPAR-γ2 polymorphism.[29] In our study, no interactions between PPAR-γ2 and licorice supplementation were observed. Anthropometric indices were decreased in the homozygote subjects for Pro more than heterozygotes independent of the intervention. Differences in race, study design, intervention, gene-gene interactions and gene –intervention interactions might lead to different findings.

In the present study, irrespective to the intervention, a significant difference in QUICKI was observed in genotype subgroups at the end of the study. Increase of QUICKI was more in subjects with Pro/Pro genotype compared to the Pro/Ala genotype. Limited clinical trials evaluated the effects of licorice on glycemic status. Tominaga *et al.* found that 1800 mg/day LFO did not change FBS and insulin concentrations in overweight subject after 12 weeks.[4] But Luan *et al.* indicated that 10 μM glabridin reduced insulin level and insulin resistance in women with polycystic ovary syndrome after 12 months.[30] Based on Wu *et al.* study, glabridin decreased FBS and insulin resistance after 28 days in diabetic mice. They suggested that antioxidative property of glabridin might lead to anti-hyperglycemic effects of glabridin in diabetic model.[13] Moreover in some studies, anti-diabetic effects of glycyrrhizin were reported.[31,32] Glycyrrihizin can elevate PPAR-γ and glucose transporter 4 proteins in skeletal muscles and modulate glycemic status.[33,34] In our study, owing to mineral corticoid actions and presser effects of Glycyrrihizin,[35] Glycyrrihizin had been reduced to <0.01. This issue might result in no significant reduction in FBS and insulin concentrations. Moreover, disease background, BMI, dosages and form

of licorice or its pure ingredients and the duration of intervention can involve in varying findings.

There are limited studies with contrasting findings on possible associations between the Pro12Ala and insulin response to calorie restriction. In contrary to our findings, Curti et al., reported that Pro12Ala polymorphism made no impact on glycemic status in responses to a low-calorie diet concurrent with exercise in Brazilians at high cardiometabolic risk.[29] Stefanski et al. found no differences in insulin resistance and insulin secretion between the genotype groups in people with long-standing type 2 diabetes (BMI ≥30 kg/m^2, a mean age of 64 years).[36] But Garaulet et al. reported a protective role for the Ala12 allele against insulin resistance in a Spanish overweight/obese population who adhered to a Mediterranean diet and physical activity program for losing weight.[23] Delahanty et al. also concluded that independent of the intervention, a significant association between the Ala12 allele at PPAR-γ was observed after short and long-term weight loss.[22]

In the present study, no participants had the Ala/Ala genotype, and previous studies have shown that Ala/Ala is found at zero frequency in many Asian populations.[37] However, results would be more reliable if a larger sample size was studied. The main mechanism in the association between the Pro12Ala genotype and insulin sensitivity was not clear. However, the protective effect of a functional variant against insulin resistance was probably due to a reduction in transcriptional activity of PPAR-γ2 by activating a ligand-independent domain in the N-terminal. The location of the Pro12Ala substitution in the N-terminal region means that it can be involved in reducing transcription, as well as its association between genotypes and increased insulin activity.[22]

The present study had some limitations. Sample size was relatively small and we did not find the Ala12Ala polymorphism in our study population. However, its frequency has often been reported as being too low in other populations. Moreover in the present study, other polymorphisms of the PPAR-γ2 gene were not evaluated. The strengths of the current study are as follows: it was double blinded and gene/intervention interaction was examined. Furthermore, the measured parameters were adjusted for some known confounding factors.

Conclusion

In Iranian obese subjects, it seems the Pro/Pro polymorphism of the PPAR-γ2 gene induce favourable effects on obesity management and insulin sensitivity. Furthermore, our findings did not support greater benefits for licorice supplementation vs. a low-calorie diet alone. Further clinical trials are needed to clarify whether PPAR-γ2 polymorphism or other obesity gene polymorphism can affect responses to obesity treatment.

Acknowledgments

We are grateful to the participants for their cooperation. The authors also would like to thank Drug Applied

Research Center, Tabriz University of Medical Sciences for funding of the project.

Ethical Issues

The present study was approved by the Ethical Committee of Tabriz University of Medical Sciences and it was registered on the Iranian Registry of Clinical Trials (IRCT registration number: IRCT2013062811288N3).

Conflict of Interest

The authors declare no conflict of interests.

References

1. Khanahmadi M, Naghdi Badi H, Akhondzadeh S, Khalighi–Sigaroodi F, Mehrafarin A, Shahriari S, et al. A Review on Medicinal Plant of Glycyrrhiza glabra L. *J Med Plant Res* 2013; 2(46): 1-12.
2. Prajapati S, Patel BR. Phyto Pharmacological Perspective of Yashtimadhu Glycyrrhiza Glabra LINN A Review. *Int J Pharm Biol Arch* 2013;4(5):833-41.
3. Kaur R, Kaur H, Dhindsa AS. Glycyrrhiza glabra: a phytopharmacological review. *Int J Pharmaceut Sci Res* 2013;4(7):2470-7. doi:10.13040/IJPSR.0975-8232.4(7).2470-2477.
4. Tominaga Y, Mae T, Kitano M, Sakamoto Y, Ikematsu H, Nakagawa K. Licorice flavonoid oil effects body weight loss by reduction of body fat mass in overweight subjects. *Int J Health Sci* 2006;52(6):672-83. doi:10.1248/jhs.52.672
5. Aoki F, Honda S, Kishida H, Kitano M, Arai N, Tanaka H, et al. Suppression by licorice flavonoids of abdominal fat accumulation and body weight gain in high-fat diet-induced obese c57bl/6j mice. *Biosci Biotech Bioch* 2007;71(1):206-14.
6. Malik ZA, Sharma PL. An ethanolic extract from licorice (glycyrrhiza glabra) exhibits anti-obesity effects by decreasing dietary fat absorption in a high fat diet-induced obesity rat model. *Int J Pharmaceut Sci Res* 2011;2(11):3010-3. doi:10.13040/IJPSR.0975-8232.2(11).3010-18.
7. Kamisoyama H, Honda K, Tominaga Y, Yokota S, Hasegawa S. Investigation of the anti-obesity action of licorice flavonoid oil in diet-induced obese rats. *Biosci Biotech Bioch* 2008;72(12):3225-31. doi:10.1271/bbb.80469
8. Nakagawa K, Kishida H, Arai N, Nishiyama T, Mae T. Licorice flavonoids suppress abdominal fat accumulation and increase in blood glucose level in obese diabetic kk-a(y) mice. *Biol Pharm Bull* 2004;27(11):1775-8.
9. Ahn J, Lee H, Jang J, Kim S, Ha T. Anti-obesity effects of glabridin-rich supercritical carbon dioxide extract of licorice in high-fat-fed obese mice. *Food Chem Toxicol* 2013;51:439-45. doi:10.1016/j.fct.2012.08.048
10. World Health Organization. Obesity and overweight fact sheet [data base on the internet] UK: WHO Media centre; 2015; cited 28 November 2015; Available from: www.who.int/mediacentre/factsheets/fs311/en.
11. Nisoli E, Carruba MO. Emerging aspects of pharmacotherapy for obesity and metabolic syndrome. *Pharmacol Res* 2004;50(5):453-69. doi: 10.1016/j.phrs.2004.02.004
12. Mirtaheri E, Namazi N, Alizadeh M, Sargheini N, Karimi S. Effects of dried licorice extract with low-calorie diet on lipid profile and atherogenic indices in overweight and obese subjects: A randomized controlled clinical trial. *Eur J Integr Med* 2015;7(3):287-93. doi: 10.1016/j.eujim.2015.03.006
13. Wu F, Jin Z, Jin J. Hypoglycemic effects of glabridin, a polyphenolic flavonoid from licorice, in an animal model of diabetes mellitus. *Mol Med Rep* 2013;7(4):1278-82. doi: 10.3892/mmr.2013.1330
14. Zhao H, Wang Y, Wu L, Yongping MA. Effect of licorice flavonoids on blood glucose, blood lipid and other biochemical indicators in type 2 diabetic rats. *China J Physiol* 2012;1:30-3.
15. Hajiaghamohammadi AA, Ziaee A, Samimi R. The efficacy of licorice root extract in decreasing transaminase activities in non-alcoholic fatty liver disease: A randomized controlled clinical trial. *Phytother Res* 2012;26(9):1381-4. doi: 10.1002/ptr.3728
16. Bell ZW, Canale RE, Bloomer RJ. A dual investigation of the effect of dietary supplementation with licorice flavonoid oil on anthropometric and biochemical markers of health and adiposity. *Lipids Health Dis* 2011;10:29. doi: 10.1186/1476-511X-10-29
17. Armanini D, De Palo CB, Mattarello MJ, Spinella P, Zaccaria M, Ermolao A, et al. Effect of licorice on the reduction of body fat mass in healthy subjects. *J Endocrinol Invest* 2003;26(7):646-50. doi: 10.1007/BF03347023
18. Gonzalez Sanchez JL, Serrano Rios M, Fernandez Perez C, Laakso M, Martinez Larrad MT. Effect of the pro12ala polymorphism of the peroxisome proliferator-activated receptor gamma-2 gene on adiposity, insulin sensitivity and lipid profile in the spanish population. *Eur J Endocrinol* 2002;147(4):495-501.
19. Passaro A, Dalla Nora E, Marcello C, Di Vece F, Morieri ML, Sanz JM, et al. Ppargamma pro12ala and ace id polymorphisms are associated with bmi and fat distribution, but not metabolic syndrome. *Cardiovasc Diabetol* 2011;10:112. doi: 10.1186/1475-2840-10-112
20. Prakash J, Srivastava N, Awasthi S, Agarwal C, Natu S, Rajpal N, et al. Association of ppar-gamma gene polymorphisms with obesity and obesity-associated phenotypes in north indian population. *Am J Hum Biol* 2012;24(4):454-9. doi: 10.1002/ajhb.22245
21. Masud S, Ye S, Group SAS. Effect of the peroxisome proliferator activated receptor-gamma

gene pro12ala variant on body mass index: A meta-analysis. *J Med Genet* 2003;40(10):773-80.

22. Delahanty LM, Pan Q, Jablonski KA, Watson KE, McCaffery JM, Shuldiner A, et al. Genetic predictors of weight loss and weight regain after intensive lifestyle modification, metformin treatment, or standard care in the diabetes prevention program. *Diabetes Care* 2012;35(2):363-6. doi: 10.2337/dc11-1328

23. Garaulet M, Smith CE, Hernandez-Gonzalez T, Lee YC, Ordovas JM. Ppargamma pro12ala interacts with fat intake for obesity and weight loss in a behavioural treatment based on the mediterranean diet. *Mol Nutr Food Res* 2011;55(12):1771-9. doi: 10.1002/mnfr.201100437

24. Mirzayi H, Golmohammadi T, Akrami M, Dusti M, Nakhjavani M, Heshmati R, et al. Assosiation between PPAR-γ2 polymorphism with obesity in Iranian population. *Iranian J Diabetes Lipid* 2006; 6(1):9-16.

25. Dumville JC, Hahn S, Miles JN, Torgerson DJ. The use of unequal randomisation ratios in clinical trials: A review. *Contemp Clin Trials* 2006;27(1):1-12. doi: 10.1016/j.cct.2005.08.003

26. Craig CL, Marshall AL, Sjöström M, Bauman AE, Booth ML, Ainsworth BE, et al. International physical activity questionnaire: 12-country reliability and validity. *Med sci sports Exerc* 2003;35(8):1381-95. doi: 10.1249/01.MSS.0000078924.61453.FB.

27. Vogels N, Mariman EC, Bouwman FG, Kester AD, Diepvens K, Westerterp-Plantenga MS. Relation of weight maintenance and dietary restraint to peroxisome proliferator-activated receptor gamma2, glucocorticoid receptor, and ciliary neurotrophic factor polymorphisms. *Am J Clin Nutr* 2005;82(4):740-6.

28. Goyenechea E, Dolores Parra M, Alfredo Martinez J. Weight regain after slimming induced by an energy-restricted diet depends on interleukin-6 and peroxisome-proliferator-activated-receptor-gamma2 gene polymorphisms. *Br J Nutr* 2006;96(5):965-72.

29. Curti ML, Rogero MM, Baltar VT, Barros CR, Siqueira-Catania A, Ferreira SR. Fto t/a and peroxisome proliferator-activated receptor-gamma pro12ala polymorphisms but not apoa1 -75 are associated with better response to lifestyle intervention in brazilians at high cardiometabolic risk. *Metab Syndr Relat Disord* 2013;11(3):169-76. doi: 10.1089/met.2012.0055

30. Luan B-G, Sun C-X. Effect of glabridinon on insulin resistance, C-reactive protein and endothelial function in young women with polycystic ovary syndrome. *Bangl J Pharmacol* 2015;10(3):681-7. doi: 10.3329/bjp.v10i3.23648.

31. Sen S, Roy M, Chakraborti AS. Ameliorative effects of glycyrrhizin on streptozotocin-induced diabetes in rats. *J Pharm Pharmacol* 2011;63(2):287-96. doi: 10.1111/j.2042-7158.2010.01217.x

32. Takii H, Kometani T, Nishimura T, Nakae T, Okada S, Fushiki T. Antidiabetic effect of glycyrrhizin in genetically diabetic kk-ay mice. *Biol Pharm Bull* 2001;24(5):484-7.

33. Xie W, Du L. Diabetes is an inflammatory disease: Evidence from traditional chinese medicines. *Diabetes Obes Metab* 2011;13(4):289-301. doi: 10.1111/j.1463-1326.2010.01336.x

34. Yaw HP, Ton SH, Chin HF, Karim MK, Fernando HA, Kadir KA. Modulation of lipid metabolism in glycyrrhizic acid-treated rats fed on a high-calorie diet and exposed to short or long-term stress. *Int J Physiol Pathophysiol Pharmacol* 2015;7(1):61-75.

35. Bayati Zadeh JB, Kor ZM, Goftar MK. Licorice (Glycyrrhiza glabra Linn) as a valuable medicinal plant. *Int J Adv Biol Biomed Res* 2013;1:1281-8.

36. Stefanski A, Majkowska L, Ciechanowicz A, Frankow M, Safranow K, Parczewski M, et al. Lack of association between the pro12ala polymorphism in ppar-gamma2 gene and body weight changes, insulin resistance and chronic diabetic complications in obese patients with type 2 diabetes. *Arch Med Res* 2006;37(6):736-43. doi: 10.1016/j.arcmed.2006.01.009

37. Namvaran F, Rahimi-Moghaddam P, Azarpira N. Genotyping of peroxisome proliferator-activated receptor gamma (ppar-gamma) polymorphism (pro12ala) in iranian population. *J Res Med Sci* 2011;16(3):291-6.

11

Lactobacillus Casei Decreases Organophosphorus Pesticide Diazinon Cytotoxicity in Human HUVEC Cell Line

Hasan Bagherpour Shamloo[1,2], **Saber Golkari**[2], **Zeinab Faghfoori**[3,4], **AliAkbar Movassaghpour**[5], **Hajie Lotfi**[6], **Abolfazl Barzegari**[6], **Ahmad Yari Khosroushahi**[7,8]*

[1] *Biotechnology Research Center, Tabriz University of Medical Sciences, Tabriz, Iran.*
[2] *Dryland Agricultural Research Institute (DARI), Agricultural Research, Education and Extension Organization (AREEO), Maragheh, Iran.*
[3] *Tuberculosis & Lung Research Center, Tabriz University of Medical Sciences, Tabriz, Iran.*
[4] *Student Research Committee, Faculty of Nutrition, Tabriz University of Medical Sciences, Tabriz, Iran.*
[5] *Hematology and Oncology Research Center, Tabriz University of Medical Sciences, Tabriz, Iran.*
[6] *Department of Medical Biotechnology, Faculty of Advanced Medical Science, Tabriz University of Medical Sciences, Tabriz 51664, Iran.*
[7] *Drug Applied Research Center, Tabriz University of Medical Sciences, Tabriz, Iran.*
[8] *Department of Pharmacognosy, Faculty of Pharmacy, Tabriz University of Medical Sciences, Tabriz, Iran.*

Keywords:
· Apoptosis
· Cytotoxicity
· Diazinon
· *Lactobacillus casei*
· Probiotic

Abstract

Purpose: Exposure to diazinon can trigger acute and chronic toxicity and significantly induces DNA damage and proapoptotic effects in different human cells. Due to the significance of probiotic bacteria antitoxin effect, this study aimed to investigate the effect of *Lactobacillus casei* on diazinon (DZN) cytotoxicity in human umbilical vein endothelial cells (HUVEC) *in vitro*.

Methods: The cytotoxicity assessments were performed by MTT (3-(4,5-dimethylthiazol-2-yl)-2,5-diphenyltetrazolium bromide) test, DAPI (4',6-diamidino-2-phenylindole) staining and flow cytometric methodologies.

Results: Cytotoxic assessments through flow cytometry/ DAPI staining demonstrated that apoptosis is the main cytotoxic mechanism of diazinon in HUVEC cells and *L. casei* could decrease the diazinon cytotoxic effects on toxicants.

Conclusion: the screen of total bacterial secreted metabolites can be considered as a wealthy source to find the new active compounds to introduce as reducing agricultural remained pesticide cytotoxicity effects on the human food chain.

Introduction

Pesticides are widely used to increase the agricultural production through the control of the harmful insects' populations. Among these pesticides, the organophosphorus pesticides accounted for 50 percent of all insecticide applications.[1,2] Diazinon, (O, O - diethyl O -2-isopropyl-6-methylpyrimidin-4-yl phosphorothioate), a broad-spectrum organophosphorus pesticide, is used on a wide range of crops such as rice, fruits, wine grapes, sugarcane, corn, and potatoes.[3] The main concern about the utilization of pesticides such as diazinon (DZN) is their residual amount in agricultural products, soil and water.[4,5] Pesticides are stored in various tissues of plants that enter the human food chain through the consumption of the edible segments. According to the commission of the European communities report, 45 percent of fruits and vegetables contain maximum residue levels of pesticides (MRLs).[6] Monitoring of pesticide residue in Brazilian fruits has indicated that 14.3% of samples exceeded European Union MRLs.[7]

DZN inhibits the acetylcholinesterase enzyme activity that hydrolyzes the neurotransmitter acetylcholine in cholinergic synapses and neuromuscular junctions.[3,8] Exposure to DZN leads to acute symptoms such as anorexia, diarrhea, generalized weakness, muscle tremors, abnormal posturing and behavior, depression and even death as well as chronic effects including genotoxicity, immunotoxicity, effects on the reproductive system, damage to brain and intestinal cells.[3,9-11] The organophosphorus pesticides significantly induce DNA damage and pro-apoptotic effects in many different healthy cells.[12,13] Environmental protection agency (EPA) classifies DZN as "not likely a human carcinogen", but experimental studies have confirmed its carcinogenicity such as leukemia, non-Hodgkin's lymphoma besides lung, brain and prostate cancers.[14]

*Corresponding author: Ahmad Yari Khosroushahi, Email: yarikhosroushahia@tbzmed.ac.ir

Probiotic bacteria are living microorganisms and when are administered in adequate amounts, confer health benefits on the host.[15] Probiotics may have positive effects on toxic substances and performance or on toxicity of transferred drugs or toxins into the body.[16] Numerous studies have previously shown the probiotics beneficial effects on human health through their antimicrobial effects, antitoxin effects, the improvement of intestinal barrier function, the modulation of immune responses, the impacts on apoptosis and cell proliferation, and anti-oxidant function.[17,18] Several studies have assayed the viability, the colonization ability, and the binding capacity of probiotics to toxic substances.[19] *Lactobacillus casei* strain DN114001 can bind to heterocyclic aromatic amines *in vitro* and can decrease the concentration and the genotoxicity of these amines.[19] Various strains of bifidobacteria hand in hand with *Lactobacillus reuteri* strain NRRL14171 and *Lactobacillus casei* strain Shirota were able to bind to aflatoxin B$_1$ that can be attributed to the presence of these bacteria in the gastrointestinal tract which may prevent the absorption of aflatoxins.[20,21] *Lactobacillus kefir* strains (CIDCA 83115, 8321, 8345 and 8348) were able to bind to *Clostridium* difficile toxins by surface layer (s-layer) proteins.[22] By considering the aforementioned issues, this study aimed to evaluate the effects of *lactobacillus casei* secretion metabolites on the toxicity of agricultural organophosphorus pesticide (diazinon) through investigating the metabolites effects on diazinon treated/untreated human normal cell line, HUVEC *in vitro*.

Materials and Methods
Bacteria isolation
Lactobacillus casei was isolated from the traditional yogurt samples collected from East Azarbayjan, the northwest province in Iran. 5 g of each sample was suspended in 2% w/v sodium citrate solution and homogenized using the Stomacher 400 Circulator (Seward Laboratory Systems Inc, USA) for 2 min. Afterwards, 1 ml of the samples was added to 24 ml of de Man Rogosa and Sharpe (MRS, Merck, Germany) broth medium and incubated at 37 °C for 24 h. After the incubation time, the bacteria were isolated by spreading them on a de Man Rogosa and Sharpe (MRS, Merck, Germany) agar plate similar to the previous condition. Many single colonies were randomly selected and again incubated in 5 ml MRS broth for 24 h. The individual colonies were subjected to morphological evaluation. Gram positive and catalase negative bacilli colonies were stored at -80°C in MRS supplemented with glycerol 25% (v/v).

Molecular identification by 16S rDNA
Total genomic DNA was extracted from the cultures inoculated with a single colony using the previously described procedure by Drisko.[23] For this purpose, 1.5 ml of the bacterial culture, a single sub-cultured colony in MRS broth for 24 h at 37°C, was centrifuged at 10000×g

for 5 min and the cell pellet was used to isolate the DNA. All the extracted genomic DNAs of the samples, resuspended in 50 µl distilled water, were then checked and visualized via 0.8% agarose gel electrophoresis. Subsequently, the gel monitoring apparatus (Biometra, Gottingen, Germany) and spectrophotometric method were used to evaluate the quality and quantity of the extracted DNA, respectively. The PCR amplification was conducted in a thermal cycler PTC 200 (MJC research, Waltham, USA) by using a pair of LAB-specific universal primers (LABF 5′-AGATTTTGATCMTGGCTCAG-3′ and LABR 5′-TACCTTGTTAGGACTTCACC-3′). PCR amplification was performed using the following temperature profile: an initial denaturation at 94°C for 4 min, followed by 32 cycles of denaturation at 94°C for 1 min, annealing at 58°C for 1 min, extension at 72°C for 1 min, and a final extension step at 72°C for 5 min.[24] The PCR products were determined by electrophoresis in a 1% (w/v) agarose gel and were visualized through ethidium bromide staining. The PCR products were sequenced at Sinaclone Corporation, Tehran, Iran. The sequences were then analyzed using the BLAST program of the National Center for Biotechnology Information (http://www.ncbi.nlm.nih.gov/BLAST).

Acid and bile salt tolerance
The isolated cells were harvested from the cultures incubated overnight followed by centrifugation for 10 min at 6000×g and 4°C . The cell pellets were then resuspended in PBS (80 mM Na2HPO4, 1.5 M NaCl, 20 mM KH2PO4, 30 mM KCl, pH 3.0) and were incubated at 37°C for 3 h in MRS broth. The viable cells after low pH treatment were subjected to PBS (80 mM Na2HPO4, 1.5 M NaCl, 20 mM KH2PO4, 30 mM KCl, pH 7.2) containing 0.3% (w/v) of bile salt (Sigma Chemical Co., St. Louis, Mo., USA) then were incubated at 37°C for 4 h in MRS broth. Proper dilutions based on 1 h time intervals were performed, and the dilutions were centrifuged for 10 min at 6000×g and 4°C then the cell plates (acid and bile salt resistance bacteria) were incubated at 37°C in anaerobic conditions for 24 h. The survival of the bacterial cells was evaluated using log phase cultures (8 log$_{10}$CFU ml^{-1}) by plating them on MRS agar after 0, 1, 2, and 3 h of incubation in acidic (pH 3.0)/bile supplemented MRS broth at 37°C via the standard pour plate technique.

The survival rate (for both acid/bile resistance) was calculated using the following equation: survival rate (%) = (log cfu N$_1$/log cfu N$_0$) × 100, where N$_1$ corresponds to the total clones treated with extra bile salts or acids and N$_0$ corresponds to the total clones before they were incubated under harsh conditions.

Antimicrobial activity
Antibacterial activity assessments were conducted against clinically important human pathogens, including native isolate of *E. coli* (026), *Candida albicans* (PTCC 5027), *Escherichia coli* (057) (PTCC 1276), *Salmonella*

enterica subsp. *typhimurium* (ATCC 14028), *Klebsiella pneumoniae* (PTCC 1053), *Shigella flexneri* (PTCC 1234), *Pseudomonas aeruginosa* (PTCC 1181), *Serratia marcesens* (PTCC 1187), *Staphylococcus aureus* (ATCC 25923), *Bacillus cereus* subsp. *kenyae* (PTCC 1539), *Listeria monocytogenes* (PTCC 1163), *Enterococcus faecalis* (PTCC 1394), *Staphylococcus saprophyticus* subsp. *saprophyticus* (PTCC 1440), and *Streptococcus mutans* (PTCC 1683). The overnight cultured isolated strains in MRS broth medium at 37 °C were filtered through 0.2 µm filter, and then 50 µl of each filtrate was added to 7 mm diameter wells on the indicator growth medium agar, which were previously incubated overnight by indicator pathogens at 37 °C. The pH of the isolated fresh supernatants was adjusted to the pH of the each indicator pathogens growth media (Table 1). After the overnight incubation of plates at 37 °C, the clear zones around of each well were measured and considered as positive antibacterial activity. Based on the diameter of the inhibition zone, anti-pathogen activities were divided to strong (diameter $\geq$ 20 mm), moderate (20 mm $\leq$ diameter $\geq$ 10 mm), and weak (diameter $\leq$ 10 mm).[25]

Table 1. Indicator microorganisms and their growth condition

Indicator microorganism	Growth condition
Candida albicans (PTCC 5027)	Yeast mold agar, pH 6.2 ± 0.2
E. coli (026)	Nutrient agar, pH 7.0
Escherichia coli (057)	Nutrient agar, pH 7.0
Salmonella enterica subsp. *typhimurium* (ATCC 14028)	Nutrient agar, pH 7.0
Shigella flexneri (PTCC 1234)	Nutrient agar, pH 7.0
Serratia marcesens (PTCC 1187)	Nutrient agar, pH 7.07.0
Staphylococcus aureus (ATCC 25923)	Micrococcus medium, FDA, pH 7.2
Staphylococcus saprophyticus subsp. *saprophyticus* (PTCC 1440)	Nutrient agar, pH 7.0
Streptococcus mutans (PTCC 1683)	Blood agar, Difco 0045
Klebsiella pneumoniae (PTCC 1053)	Nutrient agar, pH 7.0
Pseudomonas aeruginosa (PTCC 1181)	Nutrient agar, pH 7.0
Bacillus cereus subsp. *kenyae* (PTCC 1539)	Nutrient agar, pH 7.0
Listeria monocytogenes (PTCC 1163)	Blood agar, Difco 0045
Enterococcus faecalis (PTCC 1394)	Blood agar, Difco 0045

Antibiotic susceptibility

To determine the antibiotic susceptibility, the disc diffusion method against some clinically important antibiotics such as chloramphenicol (30 µg), vancomycin (30 µg), tetracycline (30 µg), erythromycin (15 µg), Ampicillin (10 µg), gentamycin (10 µg), clindamycin (2µg), sulfamethoxazol (25µg) and penicillin (10,000 units) was used. The isolated bacteria were completely incubated on the Mueller-Hinton agar plate and then the antibiotic disks (Padtan Teb Co., Tehran, Iran) were manually placed on plates by using the sterile forceps and after 24 h incubation at 37 °C, the clear zones were measured according to disks producer's guidelines. Based on the areola size, the isolates were classified to sensitive, intermediate and resistant groups through the analysis of data.

Cell culture

The Human umbilical vein endothelial cells (HUVEC) were obtained from Pasteur Institute, National Cell Bank of Iran. The cells were cultured into 25 cm² T-flask with cell density (1×10^6 cell/ml) in RPMI 1640 (GIBCO, Uxbridge, UK) medium containing 10% fetal bovine serum (HyClone, Logan, UT, USA) inactivated at 45 °C for 1 h, 100 U/ml penicillin and 100 µg/ml streptomycin

(Sigma, St. Louis, MO, USA) were incubated at 37°C in a humidified atmosphere with 5% CO2. The media of t-flasks were renovated each 48 h intervals. For the cell passage, all cells were detached using 0.025% trypsin-0.02% EDTA (Sigma, St. Louis, MO, USA).

Cell treatment

Lactobacillus casei was cultured overnight in de Man Rogosa (MRS) broth medium (Merck, Darmstadt, Germany). To prepare cell free supernatant, the culture was centrifuged at 4000 rpm for 5 min and the supernatant's pH was adjusted to 7.2 before sterilizing through filtering using 0.2 µm membrane filter (Millipore, Eschborn, Germany). The filtered supernatant was used for the treatment of HUVEC cell line (treated with median-lethal concentration of DZN (IC_{50}: 70 µg/ml) or the untreated control). Diazinon was purchased from Merck (Merck, Darmstadt, Germany) and stored at 25 °C and kept in dark condition. Dissolved DZN in dimethyl sulfoxide (DMSO), in which DMSO was <1% (safe concentration for human cells at *in vitro* condition), with final concentration 100 µg/ml was sterilized using a 0.2 µm filter (Millipore, Eschborn, Germany). Ten concentrations of supernatant, 10-100 µg/ml with 10 intervals, were prepared to determine of DZN IC_{50}.

HUVEC cells (with seeding density 1.2×10^4 cells/well) were directly treated by the formerly-prepared concentrations of DZN with six repetitions for each concentration in 96-well microplates and were incubated for 24 hours at 37 °C and 5% CO_2. After incubation time the treated/untreated HUVEC cell line, cultured in microplate, was used to MTT [3-(4,5-dimethylthiazole-2-yl)-2,5-diphenyl tetrazolium bromide] (Sigma, St. Louis, MO, USA) assay.

50 μl of MTT solution (2 mg/ml in phosphate buffer saline) was added to each well after replacing the previous media with 150 μl of fresh culture medium, then these cells were incubated for 4 h similar to the culture condition. After that, the medium containing MTT was completely removed from each well; subsequently, 200 μl DMSO plus 25 μl of Sorenson's glycine buffer (0.1 M glycine, 0.1 M NaCl, pH 10.5) were added into each well and the microplates were incubated for 25 min at room temperature and finally the absorbance was measured by employing a microplate reader (Biotek, ELx 800, USA) at 570 nm.

DAPI staining

All treated/untreated HUVEC cells' culture medium was removed from the 6 well plates and the attached cells were washed twice by PBS (pH=7.2). The washed cells were fixed by 500 μl of 1% paraformaldehyde for 5 min. To increase the permeability of fixed cells, paraformaldehyde was replaced with 500 μl of 0.1% Triton X-100 and incubated for 10 min at room temperature. The permeabilized cells were subjected to 100 μl of 4', 6-Diamidino-2-phenylindole (DAPI; Vector Laboratories, Burlingame, CA) solution (250 ng/ml for each well) and then were incubated for 10 min at room temperature. The morphological changes were analyzed using a fluorescent microscope (Olympus BX64, Olympus, Japan) equipped with a U-MWU2 fluorescence filter (excitation filter BP 330e385, dichromatic mirror DM 400, and emission filter LP 420).

Flow cytometric analysis

To remove RPMI medium, the detached all treated/untreated control HUVEC cells were centrifuged at 335 ×g for 10 min and the cell plates were washed with PBS (pH=7.2) then were centrifuged again similar to previous condition. During the next phase, the cells were re-suspended in 100 μl binding buffer (1×10^6 cells/ml) of Annexin V-FITC kit (eBioscience, San Diego, CA). The binding buffer containing cells were mixed with 5 μl Annexin V-FITC, next 10 μl propidium iodide solution was added to the cell suspension and were kept in a 5 ml culture tube for 15 min at room temperature in dark conditions. Binding buffer (400 μl) was again added to each culture tube and assessments were conducted using a FACS Calibur flow cytometer (BD Biosciences, San Jose, CA, USA). The analysis on 100,000 cells was accomplished at a rate of 1000 cells/s. Quadrant setting was conducted using the untreated cell line as the negative control. Data analysis was performed using CellQuest Pro software (BD Biosciences, San Jose, CA, USA). Flow cytometry assessments were conducted thrice with three repetitions for each time.

Statistical Analysis

The statistical analysis was performed by SPSS software version 18.0 (SPSSInc, Chicago, IL, USA). The normal distribution of data was tested by Kolmogorov-Smirnov test. ANOVA and Tukey's post hoc test were used for analyzing data and multiple mean comparisons, respectively. Statistical significance was considered a value of P≤ 0.05 and quantitative data were reported as mean ± SD. All experiments were repeated three times with six replicates for each experiment.

Results

Isolation and identification

A total of 22 grown hemispherical white or achromatic colonies was separately propagated for further assessments. The presence of lactic acid bacteria strains in the isolated samples were confirmed by amplifying the 16S rDNA gene using gene-specific primers. Sequences of 16S rDNA gene 1500 bp fragments were blasted with the deposited sequences in GenBank. Isolates with 99% to 100% homology were identified by considering the threshold values of taxonomical studies (97%).[26] These 22 colonies belonged to *Lactobacillus casei* strain YSH, *Lactobacillus paracasei* strain YJ, *Lactobacillus rhamnosus* strain YI, *Lactobacillus fermentum* strain YAL, *Lactobacillus plantarum* strain YSH1, and *Lactobacillus delbrueckii* strain YJI.

Resistance to acid and bile salt

The survival rates of the six isolated LAB strains after incubating for 3 h at pH 3 and in 0.3% bile salt (oxgall; Sigma Chemical Co., St. Louis, Mo., USA) are shown in Table 2. Based on the results, all six selected strains retained their viability at the mentioned harshness condition where the tolerance to acidic/high bile salt conditions was strain specific. The survival rates ranging from 73% to 85% were observed in *Lactobacillus* strains at acidic condition, whereas the survival rates, ranging from 92% to 98%, were observed in bile salt condition. The strains with the most efficient tolerance to acidic conditions were *L. plantarum* strain YSH1, *L. rhamnosus* strain YI, *L. delbrueckii* strain YJI, and *L. casei* strain YSH with survival rates of 85%, 82%, 81%, and 78%, respectively. Meanwhile, the six isolates showed high survival rates with >90% under high bile conditions. The strains with the highest tolerance to 0.3% oxgall were *L. casei* strain YSH, *L. fermentum* strain YAL, *L. rhamnosus* strain YI with the survival rates of 98%, 98%, and 96%, respectively.

Antimicrobial activity

Table 3 shows the 6 isolated strains, including *L. casei* strain YSH, *L. paracasei* strain YJ, *L. rhamnosus* strain YI, *L. fermentum* strain YAL, *L. plantarum* strain YSH1, and *L. delbrueckii* strain YJI displayed significant anti-pathogenic activities against indicator microorganisms. *Lactobacillus* species, particularly *L. casei* strain YSH, showed the most efficient antagonistic activity and inhibited the growth of 13 indicator pathogens among the isolated bacteria. Meanwhile, *L. rhamnosus* strain YI, and *L. paracasei* strain YJ exhibited an overall good antagonistic activity and inhibited the growth of indicator pathogens.

Table 2. The survival rates of isolated LAB after 3 h incubation at pH 3 and 0.3% bile salts

Bacteria	pH 3 Final counts (log cfu/ml) after incubation at:					0.3% bile salt Final counts (log cfu/ml) after incubation at:				
	0 h	1h	2h	3 h	SR(%)	0h	1h	2h	3 h	SR(%)
L. paracasei strain YJ	8.873	8.754	7.124	6.743	76	8.768	8.754	8.124	8.066	92
L. plantarum strain YSH1	8.401	8.112	7.325	7.14	85	8.783	8.712	8.325	8.256	94
L. delbrueckii strain YJI	8.974	8.589	7.412	7.268	81	8.875	8.789	8.512	8.431	95
L. fermentum strain YAL	8.900	8.613	6.704	6.497	73	8.687	8.613	8.604	8.513	98
L. casei strain YSH	8.683	8.454	7.012	6.772	78	8.434	8.354	8.312	8.265	98
L. rhamnosus strain YI	8.291	8.004	6.918	6.798	82	8.394	8.304	8.118	8.058	96

SR: Survival Rate

Table 3. The inhibitory effect of isolated strains against pathogenic microorganisms

Pathogens	Diameter of inhibition zone (mm)					
	YJ	YSH	YI	YAL	YSH1	YJI
P. aeruginosa	13.3±1.2	12.3±0.3	14.0±1.0	15.3±0.7	16.7±0.3	16.0±0.6
C. albicans	0.0±0.0	11.0±0.0	12.3±0.3	0.0±0.0	15.0±0.0	0.0±0.0
S. marcesens	13.7±0.3	18.3±0.0	14.7±0.3	13.0±0.6	14.0±1.0	13.0±0.0
E. faecalis	0.0±0.0	11.0±0.0	12.0±0.0	0.0±0.0	15.3±1.2	0.0±0.0
S. saprophyticus	0.0±0.0	12.3±0.7	0.0±0.0	14.0±0.6	0.0±0.0	0.0±0.0
S. mutans	12.0±0.0	18.3±0.6	0.0±0.0	0.0±0.0	0.0±0.0	13.3±1.2
E. coli (0157)	14.7±1.2	11.0±0.0	12.0±1.0	0.0±0.0	15.3±0.3	15.0±0.0
S. typhimurium	0.0±0.0	13.3±1.2	12.3±1.2	0.0±0.0	13.3±0.3	0.0±0.0
S. aureus	0.0±0.0	12.7±0.3	15.7±0.3	0.0±0.0	15.0±0.0	15.7±1.2
E. coli (026)	0.0±0.0	13.3±0.7	13.3±0.6	0.0±0.0	15.7±0.3	0.0±0.0
B. cereus	0.0±0.0	11.0±0.0	0.0±0.0	0.0±0.0	0.0±0.0	0.0±0.0
L. monocytogenes	0.0±0.0	14.7±0.9	16.7±0.7	0.0±0.0	17.0±0.0	0.0±0.0
K. pneumoniae	14.3±0.7	13.0±0.6	12.3±0.7	12.7±1.2	13.3±1.2	13.0±1.0
S. flexneri	14.0±0.0	13.0±0.0	13.0±0.0	12.0±0.0	14.0±0.6	13.3±0.7

Notes: values are mean ± standard error
S (strong *r* ≥20 mm), M (moderate *r*<20 mm and >10 mm), and W (weak ≤10 mm)
Lactobacillus casei strain YSH, *Lactobacillus paracasei* strain YJ, *Lactobacillus rhamnosus* strain YI, *Lactobacillus fermentum* strain YAL, *Lactobacillus plantarum* strain YSH1, and *Lactobacillus delbrueckii* strain YJI

Antibiotic susceptibility

The antibiotic susceptibility of the isolated bacteria against the high consumption antibiotics was evaluated using the measurements of inhibition zone diameter. The antibiotic susceptibility results of the six isolated LAB against clinically important antibiotics are presented in Table 4. Based on our findings, all six isolated bacteria were sensitive or semi-sensitive to tetracycline and clindamycin. *Lactobacillus* strains generally displayed the highest susceptibility to the majority of antibiotics. *L.* *casei* strain YSH displayed the best results and was sensitive or semi-sensitive to all antibiotics.

The effect of L. casei on diazinon toxicity

The effect of different concentrations of DZN on cell proliferation was measured by MTT assay. DZN at concentration of 70 μg/ml reduced the viability of HUVEC cell lines by 50.97% in a dose-response manner, so, this concentration was selected as IC50 of diazinon in this study and used in other treatments. Among the other strains, *L. casei* cell free supernatant

(50 µg/ml) significantly increased the cell viability compared with control (p≤0.01) while DZN IC$_{50}$ increased cell death at a concentration of 70 µg/ml (p≤ 0.01).The treatment of HUVEC cell line with IC50 of

diazinon and *L. casei* secreted metabolites showed a significant decrease in the cytotoxicity of DZN on HUVEC cell lines (Figure 1).

Table 4. Antibiotic susceptibility of isolated LAB against the high consumption antibiotics by disc diffusion assay

Isolated Strains	Diameter of inhibition zone (mm)								
	C	TE	ER	AM	GE	CC	SLX	P	V
L. casei strain YSH	30S	30S	23I	32S	15S	26S	22S	23S	22S
L. plantarum strain YSH1	20S	20S	20I	40S	11S	18S	25S	40S	0R
L. delbrueckii strain YJI	23S	25S	25S	28S	25S	27S	0R	23S	0R
L. fermentum strain YAL	28S	18S	26S	26S	18S	27S	0R	15I	24S
L. paracasei strain YJ	20S	20S	0R	24S	13S	30S	15I	24S	30S
L. rhamnosus strain YI	22S	30S	20I	25S	12S	20S	22S	24S	15S

chloramphenicol; TE: tetracycline; ER: erythromycin; AM: Ampicillin; GE: gentamycin; CC: clindamycin; SLX: sulfamethoxazol; P: penicillin; V: vancomycin
Erythromycin results based on R ≤13 mm; I: 13–23 mm; S≥23 mm.
Gentamycin results based on R ≤6 mm; I: 7–9 mm; S≥10 mm.
Vancomycin results based on R ≤12 mm; I: 12–13 mm; S≥13 mm.
I: intermediate (zone diameter, 12.5–17.4mm); R: resistant (zone diameter, ≤12.4mm); S: susceptible (zone diameter, ≥17.5).

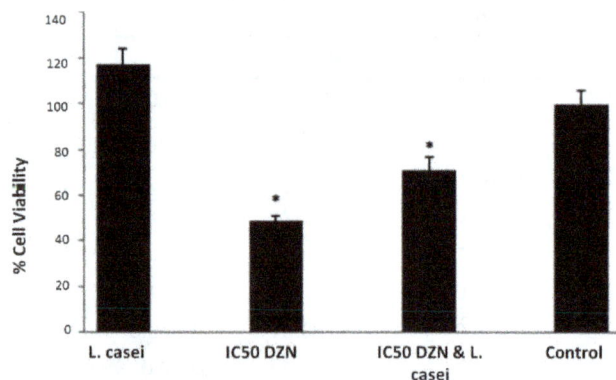

Figure 1. The effect of *L. casei* on diazinon toxicity. Error bares represent standard deviations. *P≤0.05

Apoptosis assessment

To analyze the apoptosis incidence in DZN treated cells and prove the effect of *L. casei* on the viability of HUVEC cells, the latter was exposed to 50 µg/ml of filtered supernatant of late stationary phase growth of *L. casei* after 24 h incubation to visualize the apoptosis using Dapi staining and observation by fluorescent microscopy (Olympus BX64, Olympus, Japan).

The intact viable cells displayed a plenary health nucleus (Figure 2B), whereas the apoptotic cells were characterized by shrinking cells with condensed (early apoptosis) or fragmented (late apoptosis) nuclei (Figure 2A). The DZN treated HUVEC cells illustrated the very distinctive signs of apoptosis, including the formation of micronuclei, cell shrinkage, membrane blebbing, nucleus fragmentation, and apoptotic bodies (Figure 2A). None of these signals were observed in untreated HUVEC cells (Figure 2C). The *L. casei* secretion metabolites could decrease the apoptosis-related signals in DZN-treated HUVEC cells (Figure 2D).

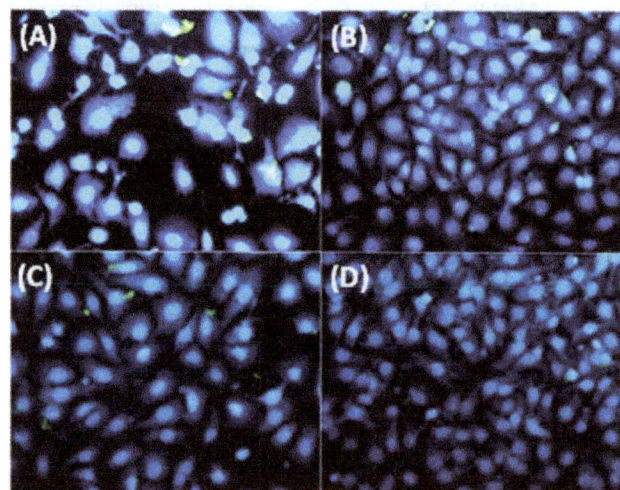

Figure 2. Nuclear morphology analysis using DAPI of HUVEC cell line, **A)** HUVEC cells treated with IC50 dose of diazinon, **B)** Untreated HUVEC cells, **C)** HUVEC cells treated with *L. casei* and **D)** HUVEC cells treated with *L. casei* and IC50 dose of diazinon

Annexin V-FITC/PI flow cytometry analysis was performed to confirm the metabolite secreted from selected *L. casei* strain effects on apoptosis of HUVEC cells. These cells were treated with 50 µg/ml *L. casei* supernatant for 24 h. The dual parameter fluorescent dot blots revealed the viable cell population in the lower left quadrant (annexin V^{-}/PI^{-}), the cells at the early apoptosis are in the lower right quadrant (annexin V^{+}/PI^{-}), and the cells at the late apoptosis are in the upper right quadrant (annexin V^{+}/PI^{+}). Figures 3A to 3C show that 0.53 percent of the cells was annexin V^{+}/PI^{-} in untreated cells after 24 h of post seeding. Our findings indicated that the cytotoxicity of DNZ on HUVEC cells occurred during apoptosis. A total of 18.3% and 11.6% of the treated cells was induced at early and late stages of apoptosis after 24 of incubation. These results revealed that significant differences existed in apoptotic induction by DNZ. The cells stained by PI alone (V^-/PI^+) underwent necrosis. As shown in Figure 3, the DZN-treated cells demonstrated an increase in the necrotic population (6.2%) shown in the upper left quadrant whereas the toxin treated cells exposed to *L. casei* supernatant showed a slight increase in necrotic cells (0.32%) compared to the untreated cells (0.04%). These findings proved that *L. casei* secretion metabolites could decrease the DZN cytotoxicity effects on human normal cells (HUVEC) at *in vitro*.

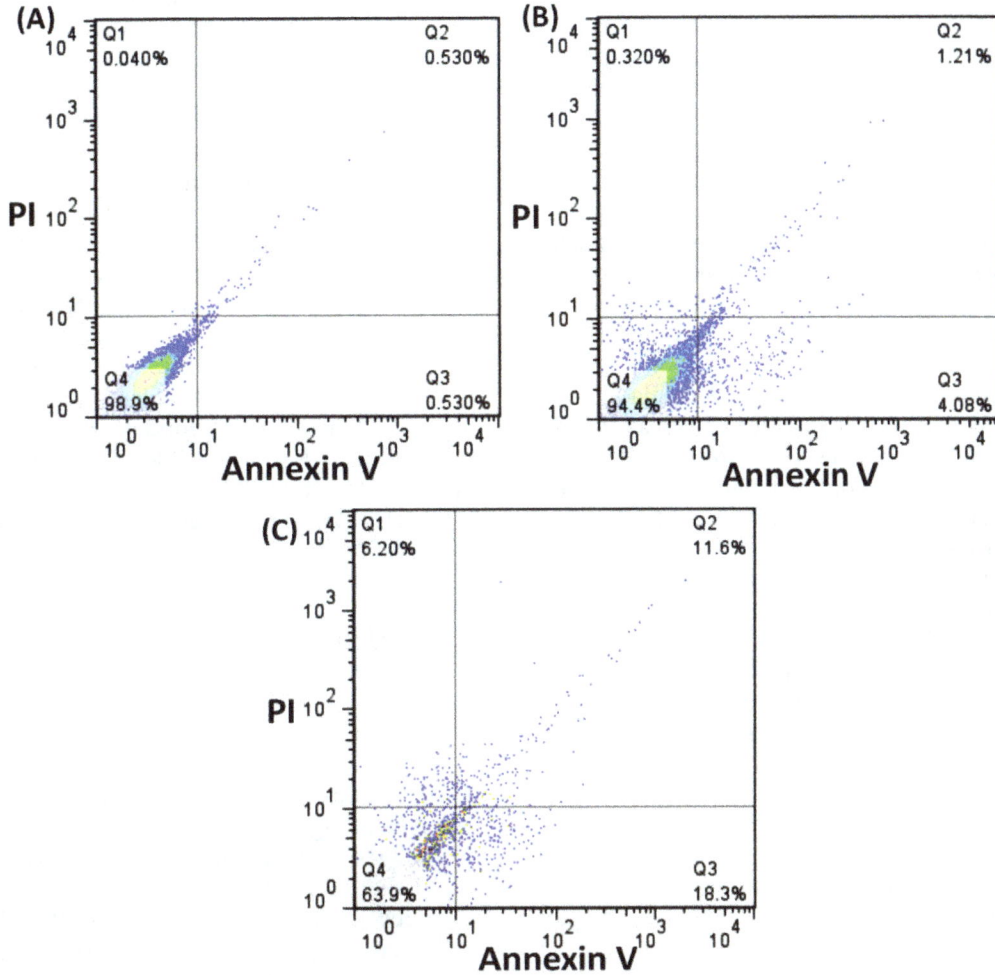

Figure 3. The flow cytometry assessment on HUVEC cell line, **A)** Untreated HUVEC cells, **B)** HUVEC cells treated with *L. casei* and IC50 dose of diazinon. **C)** HUVEC cells treated with IC50 dose of diazinon, Lower left column: Annexin V/PI (viable cells), lower right column: Annexin V^+/PI (early apoptotic cells), upper right column: Annexin V^+/P^+ (late apoptotic cells) and upper left column Annexin V/P^+ (necrotic cells).

Discussion

The results of the present study indicated the treatment of human poisoned cells with *L. casei* showed the protective effects against DZN induced cytotoxicity at *in vitro*. Human and animal studies have shown the toxicity of DZN in different tissues such as hematological disorders,[27] cardiotoxicicty,[27] hepatotoxicity,[28] nephrotoxicity,[29] neurotoxicity,[30] and both female and male reproductive toxicity.[29] The exposure of the NTera2/D1 (NT2) cell line to diazinon at concentrations ranging between 10^{-4} and 10^{-5} M enhanced cell death with a number of special features of apoptosis including membrane and mitochondrial potential changes.[31] Slotkin and Seidler indicated that the target genes of the organophosphates including chlorpyrifos and diazinon are the cell cycle and apoptosis-regulating genes in the developing brain and in neuronotypic cells *in vitro*.[32]

In our study, the co-treatment of the HUVEC cells with *L. casei* supernatant and diazinon decreased cell death and apoptosis induced by diazinon. The previous studies have suggested that some probiotics may regulate apoptosis.[33] The activation of the antiapoptotic Akt/protein kinase B and inhibition of the activation of proapoptotic p38/mitogen-activated protein kinase by probiotic bacteria were suggested to prevent apoptosis in the colon epithelial cells.[34,35] Also, probiotics possess the antitoxin effects through binding to the toxins ;thus, can protect cells against both membrane and DNA-damaging toxins.[36]

Although the main mechanism of DZN toxic effects on target and non-target organisms is the inhibition of acetylcholinesterase,[37] the researchers have shown that it is not in charge of all of toxic effects and several studies suggest that DZN induces oxidative stress and produces free radicals in biological systems which is the main mechanism of chronic organophosphates (Ops) toxicity.[38] The chronic Ops elevate the level of reactive oxygen species which is a major apoptotic stimulant in different organs.[31] Indeed, apoptosis is a common outcome for the exposures to toxicant that evoke oxidative stress.[2,5,28,39] Diazinon increase lipid peroxidation and decrease antioxidant biomarkers including reduced glutathione, glutathione peroxidase, superoxide dismutase, catalase and total antioxidant capacity in male wistar albino rats.[29] The injection of DZN at high doses has increased the level of malondialdehyde, superoxide dismutase and glutathione S-transferase activities and has decreased glutathione (GSH) level, lactate dehydrogenase, and cholinesterase activities in the brain, heart, and spleen of female Wistar and Norway rats.[38] Sub-acute exposure to DZN has induced oxidative stress-mediated apoptosis in rat liver through the activation of caspases-9 and -3, and increasing Bax/Bcl-2 expression ratio.[28]

Probiotics with antioxidant effects, *Lactobacillus acidophilus,* could decrease malondialdehyde and could increase the levels of antioxidants, glutathione reductase, superoxide dismutase, and glutathione peroxidase in Sprague–Dawley rats.[40] Therefore, it seems that anti-apoptotic effects of *L. casei* in HUVEC cells treated with DZN probably due to a decrease in oxidative stress and anti-oxidant effects.

Conclusion
The results of the present study reveal that diazinon has cytotoxic effects on normal cells and apoptosis is the main cytotoxic mechanism of diazinon; however, *L. casei* secretions is able to decrease its cytotoxic effects. Although the exact mechanism of anti-toxic effects of *L. casei* is not clear but the reduction of DZN cytotoxicity on human normal cells is because of its anti-apoptotic mechanisms, antitoxin effects and/or via decreasing the oxidative stress.

Ethical Issues
No ethical issues to be promulgated.

Conflict of Interest
The authors declare that there are no conflicts of interests.

References
1. Mosaddegh MH, Emami F, Asghari G. Evaluation of residual diazinon and chlorpiryfos in children herbal medicines by headspace-spme and GC-FID. *Iran J Pharm Res* 2014;13(2):541-9.

2. Slotkin TA, Seidler FJ. Does mechanism matter? Unrelated neurotoxicants converge on cell cycle and apoptosis during neurodifferentiation. *Neurotoxicol Teratol* 2012;34(4):395-402. doi: 10.1016/j.ntt.2012.04.008

3. Aggarwal V, Deng X, Tuli A, Goh KS. Diazinon-chemistry and environmental fate: A california perspective. *Rev Environ Contam Toxicol* 2013;223:107-40. doi: 10.1007/978-1-4614-5577-6_5

4. Boobis AR, Ossendorp BC, Banasiak U, Hamey PY, Sebestyen I, Moretto A. Cumulative risk assessment of pesticide residues in food. *Toxicol Lett* 2008;180(2):137-50. doi: 10.1016/j.toxlet.2008.06.004

5. Razavi BM, Hosseinzadeh H, Movassaghi AR, Imenshahidi M, Abnous K. Protective effect of crocin on diazinon induced cardiotoxicity in rats in subchronic exposure. *Chem Biol Interact* 2013;203(3):547-55. doi: 10.1016/j.cbi.2013.03.010

6. Mundargi RC, Babu VR, Rangaswamy V, Patel P, Aminabhavi TM. Nano/micro technologies for delivering macromolecular therapeutics using poly(d,l-lactide-co-glycolide) and its derivatives. *J Control Release* 2008;125(3):193-209. doi: 10.1016/j.jconrel.2007.09.013

7. Ciscato CH, Bertoni Gebara A, Henrique Monteiro S. Pesticide residue monitoring of brazilian fruit for export 2006-2007. *Food Addit Contam Part B Surveill* 2009;2(2):140-5. doi: 10.1080/19440040903330326

8. Pomeroy-Black M, Ehrich M. Organophosphorus compound effects on neurotrophin receptors and intracellular signaling. *Toxicol In Vitro* 2012;26(5):759-65. doi: 10.1016/j.tiv.2012.03.008

9. Ahmed MA, Ahmed HI, El-Morsy EM. Melatonin protects against diazinon-induced neurobehavioral changes in rats. *Neurochem Res* 2013;38(10):2227-36. doi: 10.1007/s11064-013-1134-9

10. Lecoeur S, Videmann B, Mazallon M. Effect of organophosphate pesticide diazinon on expression and activity of intestinal P-glycoprotein. *Toxicol Lett* 2006;161(3):200-9. doi: 10.1016/j.toxlet.2005.09.003

11. Guizzetti M, Pathak S, Giordano G, Costa LG. Effect of organophosphorus insecticides and their metabolites on astroglial cell proliferation. *Toxicology* 2005;215(3):182-90. doi: 10.1016/j.tox.2005.07.004

12. Calviello G, Piccioni E, Boninsegna A, Tedesco B, Maggiano N, Serini S, et al. DNA damage and apoptosis induction by the pesticide mancozeb in rat cells: Involvement of the oxidative mechanism. *Toxicol Appl Pharmacol* 2006;211(2):87-96. doi: 10.1016/j.taap.2005.06.001

13. Carlson K, Jortner BS, Ehrich M. Organophosphorus compound-induced apoptosis in sh-sy5y human neuroblastoma cells. *Toxicol Appl Pharmacol* 2000;168(2):102-13. doi: 10.1006/taap.2000.8997

14. Zhang X, Wallace AD, Du P, Lin S, Baccarelli AA, Jiang H, et al. Genome-wide study of DNA

methylation alterations in response to diazinon exposure in vitro. *Environ Toxicol Pharmacol* 2012;34(3):959-68. doi: 10.1016/j.etap.2012.07.012

15. Salminen S, Nybom S, Meriluoto J, Collado MC, Vesterlund S, El-Nezami H. Interaction of probiotics and pathogens--benefits to human health? *Curr Opin Biotechnol* 2010;21(2):157-67. doi: 10.1016/j.copbio.2010.03.016

16. Oliveira Silva E, Cruz de Carvalho T, Parshikov IA, Alves dos Santos R, Silva Emery F, Jacometti Cardoso Furtado NA. Cytotoxicity of lapachol metabolites produced by probiotics. *Lett Appl Microbiol* 2014;59(1):108-14. doi: 10.1111/lam.12251

17. Uccello M, Malaguarnera G, Basile F, D'Agata V, Malaguarnera M, Bertino G, et al. Potential role of probiotics on colorectal cancer prevention. *BMC Surg* 2012;12 Suppl 1:S35. doi: 10.1186/1471-2482-12-S1-S35

18. Butel MJ. Probiotics, gut microbiota and health. *Med Mal Infect* 2014;44(1):1-8. doi: 10.1016/j.medmal.2013.10.002

19. Nowak A, Libudzisz Z. Ability of probiotic *lactobacillus casei* dn 114001 to bind or/and metabolise heterocyclic aromatic amines *in vitro*. *Eur J Nutr* 2009;48(7):419-27. doi: 10.1007/s00394-009-0030-1

20. Oatley JT, Rarick MD, Ji GE, Linz JE. Binding of aflatoxin B1 to bifidobacteria *in vitro*. *J Food Prot* 2000;63(8):1133-6.

21. Hernandez-Mendoza A, Guzman-de-Pena D, Garcia HS. Key role of teichoic acids on aflatoxin b binding by probiotic bacteria. *J Appl Microbiol* 2009;107(2):395-403. doi: 10.1111/j.1365-2672.2009.04217.x

22. Carasi P, Trejo FM, Perez PF, De Antoni GL, Serradell Mde L. Surface proteins from *lactobacillus kefir* antagonize in vitro cytotoxic effect of *clostridium* difficile toxins. *Anaerobe* 2012;18(1):135-42. doi: 10.1016/j.anaerobe.2011.11.002

23. Drisko J, Bischoff B, Giles C, Adelson M, Rao RV, McCallum R. Evaluation of five probiotic products for label claims by DNA extraction and polymerase chain reaction analysis. *Dig Dis Sci* 2005;50(6):1113-7. doi: 10.1007/s10620-005-2931-z

24. Dubernet S, Desmasures N, Gueguen M. A PCR-based method for identification of lactobacilli at the genus level. *FEMS Microbiol Lett* 2002;214(2):271-5. doi: 10.1111/j.1574-6968.2002.tb11358.x

25. Haghshenas B, Abdullah N, Nami Y, Radiah D, Rosli R, Khosroushahi AY. Different effects of two newly-isolated probiotic *lactobacillus plantarum* 15HN and *lactococcus lactis* subsp. *Lactis* 44lac strains from traditional dairy products on cancer cell lines. *Anaerobe* 2014;30:51-9. doi: 10.1016/j.anaerobe.2014.08.009

26. Deng W, Xi D, Mao H, Wanapat M. The use of molecular techniques based on ribosomal RNA and DNA for rumen microbial ecosystem studies: A review. *Mol Biol Rep* 2008;35(2):265-74. doi: 10.1007/s11033-007-9079-1

27. Hariri AT, Moallem SA, Mahmoudi M, Hosseinzadeh H. The effect of crocin and safranal, constituents of saffron, against subacute effect of diazinon on hematological and genotoxicity indices in rats. *Phytomedicine* 2011;18(6):499-504. doi: 10.1016/j.phymed.2010.10.001

28. Lari P, Abnous K, Imenshahidi M, Rashedinia M, Razavi M, Hosseinzadeh H. Evaluation of diazinon-induced hepatotoxicity and protective effects of crocin. *Toxicol Ind Health* 2015;31(4):367-76. doi: 10.1177/0748233713475519

29. Abdel-Daim MM. Synergistic protective role of ceftriaxone and ascorbic acid against subacute diazinon-induced nephrotoxicity in rats. *Cytotechnology* 2016;68(2):279-89. doi: 10.1007/s10616-014-9779-z

30. Colovic MB, Vasic VM, Avramovic NS, Gajic MM, Djuric DM, Krstic DZ. In vitro evaluation of neurotoxicity potential and oxidative stress responses of diazinon and its degradation products in rat brain synaptosomes. *Toxicol Lett* 2015;233(1):29-37. doi: 10.1016/j.toxlet.2015.01.003

31. Aluigi MG, Guida C, Falugi C. Apoptosis as a specific biomarker of diazinon toxicity in NTera2-D1 cells. *Chem Biol Interact* 2010;187(1-3):299-303. doi: 10.1016/j.cbi.2010.03.031

32. Slotkin TA, Seidler FJ. Developmental neurotoxicity of organophosphates targets cell cycle and apoptosis, revealed by transcriptional profiles *in vivo* and *in vitro*. *Neurotoxicol Teratol* 2012;34(2):232-41. doi: 10.1016/j.ntt.2011.12.001

33. Iyer C, Kosters A, Sethi G, Kunnumakkara AB, Aggarwal BB, Versalovic J. Probiotic *lactobacillus* reuteri promotes TNF-induced apoptosis in human myeloid leukemia-derived cells by modulation of NF-kappab and mapk signalling. *Cell Microbiol* 2008;10(7):1442-52. doi: 10.1111/j.1462-5822.2008.01137.x

34. Ng SC, Hart AL, Kamm MA, Stagg AJ, Knight SC. Mechanisms of action of probiotics: Recent advances. *Inflamm Bowel Dis* 2009;15(2):300-10. doi: 10.1002/ibd.20602

35. Aureli P, Capurso L, Castellazzi AM, Clerici M, Giovannini M, Morelli L, et al. Probiotics and health: An evidence-based review. *Pharmacol Res* 2011;63(5):366-76. doi: 10.1016/j.phrs.2011.02.006

36. Oelschlaeger TA. Mechanisms of probiotic actions - a review. *Int J Med Microbiol* 2010;300(1):57-62. doi: 10.1016/j.ijmm.2009.08.005

37. Jameson RR, Seidler FJ, Slotkin TA. Nonenzymatic functions of acetylcholinesterase splice variants in the developmental neurotoxicity of organophosphates: Chlorpyrifos, chlorpyrifos oxon, and diazinon. *Environ Health Perspect* 2007;115(1):65-70. doi: 10.1289/ehp.9487

38. Jafari M, Salehi M, Ahmadi S, Asgari A, Abasnezhad M, Hajigholamali M. The role of oxidative stress in diazinon-induced tissues toxicity in wistar and norway rats. *Toxicol Mech Methods* 2012;22(8):638-47. doi: 10.3109/15376516.2012.716090

39. Hariri AT, Moallem SA, Mahmoudi M, Memar B, Hosseinzadeh H. Sub-acute effects of diazinon on biochemical indices and specific biomarkers in rats: Protective effects of crocin and safranal. *Food Chem Toxicol* 2010;48(10):2803-8. doi: 10.1016/j.fct.2010.07.010

40. Verma A, Shukla G. Synbiotic (*lactobacillus rhamnosus+lactobacillus acidophilus*+inulin) attenuates oxidative stress and colonic damage in 1,2 dimethylhydrazine dihydrochloride-induced colon carcinogenesis in sprague-dawley rats: A long-term study. *Eur J Cancer Prev* 2014;23(6):550-9. doi: 10.1097/CEJ.0000000000000054

Anti-Inflammatory and Anti-Angiogenesis Effects of Verapamil on Rat Air Pouch Inflammation Model

Tahereh Eteraf-Oskouei[1], Sevda Mikaily Mirak[2], Moslem Najafi[1]*

[1] *Department of Pharmacology and Toxicology, Faculty of Pharmacy, Tabriz University of Medical Sciences, Tabriz, Iran.*
[2] *Student Research Committee, Faculty of Pharmacy, Tabriz University of Medical Sciences, Tabriz, Iran.*

Keywords:
· Verapamil
· Air-Pouch
· Inflammation
· Angiogenesis
· VEGF
· IL-1β

Abstract
Purpose: In the present study, the effects of verapamil on inflammation and angiogenesis in air pouch model were studied.
Methods: To create a model of inflammation in the rats, on days 1 and 3 sterile air, and on the sixth day, carrageenan was injected into the pouch subcutaneously. Normal saline as control, diclofenac sodium and dexamethasone as standards and verapamil (0.05, 0.1 and 0.2mg/rat) was injected into the pouch simultaneously with carrageenan and as well as 24 and 48 hours later. After 72 hours, volume of exudate, the leukocytes count, concentration of VEGF and IL-1ß, granulomatous tissue weight, histopathological changes and angiogenesis were considered.
Results: Verapamil significantly reduced leukocyte accumulation in all doses, but effect of 0.1mg/rat was more significant (P<0.001). The exudate volume and granulomatous tissue weight was reduced with all doses, especially 0.1mg/rat (P<0.01). Doses 0.05, 0.1 and 0.2mg/rat of verapamil compared with the control group (carrageenan) led to a reduction in the amount of hemoglobin in the tissue as the angiogenesis indicator (P<0.001, P<0.01 and P<0.05, respectively). VEGF level of exudate was reduced by doses of 0.05 and 0.1mg/rat (P<0.05). In addition, IL-1β concentration was lowered by 0.1mg/rat of verapamil (P<0.05). Histopathological changes, severity of granulomatous inflammation, granulomatous tissue cell density and angiogenesis in verapamil group were markedly lower compared to carrageenan group.
Conclusion: Verapamil has significant anti-inflammatory and anti-angiogenesis effects in the air pouch model probably due to attenuation effects of verapamil on IL-1β and VEGF.

Introduction

Inflammation is immune response to infection or tissue injury and plays a major role in the pathogenesis of diseases such as arthritis, cancer, cardiovascular and neurodegenerative diseases.[1] Inflammation leads to activation of local tissues and release of intermediates of them that ultimately causes vasodilatation and increased vascular permeability, swelling and pain fibers activity.[2] Induction of acute inflammation is the main method employed by the innate immunity system to fight against infections and tissue damages that can be created within minutes to hours and continues to days. Proinflammatory TNF-α, IL-1 and IL-6 cytokines play an important role in activating the inflammatory cells.[3] If the infection is not removed or the tissue damage is prolonged, chronic inflammation continues after acute inflammation.[4] Chronic inflammation sites often undergo tissue regeneration along with angiogenesis and fibrosis.[5] Glucocorticosteroids and non-steroidal anti-inflammatory drugs (NSAIDs) are the most common anti-inflammatory drugs,[6] but cause serious side effects in long-term use. So today, attempts are made to provide drugs, in addition to suitable anti-inflammatory effects of which, cause the least side effects.[7]

Calcium ions play an important role in the synthesis and release of chemical mediators of inflammation.[8] Calcium leads to the activation of nitric oxide synthase, phospholipase A_2 (PLA_2) and phospholipase C (PLC) enzymes. PLA_2 causes a release of arachidonic acid, which is a precursor of prostaglandin synthesis, leukotrienes and thromboxanes.[9] Inflammatory leukocytes perform a wide range of functional responses such as degranulation, production of superoxide, nitric oxide (NO) and TNF-α through calcium ion. Thus, inhibition of calcium influx may be an important factor in reducing leukocyte activation.[10]

Calcium channel blockers (CCBs) such as verapamil exert their cardiovascular effects by blocking voltage-dependent L-type calcium channels.[11] Increased calcium influx through type L calcium channels causes the activation of various signaling cascades, such as reactive oxygen and nitrogen species and activation of proinflammatory cytokines.[12] According to previous

---

studies, verapamil can inhibit the production of inflammatory cytokines such as TNF-α, IL-1 and IL-6 and increase plasma levels of inflammatory cytokines such as IL-10.[13,14]

There is no report on exact effects of verapamil on the inflammatory and angiogenesis parameters in the air pouch model, so the possible anti-inflammatory and anti-angiogenesis effects of this drug were studied in rats in this study.

Materials and Methods
Animals
In this study, male Wistar rats (200-250g) were used. The animals had free access to food and water under standard temperature conditions of 21±3 °C and were kept in 12 hours light and 12 hours of darkness.

Air pouch model of inflammation
The hair of animals is shaved over the whole dorsal region after being anesthetized and 20ml of sterile air was injected subcutaneously. Three days later, 10ml of air was injected into the above region. One ml of 1% carrageenan solution was injected into the pouch on the sixth day after the initial air injection.

Studied groups
The rats were randomly divided into eight groups:

1&2- Normal saline control group and control carrageenan: These groups respectively received 1ml normal saline or carrageenan (intra-pouch) after creation of pouch on the sixth day. Then, 1ml normal saline was injected into the pouch immediately before and 24 and 48 hours later.

3. Diclofenac sodium positive control group: To compare the effect of verapamil with NSAIDs (as standard) drugs, this group received 1mg diclofenac at volume of 1ml on the sixth day after formation of pouch, immediately before the injection of carrageenan and 24 and 48 hours later.

4. Dexamethasone positive control group: To compare the effects of verapamil with corticosteroids (as standard), this group, similar to group 3 received 0.4mg dexamethasone (1ml, intra-pouch).

5-8. Verapamil treatment groups: These groups after pouch formation on the sixth day, immediately before the injection of carrageenan and 24 and 48 hours later, 0.05, 0.1, 0.2 and 2.5mg/rat of verapamil (1ml) was injected intra-pouch.

Studied inflammatory parameters
Determining exudate volume and counting the number of leukocytes
Three days after the injection of carrageenan, the rats were sacrificed and the inflammatory exudate was removed and its volume was measured. Some of the exudate was later poured into the test tube containing EDTA and leukocyte count was carried on by Neubauer slide after mixing and dilution under light microscope (Olympus, Japan).

Measurement of VEGF and IL-1ß in exudate
Three days after the induction of inflammation, exudate collected was centrifuged at 1000g and 4°C for 10 minutes. The cell-free supernatant was used to determine the amount of VEGF and IL-1ß using ELISA according to the manufacturer's instructions.

Angiogenesis evaluation
Angiogenesis was determined using the method described previously (Ghosh et al.) with a little change. Granulomatous tissue was initially removed, washed with PBS solution (pH=7.4) and dried. It was later cut into small pieces, then Drabkin solution (ZistChem Diagnostics, Iran) was added and homogenized at 15000 for 5 minutes at ice bed by a homogenizer (HO4 AP-Edmund Bühler, B. Braun, Germany). The homogenized tissue was centrifuged at 10000 RCF and 4°C for 30 minutes. Subsequently, 1ml of supernatant was later mixed with 4ml of Drabkin solution and after being smooth out by millipore filters (0.22μ), the amount of hemoglobin was determined as a marker of angiogenesis using hemoglobin standard curve by UV spectrophotometer at 540nm in accordance with the kit manufacturer instructions.[15]

Granulomatous tissue weighing and evaluating its histopathological changes
Three days after the injection of carrageenan, the animals were sacrificed and the outer skin of the formed cavity was cut and the pouch was isolated from the surrounding tissues and weighed. Granulomatous tissue formed around pouch was fixed in 10% formalin and was later cut by a microtome (Lieits, Germany) with diameter of 5.6 microns after paraffin dehydration and molding process and was finally placed on a slide. After deparaffinization, the slides were stained by hematoxylin-eosin and the histopathological changes, including granulomatous intensity, polymorphonuclear density, macrophage density and angiogenesis intensity were evaluated using the light microscope.

Statistical analysis of data
The results were reported as mean±SEM and SPSS v. 17 was used for statistical analysis. Independent-samples t-test was used to compare between normal saline and carrageenan control groups to ensure the validity of the formed inflammation. The other groups were compared by one-way ANOVA and post hoc LSD test. P-value of <0.05 was considered statistically significant.

Results
First, to ensure the validity of the inflammation formed in the air pouch, a comparison was made on the results obtained in the normal saline control and carrageenan groups. All studied parameters in the carrageenan control group were significantly increased compared with normal saline group (P<0.001).

Effect of verapamil on leukocyte accumulation

As can be seen in Figure 1, the total number of leukocytes in the diclofenac and dexamethasone groups was 15.35±5.18 and 1.66±0.49 million, respectively. Verapamil by doses 0.05, 0.1 and 0.2mg/rat reduced leukocytes compared with the carrageenan group (P<0.01, P<0.001 and P<0.05, respectively), but 2.5mg/rat of verapamil did not create a significant decrease. In this parameter, all verapamil doses showed significant difference with diclofenac and dexamethasone.

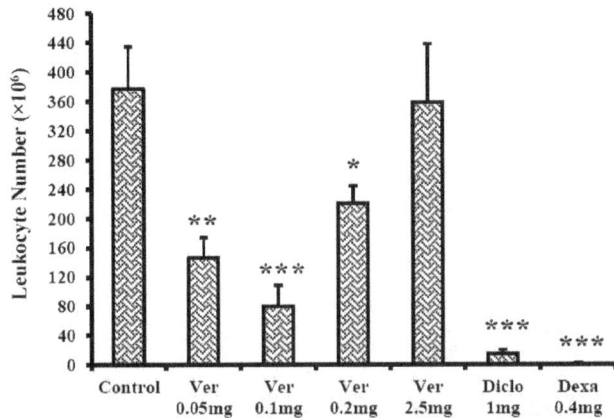

Figure 1. Effects of verapamil on the leukocyte accumulation in the pouch fluid in male rats (n≥6). Data are presented as mean±SEM. * P<0.05, ** P<0.01, *** P<0.001 compared to the control carrageenan. Ver: Verapamil, Diclo: Diclofenac sodium, Dexa: Dexamethasone.

Effect of verapamil on the volume of exudate and granulomatous tissue weight

Exudate volume in diclofenac and dexamethasone groups was 4.61±0.56 and 2.27±0.23ml, respectively. The same volume was obtained 6.65±0.66, 4.74±0.92, 6.38±0.43 and 6.54±0.37ml at verapamil doses of 0.05, 0.1, 0.2 and 2.5mg/rat, respectively. Only 0.1mg/rat of verapamil led to a significant reduction as compared to carrageenan (P<0.01). In addition, diclofenac, dexamethasone, 0.1 and 0.05mg/rat verapamil doses significantly reduced the granulomatous tissue weight compared with carrageenan (Figure 2).

Effect of verapamil on granulation tissue angiogenesis

In order to evaluate angiogenesis, tissue hemoglobin was measured as a marker of angiogenesis. Verapamil by doses of 0.05, 0.1 and 0.2 mg/rat significantly reduced angiogenesis from the carrageenan control group value (291.0±10.5) to 154.5±12.0 (P<0.001), 184.7±28.0 (P<0.01) and 241.2±18.5 mg/100g tissue (P<0.05), respectively. In addition, compared to the control group, angiogenesis was decreased by diclofenac and dexamethasone to 170.4±17.4 (P<0.001) and 32.3±7.9 (P<0.001), respectively.

Effect of verapamil on the amount of exudate VEGF

Considering the importance of VEGF protein in angiogenesis, as well as to confirm the data obtained

from angiogenesis, its amount was measured in inflammatory exudates using more effective verapamil doses. VEGF levels in the carrageenan and diclofenac groups, 0.05, 0.1mg/rat verapamil groups were 72.804±6.736, 25.563±6.027, 46.254±3.543 and 48.441±6.098ng, respectively. Diclofenac at P<0.001 and both verapamil doses at P<0.05 reduced VEGF levels compared with carrageenan group.

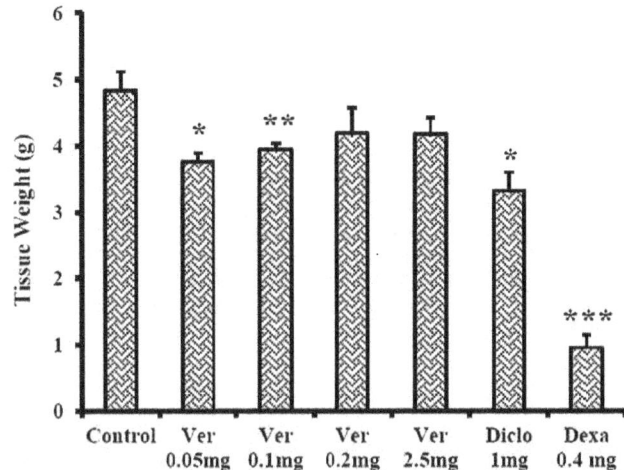

Figure 2. Effects of verapamil on the granulomatous tissue weight in male rats (n≥6). Data are presented as mean±SEM. * P<0.05, ** P<0.01, *** P<0.001 compared to the control carrageenan. Ver: Verapamil, Diclo: Diclofenac sodium, Dexa: Dexamethasone.

Effect of verapamil on the amount of exudate IL-1β

The amount of IL-1β was 7.432±0.487pg in the carrageenan group, which was reduced to 3.547±0.052pg when diclofenac was used. Also, 0.1 dose of verapamil (the most effective dose to reduce all inflammatory parameters) decreased IL-1β level to 4.683±0.622pg that was significant compared with the carrageenan group (P<0.05).

Comparative study of verapamil effects on granulation tissue angiogenesis and VEGF level

VEGF is one of the most important factors in stimulating angiogenesis and exerts its stimulatory effects by increasing migration and proliferation of endothelial cells and formation of vascular network.[16] Given the key role of VEGF in the angiogenesis process, the effects of verapamil on angiogenesis and VEGF were compared in Figure 3. Verapamil could reduce angiogenesis and VEGF level using a similar pattern.

Effect of verapamil on histopathological changes of granulomatous tissue

Granulomatous intensity, polymorphonuclear density, macrophage density and angiogenesis intensity in normal saline and carrageenan control groups was evaluated mild and very severe, respectively. In the groups treated with verapamil, anti-inflammatory and anti-angiogenesis effects were shown to be associated with significant decrease in these parameters that is comparable to the group receiving diclofenac. The most decreasing effect on these parameters was observed in the dexamethasone group. Figure 4 shows an example of histological changes in granulomatous tissue in different groups.

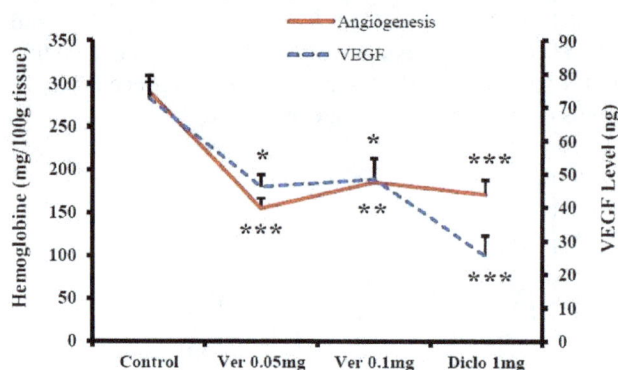

Figure 3. Comparative study of verapamil effects on granulation tissue angiogenesis and VEGF in male rats (n≥6). Data are presented as mean±SEM. * $P<0.05$, ** $P<0.01$, *** $P<0.001$ compared to the control carrageenan. Ver: Verapamil, Diclo: Diclofenac sodium.

Discussion

Calcium ions play a major role in the synthesis and release of inflammatory mediators[11] and CCBs can be used to study its inflammatory role.[9] The present study aimed to examine the effect of verapamil, as L-type calcium channel blocker, on inflammatory parameters and angiogenesis in air pouch experimental model of inflammation.

The leukocyte accumulation was significantly decreased using verapamil, especially at a dose of 0.1mg/rat. Bilici et al. in their study on the effects of mibefradil (a new CCB) on histamine-induced inflammation in the rat paw showed that the agent is able to reduce leukocyte accumulation.[17] Diltiazem is another CCB drugs that prevented inflammation induced by yeast injection into the pouch and the leukocyte accumulation.[8] The observed effects of verapamil in reducing the accumulation of leukocytes in this study was consistent with the results of two above studies.

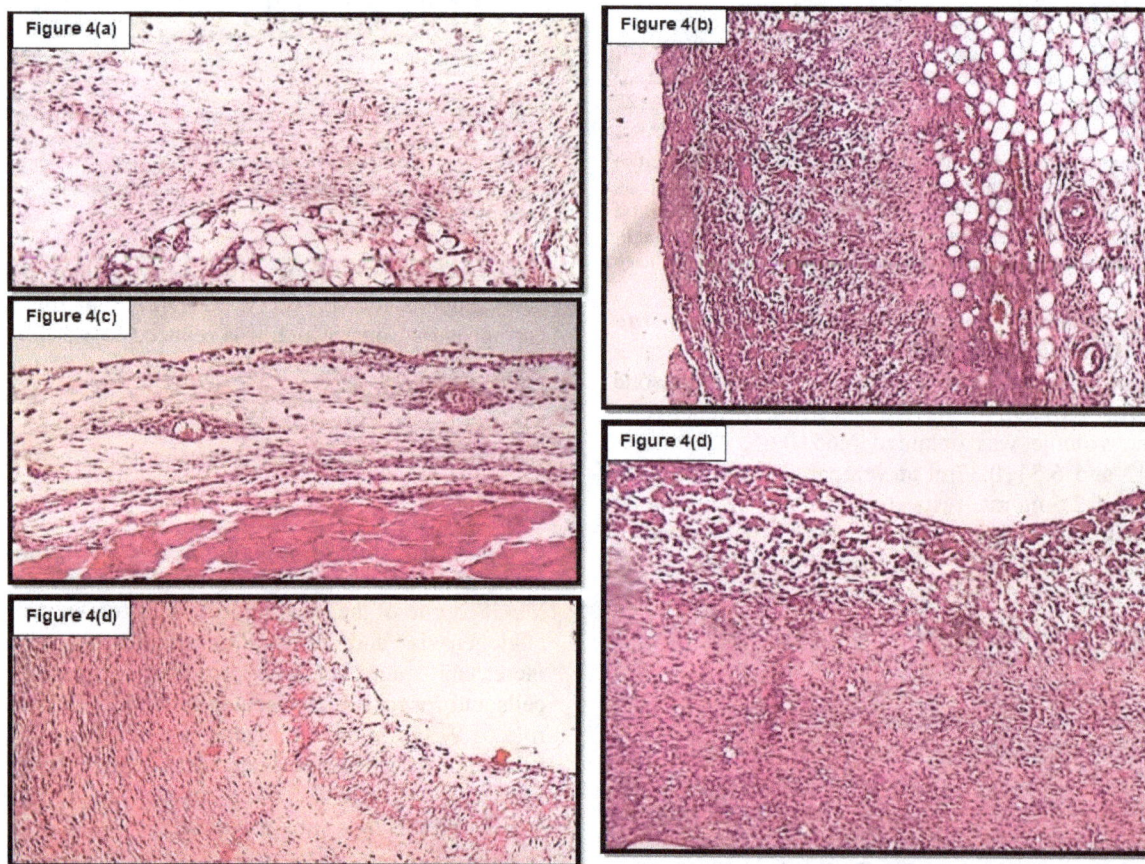

Figure 4. Histopathological changes in granulomatous tissue in different groups. 4(a): normal saline group; minimal inflammation and small cell accumulation and almost no trace of granulomatous tissue and angiogenesis. 4(b): carrageenan group; a large number of macrophages and many congested young vessels with very intense granulomatous inflammation. 4(c): dexamethasone group; the severity of granulomatosis and inflammation are clearly reduced 4(d): diclofenac group; moderate granulomatous inflammation with low macrophages and angiogenesis compared to carrageenan group. 4(e): verapamil 0.05mg; inflammation and granulomatous inflammation are reduced compared to the carrageenan group. A significant reduction in cell density and angiogenesis is also observed.

Proinflammatory cytokines, including TNF-α and IL-1 play an important role in the activation of endothelial cells by increasing the expression of adhesion molecules of ICAM-1 and VCAM-1. Mutual reactions of adhesion molecules and leukocyte ligands are very important in leukocyte recruitment.[18] In BALB/c mice that underwent an intraperitoneal injection of LPS, an inflammation-causing substance, verapamil reduced serum levels of TNF-α.[19] A study on TNF-α-stimulated human endothelial cells showed that verapamil reduced binding rate of leukocytes to endothelial cells. Also, verapamil reduced the expression of VCAM-1 in IL-1β-stimulated endothelial cells.[20] Our results showed that the concentration of IL-1β was significantly reduced when verapamil 0.1mg/rat was applied. It seems that the inhibitory effects of verapamil on serum levels of TNF-α, the expression of VCAM-1 and IL-1β in the exudates can play a role in decreasing leukocyte recruitment.

Calcium is an important biochemical mediator in the activation of macrophages, calcium channel blockers such as verapamil and nifedipine can prevent the activation of macrophages.[21] Plasminogen also plays an important role in the recruitment of macrophages to the inflammation site.[22,23] Increased intracellular calcium results in overexpression of plasminogen receptor on the surface of macrophages differentiated monocytes and verapamil or nifedipine inhibits this process.[23] PLA$_2$ enzyme needs calcium in order to exert its effect on arachidonic acid.[24] Verapamil by blocking calcium channels can prevent the release of arachidonic acid and prostaglandin synthesis and leukotriene via inhibiting PLA$_2$ activity.[24]

Following injection of carrageenan, vascular permeability is increased by the release of mediators such as histamine, serotonin, prostaglandins, leukotrienes and NO, as a result of which inflammatory exudates are formed.[25-27] Prostaglandin E$_2$ and leukotrienes C$_4$, D$_4$ and E$_4$ are involved in this process respectively through vasodilatation and increased vascular permeability.[28] In this study, verapamil reduced the volume of exudate. In another study, verapamil has been effective on inflammation caused by injecting carrageenan in the rat paw and reduced the resulting edema.[9] Studies on dihydropyridine calcium antagonists such as amlodipine and nicardipine showed that these drugs significantly reduced the edema in carrageenan-induced inflammation in the rat paw.[27] Probably, inhibition of eicosanoid synthesis by verapamil prevents the formation of inflammatory exudates.

Granulation tissue formation is one of the features of chronic inflammation and accumulation of fibroblasts and macrophages, collagen synthesis and angiogenesis are important characteristics of granulation tissue.[29] Calmodulin-calcium complex leads to the activation of various enzymes that are involved in the proliferation and activation of fibroblasts.[30] Maybe, verapamil prevents granulation tissue development by inhibiting the activity of fibroblasts.

In the present study, granuloma tissue weight was decreased with 0.05 and 0.1mg of verapamil. However, in Dengiz et al.'s study, verapamil (10mg/kg) did not reduce the granulomatous tissue weight in granulomatosis inflammation induced by subcutaneous implantation of cotton pellet in rat shoulder,[31] but the same dose of nicardipine caused significant weight loss in granulomatous tissue.[27] In *in vitro*, cytokines derived

from macrophages (IL-1 and TNF-α) in the formation of granulation tissue are very important. The inhibitory effect of verapamil on TNF-α[11,19,32] and IL-1 can prevent development of granulomatous tissue. Our study also showed the inhibitory effect of verapamil on the amount of IL-1β in inflammatory exudates.

Several studies have shown that NO plays an important role in inflammation induced by carrageenan.[27] In the carrageenan-induced inflammation, NO is derived from vascular endothelial cells[33] and its synthesis pathway is calcium dependent, so inhibiting the NO synthesis by verapamil is another potential mechanism to reduce the inflammatory exudates. Also, NO produced by the macrophages is effective on the formation of granulomatous tissue.[34] Studies on LPS-stimulated microglia cells showed that NO production was significantly reduced by verapamil.[11]

A distinctive feature of granulomatous tissue is angiogenesis,[29] on which the persistence of chronic inflammation depends and angiogenesis inhibition can prevent inflammation.[35] In the present study, verapamil could prevent angiogenesis of granulomatous tissue. VEGF is one of the most important factors stimulating angiogenesis and its inhibition may be a therapeutic target to decrease angiogenesis.[16] The results of this study showed that verapamil, like angiogenesis, caused significant reduction in VEGF levels of exudate. In fact, angiogenesis and VEGF reduction pattern is very similar and indicates a significant correlation between angiogenesis and VEGF. VEGF reduction by verapamil may be an important mechanism to inhibit angiogenesis. In a study, Giuglian et al. demonstrated that verapamil prevented VEGF production by fibroblasts in hypoxic conditions.[36] Inhibition of TNF-α,[11,19,32] decreased NO production by macrophages,[11] inhibition of prostaglandin E$_2$ synthesis,[24] and decreased matrix metalloproteinase activity in blood mononuclear cells[37] are all the possible mechanisms of verapamil that are involved in decreasing angiogenesis in addition to reducing VEGF levels.

Verapamil reduction pattern was just bell-shape in the case of inflammatory parameters and angiogenesis so that the maximum effect was observed at the middle dose and the anti-inflammatory effect was reduced in higher and lower doses. Such bell-shaped dose-response curve was previously reported for verapamil in cardiovascular system,[38] including in the treatment of ischemic arrhythmias.[39,40] The mechanism of such dose-response curve is unknown, but probably reflects the complex pharmacology of verapamil.[41]

Conclusion

The findings of this study showed that verapamil had significant anti-inflammatory and anti-angiogenesis effects in the air pouch model of inflammation, which is likely due to attenuation effects of verapamil on IL-1β and VEGF.

Acknowledgments
This study was supported by Student Research Committee, Tabriz University of Medical Sciences, Tabriz, Iran. The authors would like to thank Drug Applied Research Center, Tabriz University of Medical Sciences for providing laboratory facilities and supporting this work. Verapamil was gifted by Alborz Daru Pharmaceutical Company, Iran.

Ethical Issues
This study was carried out in accordance with the principles and rules maintenance and use of laboratory animals approved by the Ethics Committee of Tabriz University of Medical Sciences.

Conflict of Interest
No potential conflicts of interest were disclosed.

References
1. Ricciotti E, FitzGerald GA. Prostaglandins and inflammation. *Arterioscler Thromb Vasc Biol* 2011;31(5):986-1000. doi: 10.1161/ATVBAHA.110.207449
2. Bishop-Bailey D, Bystrom J. Emerging roles of peroxisome proliferator-activated receptor-β/δ in inflammation. *Pharmacol Ther* 2009;124(2):141-50. doi: 10.1016/j.pharmthera.2009.06.011
3. Khan FA, Khan MF. Inflammation and acute phase response. *Int J Appl Biol Pharm Technol* 2010;1(2):312-21.
4. Sharma RA, Dalgleish AG, Steward WP, O'Byrne KJ. Angiogenesis and the immune response as targets for the prevention and treatment of colorectal cancer (review). *Oncol Rep* 2003;10(5):1625-31. doi: 10.3892/or.10.5.1625
5. Koch AE. Review: Angiogenesis: Implications for rheumatoid arthritis. *Arthritis Rheum* 1998;41(6):951-62.
6. Katzung BG, Masters SB, Trevor AJ. Basic & clinical pharmacology. 11th ed. United States: McGraw-Hill; 2009.
7. Davies NM, Reynolds JK, Undeberg MR, Gates BJ, Ohgami Y, Vega-Villa KR. Minimizing risks of NSAIDs: Cardiovascular, gastrointestinal and renal. *Expert Rev Neurother* 2006;6(11):1643-55. doi: 10.1586/14737175.6.11.1643
8. EL-Halawany SA, Khorshid OA, Rashed LA, Ibrahim E. Role of calcium as a modulator of inflammation an expermintal study in albino rats. *Med J Cairo Univ* 2011;79(2):105-13.
9. Khaksari M, Mahani SE, Mahmoodi M. Calcium channel blockers reduce inflammatory edema in the rat: Involvement of the hypothalamus-pituitary-adrenal axis. *Indian J Pharmacol* 2004;36(6):351-4.
10. Lucas R, Alves M, del Olmo E, San Feliciano A, Paya M. LAAE-14, a new in vitro inhibitor of intracellular calcium mobilization, modulates acute and chronic inflammation. *Biochem Pharmacol* 2003;65(9):1539-49. doi: 10.1016/S0006-2952(03)00120-5
11. Liu Y, Lo YC, Qian L, Crews FT, Wilson B, Chen HL, et al. Verapamil protects dopaminergic neuron damage through a novel anti-inflammatory mechanism by inhibition of microglial activation. *Neuropharmacology* 2011;60(2-3):373-80. doi: 10.1016/j.neuropharm.2010.10.002
12. Kalonia H, Kumar P, Kumar A. Attenuation of proinflammatory cytokines and apoptotic process by verapamil and diltiazem against quinolinic acid induced huntington like alterations in rats. *Brain Res* 2011;1372:115-26. doi: 10.1016/j.brainres.2010.11.060
13. Nemeth ZH, Hasko G, Szabo C, Salzman AL, Vizi ES. Calcium channel blockers and dantrolene differentially regulate the production of interleukin-12 and interferon-γ in endotoxemic mice. *Brain Res Bull* 1998;46(3):257-61. doi: 10.1016/s0361-9230(98)00005-7
14. Li G, Qi XP, Wu XY, Liu FK, Xu Z, Chen C, et al. Verapamil modulates LPS-induced cytokine production via inhibition of NF-kappa B activation in the liver. *Inflamm Res* 2006;55(3):108-13. doi: 10.1007/s00011-005-0060-y
15. Ghosh AK, Hirasawa N, Niki H, Ohuchi K. Cyclooxygenase-2-mediated angiogenesis in carrageenin-induced granulation tissue in rats. *J Pharmacol Exp Ther* 2000;295(2):802-9.
16. Salehi E, Amjadi FS, Khazaei M. Angiogenesis in health and disease: Role of vascular endothelial growth factor (VEGF). *J Isfahan Med Sch* 2011;29(132):312-26.
17. Bilici D, Akpinar E, Gursan N, Dengiz Go, Bilici S, Altas S. Protective effect of t-type calcium channel blocker in histamine-induced paw inflammation in rat. *Pharmacol Res* 2001;44(6):527-31. doi: 10.1006/phrs.2001.0877
18. Abbas AK, Lichtman AH, Pillai S. Cellular and molecular immunology. 7th ed. Philadelphia: Elsevier Health Sciences; 2012.
19. Szabo C, Hasko G, Nemeth ZH, Vizi ES. Calcium entry blockers increase interleukin-10 production in endotoxemia. *Shock* 1997;7(4):304-7. doi: 10.1097/00024382-199704000-00011
20. Yamaguchi M, Kuzume M, Nakano H, Kumada K. Verapamil suppressed lymphocyte adhesion to vascular endothelial cells via selective inhibition of VCAM-1 expression. *Transplant Proc* 1998;30(7):2955. doi: 10.1016/S0041-1345(98)00885-9
21. Wright B, Zeidman I, Greig R, Poste G. Inhibition of macrophage activation by calcium channel blockers and calmodulin antagonists. *Cell Immunol* 1985;95(1):46-53. doi: 10.1016/0008-8749(85)90293-x
22. Ploplis VA, French EL, Carmeliet P, Collen D, Plow EF. Plasminogen deficiency differentially affects

recruitment of inflammatory cell populations in mice. *Blood* 1998;91(6):2005-9.

23. Das R, Burke T, Van Wagoner DR, Plow EF. L-type calcium channel blockers exert an antiinflammatory effect by suppressing expression of plasminogen receptors on macrophages. *Circ Res* 2009;105(2):167-75. doi: 10.1161/CIRCRESAHA.109.200311

24. Seale JP, Ozols S, Compton MR, Shaw J. Effects of verapamil on activation of arachidonic acid metabolism in guinea-pig lungs. *Eur J Pharmacol* 1986;120(3):329-34. doi: 10.1016/0014-2999(86)90473-5

25. Di Rosa M. Biological properties of carrageenan. *J Pharm Pharmacol* 1972;24(2):89-102. doi: 10.1111/j.2042-7158.1972.tb08940.x

26. Morris CJ. Carrageenan-induced paw edema in the rat and mouse. *Methods Mol Biol* 2003;225:115-21. doi: 10.1385/1-59259-374-7:115

27. Suleyman H, Halici Z, Hacimuftuoglu A, Gocer F. Role of adrenal gland hormones in antiinflammatory effect of calcium channel blockers. *Pharmacol Rep* 2006;58(5):692-9.

28. Kumar V, Abbas AK, Fausto N, Mitchell R. Robbins Basic Pathology. 8th Ed. Philadelphia: Saunders Elsevier; 2007.

29. Sato K, Komatsu N, Higashi N, Imai Y, Irimura T. Granulation tissue formation by nonspecific inflammatory agent occurs independently of macrophage galactose-type c-type lectin-1. *Clin Immunol* 2005;115(1):47-50.

30. Kang Y, Lee DA, Higginbotham EJ. In vitro evaluation of antiproliferative potential of calcium channel blockers in human tenon's fibroblasts. *Exp Eye Res* 1997;64(6):913-25. doi: 10.1006/exer.1997.0285

31. Dengiz GO, Akpinar G. Anti-inflammatory effects of L-type calcium channel blockers. *Turkiye Klinikleri J Med Sci* 2007;27(3):328-34.

32. Matsumori A, Nishio R, Nose Y. Calcium channel blockers differentially modulate cytokine production by peripheral blood mononuclear cells. *Circ J* 2010;74(3):567-71. doi: 10.1253/circj.cj-09-0467

33. Sautebin L, Ialenti A, Ianaro A, Di Rosa M. Endogenous nitric oxide increases prostaglandin biosynthesis in carrageenin rat paw oedema. *Eur J Pharmacol* 1995;286(2):219-22. doi: 10.1016/0014-2999(95)00581-5

34. Iuvone T, Carnuccio R, Di Rosa M. Modulation of granuloma formation by endogenous nitric oxide. *Eur J Pharmacol* 1994;265(1-2):89-92. doi: 10.1016/0014-2999(94)90227-5

35. Ghosh AK. Regulation by prostaglandin E2 and histamine of angiogenesis in inflammatory granulation tissue. *Yakugaku Zasshi* 2003;123(5):295-303.

36. Giugliano G, Pasquali D, Notaro A, Brongo S, Nicoletti G, D'Andrea F, et al. Verapamil inhibits interleukin-6 and vascular endothelial growth factor production in primary cultures of keloid fibroblasts. *Br J Plast Surg* 2003;56(8):804-9. doi: 10.1016/s0007-1226(03)00384-9

37. Hajighasemi F, Kakadezfuli N. Suppression of gelatinase activity in human peripheral blood mononuclear cells by verapamil. *Cell J* 2014;16(1):11-6.

38. Fagbemi O, Kane KA, McDonald FM, Parratt JR, Rothaul AL. The effects of verapamil, prenylamine, flunarizine and cinnarizine on coronary artery occlusion-induced arrhythmias in anaesthetized rats. *Br J Pharmacol* 1984;83(1):299-304. doi: 10.1111/j.1476-5381.1984.tb10146.x

39. Curtis MJ, Walker MJ. The mechanism of action of the optical enantiomers of verapamil against ischaemia-induced arrhythmias in the conscious rat. *Br J Pharmacol* 1986;89(1):137-47. doi: 10.1111/j.1476-5381.1986.tb11129.x

40. Curtis MJ, Walker MJ, Yuswack T. Actions of the verapamil analogues, anipamil and ronipamil, against ischaemia-induced arrhythmias in conscious rats. *Br J Pharmacol* 1986;88(2):355-61. doi: 10.1111/j.1476-5381.1986.tb10211.x

41. Nayler WG, Sturrock WJ. An inhibitory effect of verapamil and diltiazem on the release of noradrenaline from ischaemic and reperfused hearts. *J Mol Cell Cardiol* 1984;16(4):331-43. doi: 10.1016/S0022-2828(84)80604-5

13

Gellified Emulsion of Ofloxacin for Transdermal Drug Delivery System

Swati Jagdale*, Saylee Pawar

MAEER's Maharashtra Institute of Pharmacy, MIT campus, Kothrud, Pune (MS) 411038, Savitribai Phule Pune University, India.

Keywords:
· Emulgel
· Transdermal
· Delivery
· Ofloxacin
· Antimicrobial
· Emulsion

Abstract

Purpose: Ofloxacin is a fluoroquinolone with broad-spectrum antibacterial action, used in treatment of systemic and local infections. Ofloxacin is BCS class II drug having low solubility, high permeability with short half-life. The present work was aimed to design, develop and optimize gellified emulsion of Ofloxacin to provide site targeted drug delivery. Transdermal drug delivery will enhance the bioavailability of the drug giving controlled drug release.

Methods: Transdermal drug delivery system was designed with gelling agent (Carbopol 940 and HPMC K100M), oil phase (oleic acid) and emulsifying agent (Tween 80: Span 80). Effect of concentration of gelling agent on release of drug from transdermal delivery was studied by 3^2 factorial design. Emulgel was evaluated for physical appearance, pH, drug content, viscosity, spreadability, antimicrobial activity, *in- vitro* diffusion study and *ex-vivo* diffusion study.

Results: FE-SEM study of the emulsion batch B5 has revealed formation of emulsion globules of approximately size 6-8 μm with -11.2 mV zeta potential showing good stability for the emulsion. Carbopol 940 had shown greater linear effect on drug release and viscosity of the formulations due to its high degree of gelling. *In-vitro* diffusion study through egg membrane had shown 88.58±1.82 % drug release for optimized batch F4. *Ex-vivo* diffusion study through goat skin indicated 76.68 ± 2.52% drug release.

Conclusion: Controlled release Ofloxacin emulgel exhibiting good *in-vitro and ex-vivo* drug release proving good antimicrobial property was formulated.

Introduction

Formulations that are applied to the skin or to mucus membrane are referred as transdermal or topical. Drugs administered through the topical route may have both local and systemic effects, depending on where the application is made and on how the formulation is been constructed. Three different functions may be achieved via application of the formulations to human skin.[1] First function is the desirability to make the active remain on the surface of the skin, E.g. dermal insect repellents, skin infections, and cosmetics for skin decoration. These pharmaceuticals or cosmetics are called epidermal formulations. The second function is for those topical formulations which are designed for dermal penetration of their actives into the deeper regions of the skin such as the viable epidermis and dermis. These are called as endodermal or diadermal formulations. These formulations are not aimed to get absorbed into systemic circulation. Third function aimed to get the systemic action by transdermal application. Local reactions are undesired in this case. When a systemic effect is sought, topical administration can offer many advantages over oral or parenteral administration. The main advantage includes no first pass effect, the risks and inconveniences of parenteral administration are ignored and large variations in the pH in gastric emptying are avoided. Oppositely, if a local effect is sought; many adverse effects associated with an oral administration can be avoided when the topical route is used.[2]

Emulgels are the one which combine gels and emulsions together. Gelling agent in the water phase converts emulsion into an emulgel. Oil-in-water systems are designed to entrap lipophilic drugs whereas water-in-oil systems are used to encapsulate hydrophilic drugs. Emulsions possess certain degree of elegance and get easily washed off. Emulsions have a high ability to penetrate the skin. Emulgels had many advantages as a pleasing appearance, greaseless, high spreadability, easily washable, thixotropic, emollient, nonstaining, longer shelf life, bio-friendly and transparent.[3,4]

Ofloxacin is fluoroquinolone with broad-spectrum antibacterial activity. Ofloxacin is active on both actively dividing as well as dormant bacteria. The mechanism is by inhibition of bacterial DNA gyrase. Ofloxacin has a wide range of antibacterial activity for the treatment of systemic as well as local infection. The half-life of Ofloxacin is 6-7 hrs. Ofloxacin is slightly soluble in water and methanol. It belongs to BCS class II drug with low solubility and high permeability. Present work was aimed to design emulgel which can enhance the bioavailability of drug and give site

*Corresponding author: Swati Jagdale, Emails: jagdaleswati@rediffmail.com ; swati.jagdale@mippune.edu

targeted delivery. The objective was to optimize controlled release emulgel delivery and to investigate the influence of concentration of gelling agents (HPMC K100M and Carbopol 940) on the drug delivery.

Materials and Methods

Ofloxacin was gift sample from Mercury laboratories Ltd. HPMC K100M was a gift sample from Colorcon Asia Pvt. Ltd. Oleic acid and Span 80 were purchase from Merck specialties private Ltd. Tween 80 and propylene glycol 400 were obtained from Ranbaxy laboratories Ltd. Carbopol 940 was obtained from Analab fine chemicals. All other chemicals were of analytical grade.

Drug – excipient compatibility study

Ofloxacin and excipient (HPMC K100M, Carbopol 940) were mixed in 1:1 ratio. As per ICH guidelines samples were kept in the stability chamber (Thermo Lab) for 1 month at $40 \pm 2°C/75 \pm 5\%$ RH. After one month the samples were evaluated by FTIR, UV spectrophotometer and DSC study.[5]

DSC thermogram was recorded using differential scanning calorimeter (DSC-60, Shimadzu Corporation, Japan). Samples were analyzed at a heating rate of 10°C/min under nitrogen atmosphere over a range of 50-300°C.[6]

Screening of oils, surfactants and co-surfactants for emulsion formation:

For selecting solvents with good solubilizing capacity for Ofloxacin, the saturation solubility of Ofloxacin in various oils such as oleic acid, vegetable oil, light liquid paraffin, olive oil, castor oil, linseed oil; surfactants such as span 80, tween 80, span 20, tween 20 and co-surfactants such as propylene glycol, propylene glycol 400 were determined. Excess drug was added to 5 ml of oil, surfactant and co-surfactant in a rubber capped vial. They were stirred for 24 hrs on magnetic stirrer at 200 rpm and then the suspension was centrifuged at 5000 rpm. Clear supernatant liquid was separated and filter through Whatman filter paper. Solubility of Ofloxacin was determined by UV spectrophotometer at 287 nm.

Different concentrations of oils were evaluated for preparation of emulsion. Oil was selected on basis of solubility of drug. Batch A2 with composition of Oleic acid (2): Water (8): Tween 80 (0.42): Span 80(0.32) was selected for further study based on its globule size (0.2-0.5 μ).

Changing concentration of co-surfactant i.e. propylene glycol 400 from 0.1 to 0.5ml in batch A2, it was found that batch B5 containing 0.1 ml of propylene glycol 400 to A2 batch gave globule size **in** range of 0.2-0.5 μ, therefore it was selected for further study.

Preparation of gel phase

Five polymers varying their concentrations namely, carbopol 940 (1 to 5%), HPMC K100M (0.5 to 4%),

xanthan gum (2 and 3%), guar gum (1 to 3%) and sodium alginate (2 and 3%), were selected for preparation of gel phase. The carbopol gel was prepared by dispersing carbopol 940 and HPMC K100M separately in sufficient amount of warm water (40-50°C) with constant stirring at a moderate speed. Both gels were mixed in 1:1 ratio using homogenizer. The dispersion was neutralized with triethanolamine (TEA) to adjust pH in between 6-7. The gel with guar gum and HPMC K100M were prepared by dispersing the required amount of guar gum and HPMC K100M separately in warm water with constant stirring at moderate speed until gel is formed. Both gels were mixed in 1:1 ratio using homogenizer and by neutralizing the dispersion with triethanolamine, pH in between 6-7 was adjusted. Same procedure was followed for different combinations of carbopol 940 + guar gum, guar gum + xanthan gum, sodium alginate + HPMC K100M, HPMC K100M + xanthan gum.

Combination of carbopol 940 and HPMC K100M were selected to design factorial design.

Preparation of Emulgel

Ofloxacin (0.3%) was dissolved in oleic acid and stirred for 10 min on magnetic stirrer at 400-500 rpm. Span 80 was added in with stirring on magnetic stirrer at 400-500 rpm. The aqueous phase was prepared by taking required quantity of distilled water. Tween 80 and PEG 400 were dissolved in an aqueous phase with stirring on magnetic stirrer at 400-500 rpm. Oil and aqueous phase were heated separately at 70 -80°C. Then the oil phase was mixed with aqueous phase with continuous stirring. Carbopol gel was prepared by dispersing Carbopol 940 in purified water with constant stirring at a moderate speed. The gel was obtained by neutralizing the dispersion with triethanolamine. pH was adjusted to 5-7. In case of HPMC K100M gel, it was prepared by dispersing HPMC K100M in warm distilled water (40°C). The dispersion was cooled and kept overnight. The obtained emulsion was mixed with gel in 1:1 ratio to get an emulgel using homogenizer.

Experimental design

Concentration of the polymers was decided based on results of trial batches. 3^2 factorial design was applied. Concentration of carbopol 940 and HPMC K100M was indepenant variables and % cumulative drug release at 8 hrs and viscosity was dependent variables. In Table 1a independent variables are listed and batches were prepared according to the experimental design as per Table 1b.

Table 1 a. Selection of variables

Independent variables	Variables (levels)		
	High(+1)	Medium(0)	Low (-1)
Concentration of Carbopol 940 (%)	5%	4%	3%
Concentration of HPMC K100M (%)	3%	2%	1%

Table 1 b. Factorial Design

Ingredients (%w/w)	F1	F2	F3	F4	F5	F6	F7	F8	F9
Ofloxacin	0.3	0.3	0.3	0.3	0.3	0.3	0.3	0.3	0.3
Oleic acid	20	20	20	20	20	20	20	20	20
Span 80	3.2	3.2	3.2	3.2	3.2	3.2	3.2	3.2	3.2
Tween 80	4.2	4.2	4.2	4.2	4.2	4.2	4.2	4.2	4.2
PEG 400	1	1	1	1	1	1	1	1	1
Carbopol 940	3	3	3	4	4	4	5	5	5
HPMCK100M	1	2	3	1	2	3	1	2	3
TEA	q. s. adjust pH 6-7								
Water	q.s.								

Evaluation of emulsion

Globule size measurements

Droplet size measurements of optimized batch of emulsion were carried out by MOTIC microscope, Field Emission-Scanning Electron Microscopy (FEI-NOVO, NANOSEM 450) and Zetasizer.[7] In FE-SEM, the sample was prepared by drop casting method with dilution of emulsion. 1 ml of emulsion was diluted with 10 ml of distilled water, and then a drop of emulsion was taken in micropipette and placed on aluminum foil in petri dish. Petri dish was dried at room temperature for 24 hrs. Then the sample was placed in sample holder of FE-SEM and images at different parts were captured.[8]

Zeta potential measurement

Globule size and Zeta potential of optimized emulsion batch was measured by zetasizer (Malvern zetasizer, 90) with use of disposable sizing cuvette at 25.1°C. 1 ml emulsion sample was diluted with 10 ml water and result was recorded.

Dilution test, pH, Drug content, Viscosity and Centrifugation

To know type of emulsion formed, prepared emulsion was diluted with water which was external /continuous phase.[9] pH of the emulsions was measured by digital pH meter. Drug content was measured by dissolving known quantity of emulsion in methanol and stirring for 4 hrs. Absorbance was measured at 297 nm in UV/VIS spectrophotometer. Viscosity of emulsions was determined by using Brookfield's viscometer (spindle No.4). The prepared emulsion was centrifuged at ambient temperature and at 5000 rpm for 10 mins to evaluate the system for creaming or phase separation.[10]

Evaluation of Emulgel

Emulgels were evaluated by sensory evaluation for clarity, colour, homogeneity, drug content, presence of particles and fibres. pH was determined with a digital pH meter at room temperature. Viscosity was determined by using Brookfield's viscometer (spindle No.4).

Bio-adhesive strength measurement

The bioadhesion measurement was performed using a modified balance method. Two pans of physical balance were removed. Right side pan was replaced with a 100 ml beaker. On left side, a glass slide was hanged. For balancing the assembly, a weight of 20 g was hanged on the left side. Another glass slide was placed below the hanged slide. Portions of egg membrane were attached with both slides. One gram of gel was placed between two egg membrane faces. Little pressure was applied to form bioadhesion bond. Then slowly water was added on right side beaker, till the gel was separated from one face of attached egg membrane. Volume of water added was converted to mass.[11] The bioadhesive strength (grams) was calculated from equation 1.

$$\text{Bioadhesive strength} = \frac{mg}{A} \qquad \text{Equation 1}$$

Where, m = weight required to detached the slides, A = Area of rat skin attached to slides, g = Acceleration due to gravity (980 cm/s^2)

Spreadability

Spreadability was determined by an apparatus suggested by Mutimer et al. The apparatus was modified and it consists of a wooden block with pulley at one end. A rectangular ground glass plate was fixed on the block. Gel (about 2 g) was placed on the lower plate and was sandwiched between lower and upper glass plate having the same dimensions, provided with the hook. 500 mg weight was placed on the top of the two plates for 5 min to expel air and to get uniform film of gel. Excess of gel was scrapped off. Upper plate was subjected to a pull of 50 g. Time (sec) required by the upper plate to cover a distance of 10 cm was noted. The spreadability was calculated from equation 2. Shorter the time interval better the spreadability.

$$S = M \times L / T \qquad \text{Equation 2}$$

Where, S = Spreadability, M = weight tied to upper slide, L = length of the glass slide, T = time taken for plates to slide the entire length (sec).

In-vitro Diffusion Study

Cellophane membrane

A modified Franz diffusion cell was used for permeation study. Cellophane membrane was boiled in distilled water for 1 hr. Then it was soaked in phosphate buffer pH 6.8 for 24 hrs before use. Cellophane membrane was placed between the donor and receptor compartment. 1g of gel was transferred to the donor compartment. Entire surface of membrane was in contact with receptor compartment containing 25 ml of phosphate buffer pH 6.8. The cell was agitated on magnetic stirrer at 50 rpm and maintained at 37±1°C. 2 ml were withdrawn at intervals of 15, 30, 60, 120, 180, 240, 300, 360, 420 and 480 min and was replaced with equal volume of fresh phosphate buffer pH 6.8 each time. Samples were evaluated measuring their absorbance at 287 nm.[12]

Egg membrane

Procedure as that of *in-vitro* drug release study was followed. Instead of cellophane membrane egg membrane was used. A small hole was made at the bottom of raw egg to remove all its contents. The egg shell was dipped into 0.1 N HCl for 3 hrs to dissolve the egg shell. Obtained egg membrane was washed with distilled water and used for study. For each time used freshly prepared egg membrane.[13]

Ex-vivo diffusion study: Goat skin
Male Goat free from any visible sign of disease was selected. The goat dorsal skin was brought from slaughter house. It was stored in a PSS solution at 37±0.5°C. The dorsal hair was removed and skin was washed with distilled water. Dorsal skin of full thickness was excised and adhering subcutaneous fat was removed. Epidermis facing the donor compartment was mounted on the donor compartment. The receptor compartment contains phosphate buffer solution pH 6.8 at 37 ± 0.5°C. 1 g emulgel was spread. Study was carried out in the similar manner as that with cellophane membrane.[14]

Release Experiment / Model dependent method
In order to insight of the drug release mechanism from emulgel, drug release data were examined for zero order, first order, and Higuchi's model, Hixson and Crowell model, Korsmeyer and Peppas model.[15]

Flux
PCP Disso V3 software was used to study the average flux of Ofloxacin from the emulgel (F1 to F9 batches) and marketed formulation (TRIBEN-XT, skin cream) through cellophane membrane.[16]

Similarity factor
The drug release from the optimized batch (F4) of the formulation was compared to that of the marketed (TRIBEN-XT, skin cream) formulation. Comparison was carried out by determining the similarity factor. The similarity factor was calculated using the BIT-SOFT software. *In-vitro* diffusion study for the marketed formulation was carried out using the same procedure used for the permeation study through cellophane membrane.

Microbiological assay
This technique is used to study bacteriostatic or fungistatic activity of the compound. Microbiological assay was carried out on the strains of *Staphylococcus aureus* and *Escherichia coli* to study the activity of optimized batch and marketed formulation. For present study sabouraud agar medium and ditch plate technique was used (contain 40 g/liter of Dextrose, 15 g/liter of Agar, pH adjusted to approx 5.4±0.2). Concentration 100 µg/ml of optimized batch (F1 and F4), Pure drug and marketed formulation (TRIBEN-XT, skin cream) were prepared. The overnight grown culture of *Staphylococcus aureus* and *Escherichia coli* was inoculated into the sterilized agar media plates. Four Sabouraud agar medium plates were used. In each agar plate 4 wells were prepared and prepared solutions were filled into the wells. As a standard, distilled water was filled. All four agar plates were kept for incubation for 24 hrs. After 24

hrs the plates were observed and zone of inhibition was measured.[17] Percent inhibition was calculated as per equation 3.

$$\% \text{ Inhibition} = L2/L1 \times 100 \qquad \text{Equation 3}$$

Where, L1: Total length of the streaked culture, L2-: Length of inhibition.

Stability study
Stability study was carried on optimized batch F4 to assess its stability after storage using triple stability chamber. The emulgel formulation was packed in clean and dry vial and stored under the accelerated condition for period as prescribed by ICH guidelines. Storage conditions for long term stability was 30°C ± 2°C/65% ± 5% RH and for accelerated stability was 40°C ± 2°C/75% ± 5% RH. Samples were withdrawn at 1, 2, 3 months for long term stability while for accelerated stability conditions samples were withdrawn after 3 months. Samples were evaluated for physical appearance (visually inspected for any change in color and appearance), drug content and viscosity.[18]

Results and Discussion
Ofloxacin exhibited characteristic peaks as shown in Figure 1. One prominent characteristic peak was found in between 3050 and 3000 cm[-1] which was assigned to stretching vibration of OH group and intramolecular hydrogen bonding. Band also suggested NH stretching vibration of the imino-moiety of piperazinyl groups which was less prominent due to intense OH stretching vibration. Peak at 2700 cm[-1] indicated CH_3 of methyl group. 1750-1700 cm[-1] band represented the acidic carbonyl C=O stretching. 1650 to 1600 cm[-1] peak was assigned to N-H bending vibration of quinolones. Band at 1550 to 1500 cm[-1] represented CH_2 of the aromatic ring. Band at 1450-1400 cm[-1] indicated stretching vibration of CH_2 This had confirmed presence of methylene group in benzoxazine ring. Peak at 1400-1350 cm[-1] represented bending vibration of hydroxyl group. Band at 1250 to 1200 cm[-1] suggested the stretching vibration of oxo group. In addition, a strong absorption peak between 1050 and 1000 cm[-1] was assigned to C-F group. Band at 900-800 cm[-1] represented the out of plane bending vibration of double bonded 'enes' or =CH groups (as per I.P.).

Drug excipient compatibility study
After one month accelerated study, major peaks (Figure 1 A) of Ofloxacin were observed at 2936 cm[-1] (CH_2), 1714 cm[-1] (C=O), 1621 cm[-1] (NH_3), 1550 cm[-1] (CF), 1459 cm[-1] (CH_3) and 1086 cm[-1] (CH).

IR peaks (Figure 1B) for HPMC K100M were observed at 2922.59 cm[-1] (C-H), 3420.14 cm[-1] (N-H), 1058.73 (C-O) cm[-1].

IR peaks (Figure 1 C) for Carbopol 940 were observed in between 1750 and 1700 cm[-1] which indicated carbonyl C=O stretching. Band at 1450 to 1400 cm[-1] indicated C-O / O-H. Band at 1250 to 1200 cm[-1] was assigned to C-O-C of acrylates. Prominent peak at 1160 cm[-1] confirmed ethereal cross linking which represented a stretching vibration of C-O-C group. Band between 850 and 800 cm^{-1} indicated out of plane bending of C=CH, i.e., δ=C-H. The spectrum of drug + HPMC K100M is shown in the Figure 1D which showed peaks at 2936 $cm^{-1,}$ 1714 cm^{-1}, 1627 cm^{-1}, 1550 cm^{-1}, 1460 cm^{-1}, 2932 cm^{-1}, 3422 cm^{-1} and 1060 cm^{-1}.

The spectrum of drug + carbopol 940 is as shown in Figure 1E which showed peaks at 2946 cm^{-1}, 1720 cm^{-1}, 1610 cm^{-1}, 1425 cm^{-1}, 1230 cm^{-1}, 1158 cm^{-1} and 820 cm^{-1}. The spectrum of drug + HPMC K100M + Carbopol 940 is shown in Figure 1 F. The spectrum showed peaks at 2930 cm^{-1}, 1708 $cm^{-1,}$ 1635 cm^{-1}, 1555 cm^{-1}, 2940 $cm^{-1,}$ 3445 cm^{-1}, 1045 cm^{-1}, 1430 cm^{-1}, 1220 cm^{-1}, 1168 cm^{-1} and 825 cm^{-1}.

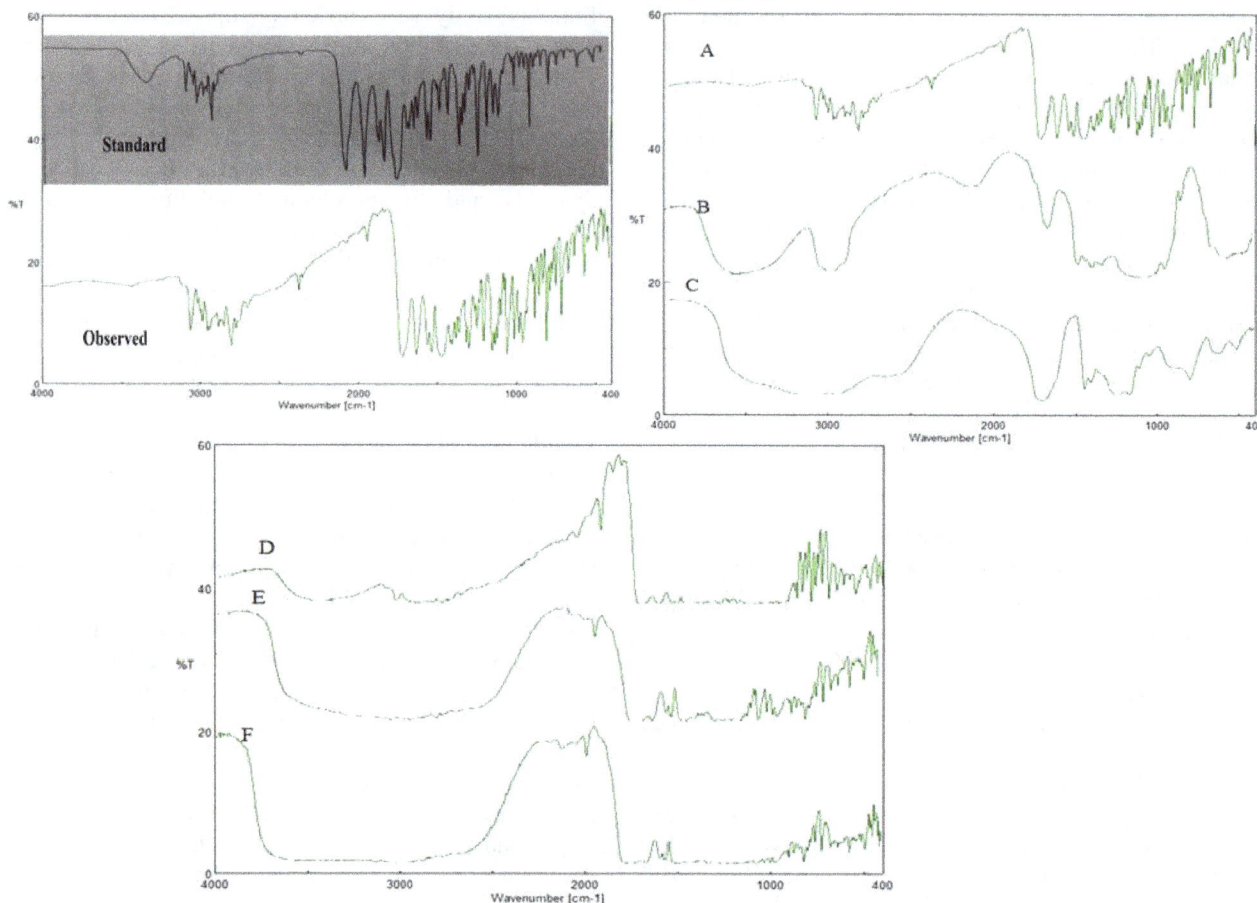

Figure 1. IR Spectrum of Ofloxacin A) Ofloxacin B) HPMC K100M C) Carbopol 940 D) Drug + HPMC K100M E) Drug + Carbopol 940 F) Drug + Carbopol 940 + HPMC K100M

The spectrum of mixtures of drug and excipients has not shown any major change in drug as well as polymer peak. Thus it was concluded that there was no chemical reaction in between drug and proposed excipients.

UV Compatibility study indicated absence of visual changes in the physical mixtures up to 4 weeks, irrespective of storage of samples at ambient conditions. The UV compatibility study indicated absence of any changes in λ max that is 287 nm which concluded that drug was compatible with the proposed excipient.

DSC spectrum of pure drug Ofloxacin indicated melting point sharp at 270.31°C (Figure 2A). Sharp peak indicated that the drug Ofloxacin is in crystalline form. HPMC K100M showed melting point at 74.4°C (Figure 2B). Carbopol 940 showed melting point at 242.6°C (Figure 2C). The mixture of plain drug, HPMC K100M and carbopol 940 showed melting point at 272.3°C, 79.4°C and 236.5°C (Figure 2D) respectively. The drug

and the excipients had shown no major change in melting points which indicated compatibility.

Screening of oil surfactant and co-surfactant

Highest solubility of Ofloxacin was obtained in oleic acid (24.88±0.24 mg/ml) amongst oils. Tween 80 (7.31±1.43 mg/ml) and Span 80 (11.88±2.38 mg/ml) amongst surfactants and propylene glycol 400 (3.50±2.10 mg/ml) amongst co-surfactants showed highest solubility. Solubility in water was 4.23±1.10 mg/ml.

From preliminary batches of emulsions, proportion oil and water phase 2:8 (A2 batch) was selected using span 80 and tween 80 as a surfactant. The other batches (A1, A3-A7) were rejected due to its phase separation and consistency of emulsion.

After that, surfactant to co-surfactant ratio 3:1 (B5 batch) was decided by using spans 80 and tween 80 as a surfactant and propylene glycol 400 as a co-surfactant. Oil and water proportion was taken as per batch A2 with span

80 and tween 80 in a beaker and then propylene glycol 400 was added into beaker drop wise with constant stirring. The emulsions were then visually inspected for

consistency. The other batches (B1-B4) were rejected due to lack of consistency of the emulsions.

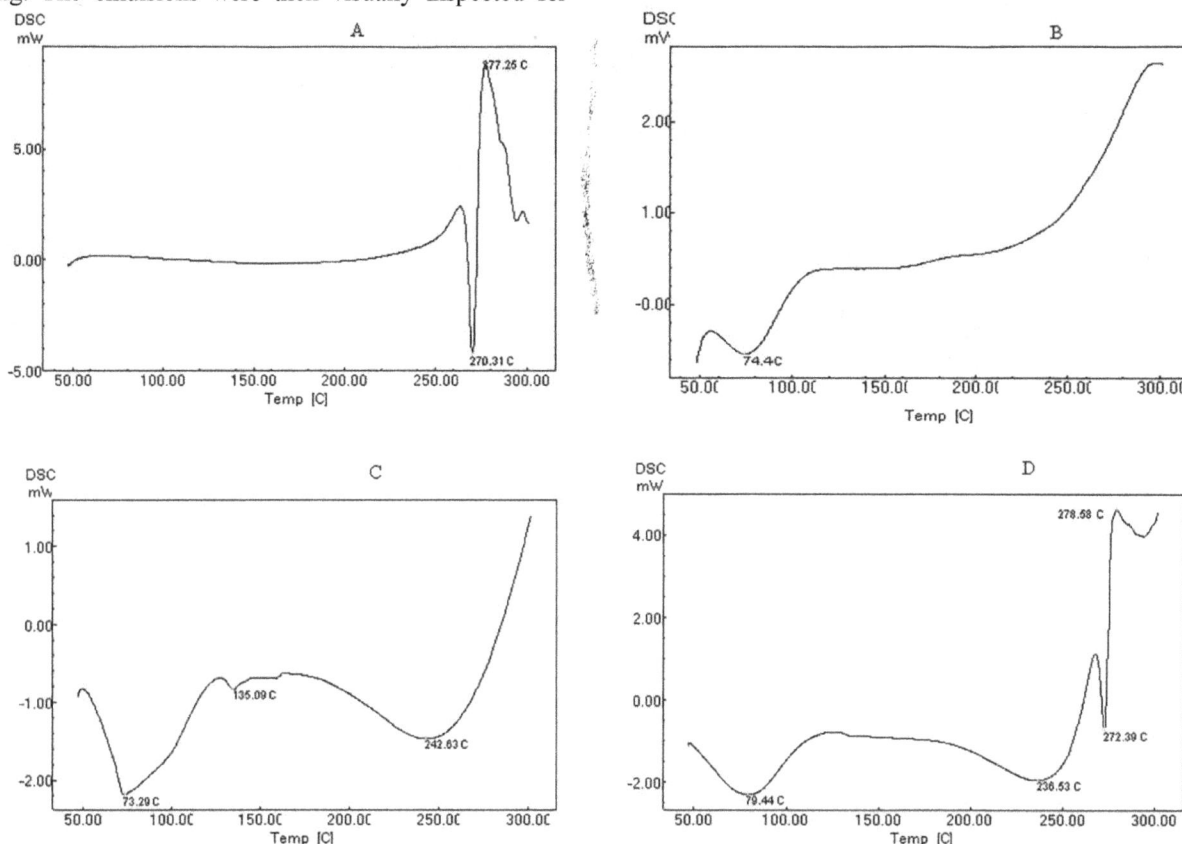

Figure 2. DSC Spectrum for A) Ofloxacin B) HPMCK100M C) Carbopol 940 D) Ofloxacin + HPMCK100M + Carbopol 940

Selection of gelling agent

From all trial batches of gels, the optimized combination of carbopol 940 and HPMC K100M polymers was selected. Batches of guar gum with HPMC and xanthan gum as well as guar gum with sodium alginate were rejected due to problem in viscosity. Also after storage for 1 week fungus formation was observed in those batches. The batches HPMC with xanthan gum because of its viscosity and spreadability.

Evaluation of emulsion

All formulation batches were found to be homogenous and milky emulsions.

Globule size measurement

Motic microscopic image of emulsion had shown spherical shape for globules in size range between 50-200 nm. Field emission-scanning electron microscope (Figure 3) indicated spherical shape for oil globules of optimized emulsion. Size range was in between 6-8 µm. This analysis of emulsion showed conformation of globule size. Globule size was found to be 206.2 nm through zetasizer. PDI is measure of particle homogeneity and it varies from 0.0 to 1.0. If PDI value closer to 0.0, it indicates narrow size distribution of the emulsion. PDI of optimized emulsion was found to be 0.749; hence it indicates

prepared emulsion is monodisperse which remains stable and not converted to micro-emulsion. Figure 4 indicates globule size and PDI of emulsion.

Zeta potential measurement

The general dividing line between stable and unstable emulsion was taken at either +30 or -30 mV. Particles with zeta potential value more positive than +30 mV or more negative than -30 mV are normally considered as stable. Zeta potential of optimized batch was found to be -11.2mV which indicated good stability of the emulsion (Figure 4).

Dilution test, pH, drug content, viscosity and Centrifugation

Dilution with water showed no phase separation indicating that optimized batch of emulsion was o/w type. pH of emulsion was 7.1, drug content 95.82 ± 1.70% and average viscosity of emulsion was found to 2000 cP. After centrifugation, no phase separation was observed which indicates that emulsion was stable.

Evaluation of emulgel

Emulgels were found to be yellowish, white viscous creamy having good appearance, spreadability and viscosity.

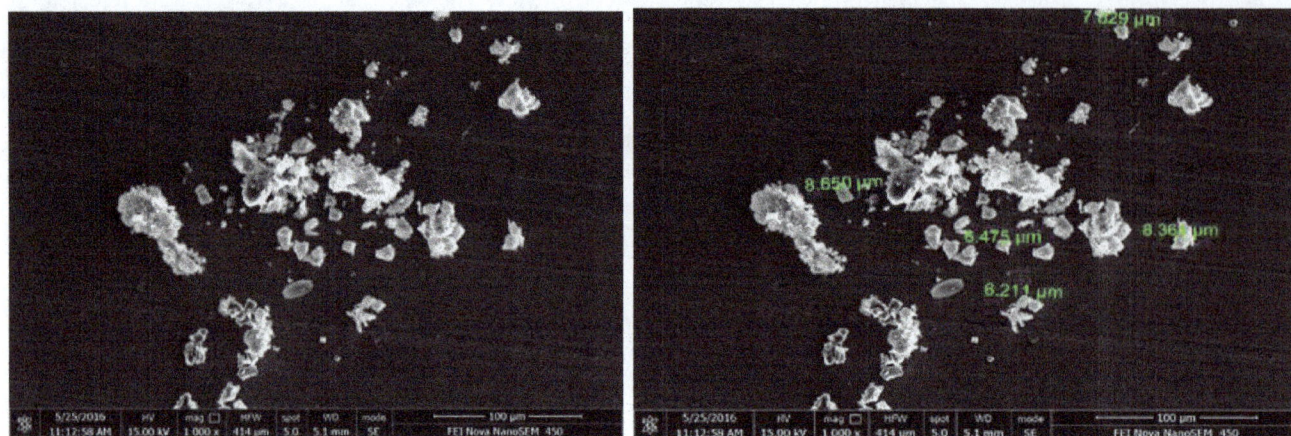

Figure 3. FE-SEM images of optimized batch of emulsion

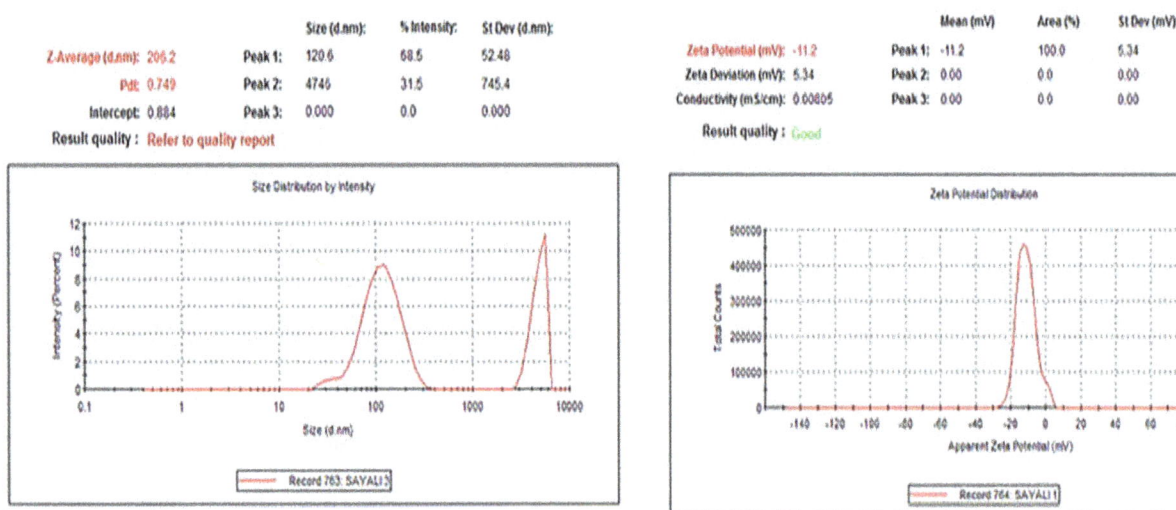

Figure 4. Zeta potential measurement

pH, Viscosity and Drug content

pH of the skin is in the range of 5.5 to 7. pH was found in range of 6.10 to 6.93 for all formulations. This indicated the compatibility of formulations to skin pH and it can show good topical delivery. Batch F6 and F7 showed higher viscosity. As the concentration of carbopol 940 increases, the viscosity of formulation was also increased. Batch F2 showed low viscosity because of low concentration of carbopol 940. The viscosity of the emulgels indicated the shear-thinning property, because as rotating speed increases, the viscosity of emulgels decreases. Batch F1 (100.90±0.37), F4 (97.45±0.61) and F7 (95.10±0.82) showed higher drug content. The drug content was within the range of 70-100%. The results indicated that the drug dispensed uniformly throughout the emulgel.

Bio-adhesive strength measurement

Bio-adhesive strength was determined in terms of detachment stress i.e. force required to detach the formulation from membrane. Results indicated that the change in concentration of Carbopol 940 and HPMC K100M showed changes in bio-adhesive strength. The gradual increase was observed in bio-adhesive strength as the level of Carbopol 940 increased, due to availability of carboxyl group. Carbopol has very high percentage of (58-68 %) of carboxyl group that undergo hydrogen bonding with sugar residues in oligosaccharide chain in membrane. Batch F4 and F7 were shows higher bio-adhesive strength 2525.36 ± 0.13dynes/cm^2 and 2703.06 ± 0.1213dynes/cm^2 respectively.

Spreadability

Spreadability of emulgel is an important parameter. With decrease in viscosity spreadability increases. Batch F1 and F4 showed highest spreadability 28.47±1.24 and 27.6±1.24 respectively. It was easily spreadable because of low viscosity. Marketed formulation showed good spreadability compare to formulated batches.

In-vitro drug diffusion study
Cellophane membrane

As shown in Figure 5A, it was found that formulation batch F1 showed 107.71 ± 2.74% and F4 showed 105.91 ± 2.74% release of drug that was faster than the other formulation due to the lower concentration of HPMC

K100M and higher concentration of Carbopol 940. As there is increase in concentration of carbopol 940 which leads to increase in viscosity of the formulation and therefore decreases the drug release,[19] Batch F9 showed $61.55 \pm 2.74\%$ was retard the drug release because the higher concentration of carbopol 940.

Egg membrane

From the diffusion study carried out with cellophane membrane and viscosity study, batch F1 and F4 were selected for further study. At the 15 min and 30 min formulations showed less drug release compare to release through cellophane membrane (Figure 5B) because of thickness of the egg membrane. After 1hr formulations showed increase in drug release compare to release through cellophane membrane. Formulations showed less drug release after 8 hrs compare to cellophane membrane. This may be due to complexity of the egg membrane.[20]

Ex-vivo drug permeation study

Ex-vivo study of F1 and F4 formulations at 15 min and 30 min showed less drug release compare to release through cellophane membrane and egg membrane (Figure 5C). After 1hr formulations showed increase in drug release but release was less after 8hrs compared to through cellophane membrane and egg membrane. This decrease in drug release may be due to the fat content and higher thickness of goat skin. F4 showed better release than F1, this may be due to the high viscosity of F1.

Kinetic study and mechanism of drug release

The release kinetics data based on correlation coefficient (R^2) indicated that the release of drug for batch F4, F6, F7 and F8 from emulgels followed Zero order kinetics. Batches F2, F3 and F5 followed Korsmeyer Peppas kinetics with release component (k) values < 0.5. Batch F1 followed Hixon Crowell kinetics. Batch F9 followed Matrix kinetic.

Experimental design (ANOVA Study)

Effect of Formulation Variables on Drug Release at 480 min

Drug Release(at 480 min)=+144.602-9.8850A-12.530B

Equation 4

Where, A: Carbopol 940 concentration, B: HPMC K100M concentration

The model terms for the drug release at 480 min. were found to be significant with high value of R^2 0.6634 which indicated the adequate fitting to a linear model. As it can be seen from the Figure 6A and B, the concentration of Carbopol 940 and concentration of HPMC K100M both has negative effect on release of drug (equation 4).

Effect of Formulation Variables on Gel Viscosity

Gel Viscosity= +9733.33+1366.667A-633.33B

Equation 5

Where, A: Carbopol 940 concentration, B: HPMC K100M concentration

The model terms for the gel viscosity was found to be significant with high value of R^2 0.9284 which indicates the adequate fitting to a linear model.

In design, as the concentration of carbopol 940 was increased, the gel viscosity also found to be increased. It was observed that higher concentration of carbopol 940 while lower the concentration of HPMC K100M produced a gel of higher viscosity as shown in Figure 6 C and B and equation 5.

Carbopol 940 showed greater linear effect on release of drug while HPMC K100M showed greater linear effect on viscosity of formulations as it having high degree of gelling capacity. Values of "Prob > F"(p value) less than 0.0500 indicate model terms were significant.

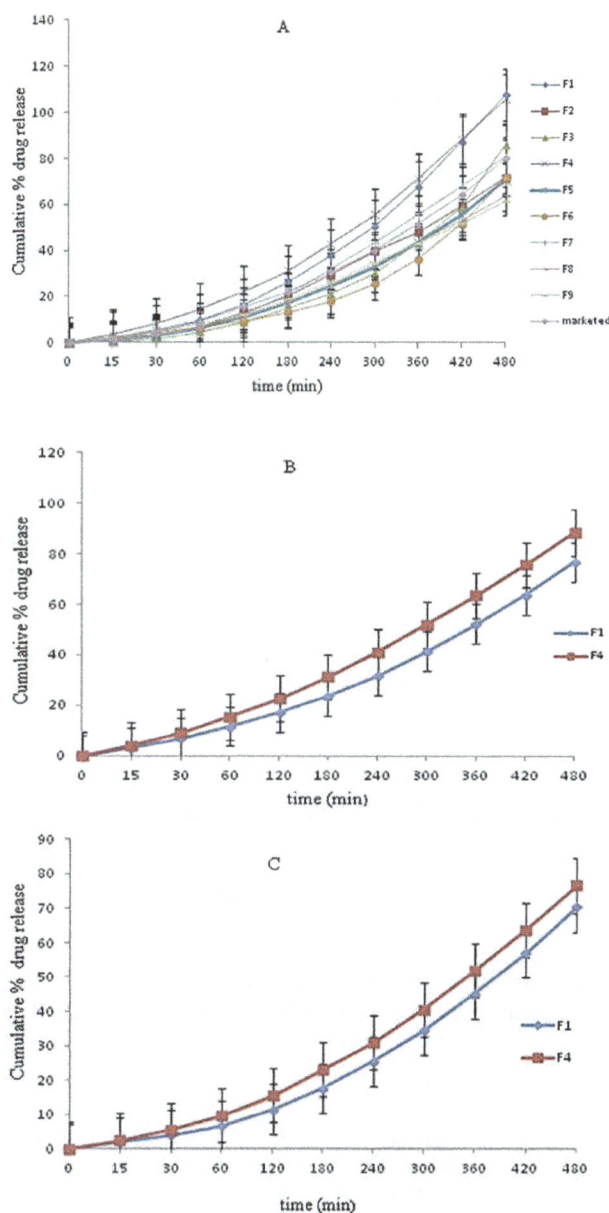

Figure 5. *In-vitro* Cumulative % drug release through A) Cellophane membrane for F1-F9 B) Egg membrane C) Goat skin

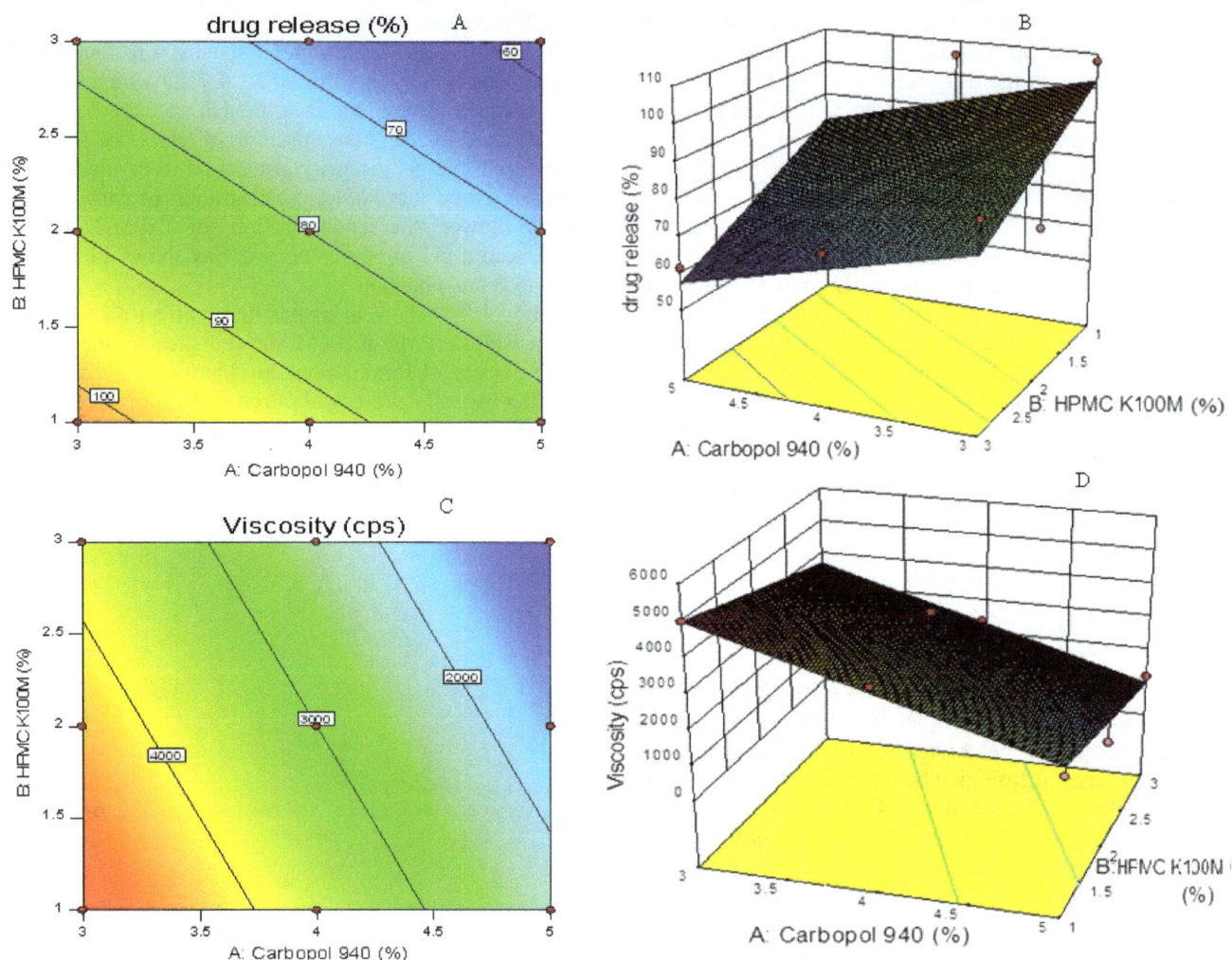

Figure 6. Contour plot (A, C) and response surface plot (B, D) showing relationship in between % drug release at 8 hrs and polymer concentration and viscosity of emulgel and polymers

Validation of statistical model
After statistical analysis by the Design expert software, optimized batch was found to be F4. Experimental values (Table 2) for the % cumulative drug release at 480 mins and viscosity were found very close to the applied and predicted values indicating successful validation for the model.

Table 2. Analysis of Variance

Sr. No.	Response Model	Sum of Squares	Df	Mean Square	F value	P value	R^2	Adequate Precision
1	**Drug Release (480 min.)**	1528.28	2	764.14	5.91	0.0381	0.6634	6.830
2	**Viscosity**	1.361E+007	2	6.807E+006	18.34	0.0028	0.8594	11.373

Flux
Diffusion flux measures the amount of substance that will flow through a small area during a small time interval. Flux was obtained from the slope values plotted for amount diffused per unit area against time. Flux of F1-F9 and marketed formulation were determined through cellophane membrane. The flux of the formulation was in the range of 0.780-1.273 $\mu g/cm^2/min$. The flux of batch F4 was found to be more than batch F1 and marketed formulation through cellophane membrane. Drug incorporation in emulgel base and use of PEG 400 as permeation enhancer were responsible for enhancement of flux.

Similarity factor
Similarity factor (f2) was found to be 39. So, it was concluded that optimized batch was not similar to the marketed formulation.

Microbiological assay
The % inhibition of pure drug found to be higher than optimized batch F1, F4 and marketed (Table 3). This may be due to slow release of drug from emulgel network.

Table 3. Zone of inhibition

Micro-organism	Formulation	L1 (cm)	L2 (cm)	Zone of inhibition (%)
Staphylococcus aureus	F1	9	3.0	33.33±1.52
	F4	9	3.1	34.44±1.74
	Marketed	9	3.5	38.88±1.50
	Pure drug	9	4.1	45.55±1.60
E .Coli	F1	9	2.0	22.22±0.80
	F4	9	2.5	27.77±1.25
	Marketed	9	3.3	36.66±1.36
	Pure drug	9	4	44.44±1.85

L1 = total length of the streaked culture (cm)

Stability Study

From the stability for batch F4, it was observed that there was no significant change on evaluation parameters before and after the study.

Conclusion

In conclusion, a stable, elegant and effective transdermal emulgel delivery for Ofloxacin has developed. The delivery was optimized using HPMC K100M and Carbopol 940 as a gelling agent. Emulgel exhibited good in-vitro drug release and viscosity. Emulgel will act as depot of drug which will release drug in controlled manner at the targeted site. Hence the optimized formulation F4 may be used to treat the topical bacterial diseases.

Acknowledgments

Authors are sincerely thankful to Mercury Laboratories Pvt. Ltd. for providing gift sample of drug. Authors would like to thank Colorcon Asia Pvt. Ltd., Mumbai, India for providing gift sample of HPMC. Authors are highly grateful to Dr. B. S. Kuchekar, Principal and management of MAEER'S Maharashtra Institute of Pharmacy, Pune, India for moral support and providing necessary infrastructure to carry out research work.

Ethical Issues

Not applicable.

Conflict of Interest

The authors declare no conflict of interests.

References

1. Trommer H, Neubert RH. Overcoming the stratum corneum: The modulation of skin penetration. A review. *Skin Pharmacol Physiol* 2006;19(2):106-21. doi: 10.1159/000091978
2. Jhawat VC, Saini V,Kambooj S, Maggon N. Transdermal drug delivery systems: approaches and advancements in drug absorption through skin. *Int J Pharm Sci Rev Res* 2013;20(1):47-56.
3. Ashara KC, Paun JS, Soniwala MM, Chavda JR, Mendapara VP, Mori NM. Microemulgel: An overwhelming approach to improve therapeutic action of drug moiety. *Saudi Pharm J* 2016;24(4):452-7. doi: 10.1016/j.jsps.2014.08.002
4. Singla V, Saini S, Joshi B, Rana AC. Emulgel: A new platform for topical drug delivery. *Int J Pharm Bio Sci* 2012;3(1):485-98.
5. Government of India. Ministry of health and welfare. Indian Pharmacopoeia, Vol. I, II. New Delhi: Controller of Publications; 2014.
6. Khunt DM, Mishra AD, Shah DR. Formulation design & development of piroxicam emulgel. Int *J Pharm Tech Res* 2012;4(3):1332-44.
7. Mulye SP, Wadkar KA, Kondawar MS. Formulation development and evaluation of indomethacin emulgel. *Der Pharmacia Sinica* 2013;4(5):31-45.
8. Singh BP, Kumar B, Jain SK, Shafaat K. Development and characterization of a nanoemulsion gel formulation for transdermal delivery of carvedilol. *Int J Drug Dev Res* 2012;4(1):151-61.
9. Srinivas S, Sagar V. Enhancing the bioavailability of simvastatin using emulsion drug delivery system. *Asian J Pharm Clin Res* 2012;5(4):134-9.
10. Fouad SA, Basalious EB, El-Nabarawi MA, Tayel SA. Microemulsion and poloxamer microemulsion-based gel for sustained transdermal delivery of diclofenac epolamine using in-skin drug depot: In vitro/in vivo evaluation. *Int J Pharm* 2013;453(2):569-78. doi: 10.1016/j.ijpharm.2013.06.009
11. Swami VJ, Kuchekar BS, Jagdale SC. Development and optimization of site targeted topical delivery of norfloxacin. *J Pharm Nanotech* 2015;3(3):22-34.
12. Thakur NK, Bharti P, Mahant S, Rao R. Formulation and characterization of benzoyl peroxide gellified emulsions. *Sci Pharm* 2012;80(4):1045-60. doi: 10.3797/scipharm.1206-09
13. Farooqui N, Singh R, Kar M. Effects of vehicle and penetration enhancer in transdermal delivery of ketorolac tromethamine. *Int J Pharm Life Sci* 2016;7(1):4872-9.
14. United State Pharmacopoeia 34 National Formulary 29. Volume 2. 2011. The United States Pharmacopoeial Convention, Rockville.1818-1822.
15. Varma VNKS, Maheshwari PV, Reddy SC, Navya M, Shivkumar HG, Gowda DV. Calcipotriol delivery into the skin as emulgels for effective permeation. *Saudi Pharm J* 2014;22(6):591-9. doi: 10.1016/j.jsps.2014.02.007
16. Jain A, Gautam SP, Gupta Y, Khambete H, Jain S. Development and characterization of Ketoconazole emulgel for topical drug delivery. *Der Pharmacia Sinica* 2010;1(3):221-31.
17. Yassin GE. Formulation and evaluation of optimised clotrimazole emulgel formulation. *Brit J Pharm Res* 2014;4(9):1014-30. doi : 10.9734/BJPR/2014/8495
18. Lombry C, Dujardin N, Preat V. Transdermal delivery of macromolecules using Skin electroporation. *J Pharm Res* 2000;17(1):32-7. doi: 10.1023/A:1007510323344

19. Jagdale SC, Khawle PS, Kuchekar BS, Chabukswar AR. Development and evaluation of pluronic lecithin organogel topical delivery of tapentadol. *American J Pharm Sci Nanotech* 2015;2(1):1-21. doi:10.7726/ajpsn.2015.1001

20. Jagdale S, Shewale N, Kuchekar BS. Optimization of thermoreversible in situ nasal gel of timolol maleate. *Scientifica* 2016;2016:6401267. doi: 10.1155/2016/6401267

14

A Survey on Phytochemical Composition and Biological Activity of *Zygophyllum fabago* from Iran

Saeid Yaripour[1,2], Mohammad-Reza Delnavazi[3], Parina Asgharian[4,5], Samira Valiyari[6], Saeed Tavakoli[3], Hossein Nazemiyeh[7,5]*

[1] Department of Drug and Food Control, Faculty of Pharmacy, Tehran University of Medical Sciences, Tehran, Iran.
[2] Department of Pharmaceutical and Food Control, Faculty of Pharmacy, Urmia University of Medical Sciences, Urmia, Iran.
[3] Department of Pharmacognosy, Faculty of Pharmacy, Tehran University of Medical Sciences, Tehran, Iran.
[4] Drug Applied Research Centre, Tabriz University of Medical Sciences, Tabriz, Iran.
[5] Department of Pharmacognosy, Faculty of Pharmacy, Tabriz University of Medical Sciences, Tabriz, Iran.
[6] Department of Medical Biotechnology, Pasteur Institute of Iran, Tehran, Iran.
[7] Research Center for Pharmaceutical Nanotechnology, Faculty of Pharmacy, Tabriz University of Medical Sciences, Tabriz, Iran.

Keywords:
· *Zygophyllum fabago* L.
· Zygophyllaceae
· Preparative HPLC
· Zygocaperoside
· MTT
· DPPH

Abstract
Purpose: *Zygophyllum fabago* L. (*Z. fabago*) is a widespread perennial herb which is used as a medicinal plant in traditional medicine of Iran, Turkey and China. The present study was a survey on phytochemical constituents and biological activities of this plant.
Methods: Methanolic extract of the roots was fractionated over a C-18 pre-packed cartridge (Sep-pak) and chromatographic separation was performed on a reversed-phase preparative HPLC. Structural elucidation of the isolated compounds was carried out using UV, ^{1}H-NMR and ^{13}C-NMR spectral analyses. Furthermore, the chemical compositions of the essential oil of the aerial parts were identified by GC-MS analysis. Antiproliferative and antioxidant activities of all extracts from aerials were determined by MTT and DPPH assays, respectively.
Results: Phytochemical investigation on the plant roots led to the isolation and identification of two the 60% methanol-water Sep-pak fraction, a prenylated flavone glycoside, 6-C-prenyl-7-O-[β -D-4'''-O-acetyl-glucopyranosyl-(1'''→2'')-β-D-glucopyranosyl] apigenin, which was named as a Zygocaperoside and also, other flavonoid, was named as the Isorhamnetin -3-O glucoside. None of the extracts showed antiproliferative effect against cancerous cells. However, among the extracts, methanolic extract indicated antioxidant activity. Moreover, essential oils of flowers and leaves of plant have high amounts of sesquiterpene hydrocarbons and diterpenoides.
Conclusion: The results of present study introduce *Z. fabago* roots as a new source of flavonoid glycosides and suggest it as an appropriate candidate for further pharmacological studies.

Introduction

Medicinal plants have always been regarded as a valuable source of new bioactive lead compounds in drug development researches. *Zygophyllum fabago* L. (*Z. fabago*) (Syrian bean-caper) belonging to the family Zygophyllaceae is a perennial herbaceous plant native to southwestern and central parts of Asia, south of Europe and north of Africa.[1] The aerial parts of *Z. fabago* have been reported internally as anti-rheumatic, anthelminthic, cathartic, anti-asthmatic, antitussive, expectorant and anti-inflammatory and externally for skin diseases, wounds, septic, and injuries.[2] In folk medicine of Iran, this species has been named as "Qeich" with known anthelmintic and cathartic properties.[3]
The plant also known as "Memeli Uzerlik" in Azerbaijan province- Iran and its roots and aerial parts are used by indigenous Azeri people (Tabriz,

Miyana, Khoy and Urmia) topically to relieve inflammatory and painful symptoms caused by insect bites (bee and scorpion). Previous pharmacological studies have shown potent butirylcholinesterase (BChE) inhibitory effects and considerable anti-fungal and anti-bacterial effects for *Z. fabago* plant.[4,5] This species has also been considered for allergenic potential of its pollen grains.[6-8] Profilin, a known allergen protein, has been recognized as responsible for this immunological reactions.[6-8] Previous phytochemical investigations on the bark and aerial parts of *Z. fabago* have reported the isolation of 27-nortriterpenoid glycosides, sulphated triterpenoid saponins (fabagoin and zygophylosides E, G, O-R) and disulfated triterpenoid derivatives.[2,9-13] Zygophylosides A, a disulphated saponin isolated from the aerial parts of *Z. fabago* has also been reported to possess a considerable inhibitory effect on Urease enzyme (87% inhibition at 0.5 mM).[2] To the best of our knowledge, there is no report on phytochemical constituents of *Z. fabago* roots and this is the first report on isolation and structure elucidation of a prenylated flavone glycoside (Zygocaperoside) from the roots of this medicinal species.

Materials and Methods
Plant Materials
The roots and aerials samples of *Z. fabago* were collected from Tabriz (East-Azarbaijan province, Iran) in July 2012. The voucher specimen of the plant was authenticated by Prof. Hossein Nazemiyeh and deposited under the code of TBZ-fph 744 at the herbarium of Faculty of pharmacy, Tabriz University of Medical Sciences (Tabriz, Iran).

Extraction and fractionation of root parts
The air-dried and powdered roots (200 g) were Soxhlet-extracted successively with *n*-hexane, dichloromethane and methanol (1.2 L each). The obtained extracts were concentrated using a rotary evaporator at 45 °C. A portion of the methanol extract (2g × 2) was fractionated on a C-18 pre-packed cartridge (Sep-pak, 10 g, Waters) by step gradient of MeOH-H$_2$O mixtures (10:90, 20:80, 40:60, 60:40, 80:20, 100:0) to get six fractions. All fractions were dried using a rotary evaporator at 45 °C.

Isolation procedure
The (40:60) and (60:40) methanolic fractions were subjected to further phytochemical analysis using preparative reversed-phase HPLC (Shimadzu, HPLC LC-8A, SPD-M10A diode array detector, Japan). The chromatographic separation was performed on ODS Column (Dr. Maisch, 250 mm × 20 mm i.d., particle size 10 µm, Germany). The mobile phase time program was as: linear gradient of 25-40% CH$_3$CN in H$_2$O during 0-50 min; linear gradient of 40-55% CH$_3$CN in H$_2$O during 50-62 min; linear gradient of 55-25% CH$_3$CN in H$_2$O during 62-75 min at flow rate of 20 mL/min to get compound 1 (4.3 mg, t_R = 17.5 min) and compound 2 (16 mg, t_R = 26.2 min). The structure of isolated compounds were elucidated using UV, ^{1}H-NMR and ^{13}C-NMR (Bruker, Germany) spectral analyses.

Extraction of aerial parts
The air-dried and ground leaves and flowers (100 g each) were individually macerated with methanol at room temperature. The obtained total methanolic extracts were concentrated using a rotary evaporator at 45 °C.

Eessential oils of aerial parts
The air-dried and comminuted leaves and flowers (100 g) were separately subjected to essential oil extraction using hydrodistillation method for 4 h by a clevenger-type apparatus. The obtained essential oils were dried over anhydrous sodium sulfate and stored at 4 °C protected from light until analysis.

GC/MS analysis
GC/MS analysis of the oil was performed on an Agilent HP-6890 gas chromatograph (Agilent Technologies, CA, USA) with a HP-5MS 5% phenyl methyl siloxane capillary column (30 m ×0.25 mm, 0.25 µm film thickness; Restek, Bellefonte, PA) equipped with an Agilent HP-5973 mass selective detector in the electron impact mode (Ionization energy: 70 eV). Oven temperature was kept at 60 °C for 3 min initially, and then raised at the rate of 3 °C/min to 250 °C. The temperatures of injector and detector were set at 220 and 290 °C, respectively. The flow rate of Helium (as carrier gas) was 1 ml/min. Aliquots of 1.0 µl of diluted samples (1/1000 in n-pentane, v/v) were injected manually into the system. The quantitative analyses data were obtained by calculation of peaks area percent. The retention indices (RI) of the compounds were calculated by injecting the homologous series of n-alkanes in conditions equal to the samples. The compositions of the essential oils were identified using computer matching with the Wiley7n.L library, and also by comparison of the retention indices and fragmentation patterns of the mass spectra with data published in the literature.

DPPH free radical-scavenging assay
Free radical-scavenging potentials of the methanolic extracts of leaves, flowers and roots were evaluated using 2, 2-diphenyl-1-picrylhydrazyl (DPPH) method. In brief, 2 ml of freshly prepared sample solutions (10 mg/ml) were serially diluted with methanol to get concentrations of 0.5 to 3.125×10^{-2} mg/ml. 2 ml of DPPH (Sigma) solution (80 µg/ml in methanol) was then added to diluted solutions. The obtained solutions were kept 30 min at 25 °C and protected from light for any reaction to take place. Then, absorbance were recorded at 517nm. Butylated hydroxytoluene (BHT) was used as a positive control.

In vitro cytotoxic activity assay
Three tumor cell lines, MCF-7 (human breast adenocarcinoma), A-549 (non-small cell line carcinoma) and HT-29 (human colon adenocarcinoma) and a normal cell line, MDBK (Madin-Darby bovine kidney) were purchased from Pasture Institute of Iran, Tehran, Iran. The cell lines were cultured in Dulbecco's Modified Eagle's Medium (DMEM) supplemented with 10% fetal bovine serum (FBS) and 1% penicillin-streptomycin in a 5% CO$_2$ incubator at 37°C. In vitro cytotoxic activities of the extracts of leaves and flowers were evaluated by MTT (3-(4, 5-dimethylthiazol-2-yl)-2, 5-diphenyltetrazolium bromide) colorimetric assay.

Cells were seeded into 96-well plates at a density of $0.5-1.5 \times 10^4$ cells/well and incubated for 24 h at 37°C. The medium was then replaced by fresh medium containing different concentrations of extracts and incubated for 72 h at 37°C. After that, the medium was replaced by fresh medium containing MTT and incubated for additional 4 h. During this period, MTT is reduced to formazan (purple dye) by living cells. Finally, the precipitated formazan crystals were dissolved in DMSO (200 µl) and absorbance was recorded at 570 nm, using a TECAN microplate reader. Cytotoxic activities of the extracts were defined as the concentrations causing a 50% reduction in viability of cells relative to the negative control which was exposed to the solvent without extract.

Results

This study was planned to the isolation of 2 compounds from the roots of Z. fabago, Zygocaperoside and Isorhamnetin-3-O glycoside (Figure 1). The chemical structure of isolated compounds were elucidated unequivocally through UV and NMR and also all spectroscopic data were in agreement with respective published data.[14-21] The data of ^{1}H-NMR and ^{13}C-NMR of the compounds are shown in Table 1 and Table 2.

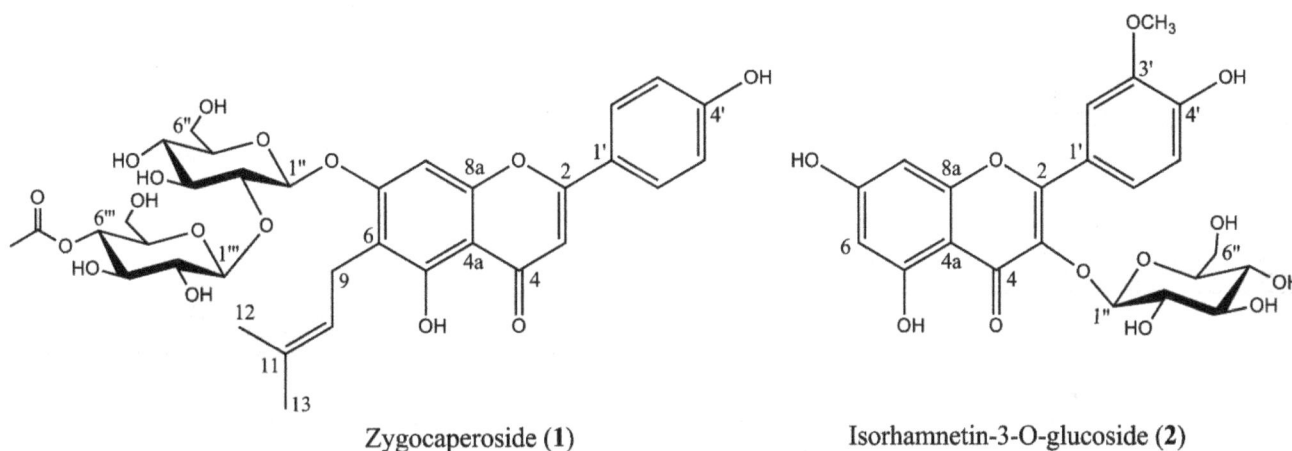

Figure 1. Chemical structures of compound 1 and 2 from the roots of Z. fabago

Spectroscopic data of compound 1
Yellow solid; On-line UV (λ max): 260, 264, 268 and 310 nm; ^{1}H-NMR (200 MHz, CD$_3$OD, δ/ppm, J/Hz). ^{1}H and ^{13}C-NMR data are shown in Table 1.

Spectroscopic data of compound 2
^{1}H and ^{13}C-NMR data are shown in Table 2.

Essential oil compositions
The hydrodistillation of Z. fabago leaves gave yellowish oil with a yield 0.1% (v/w), on dry weight basis. Five compounds representing 95.7% of the oil were identified as a result of GC/MS analysis of the leaves essential oil (Table 3). The results showed that the oil was rich in phytol (62.1%), a diterpenoid, as the main compound. Two non-terpenes, namely β-damascenone (12.6%), and β-ionone (15.9%) were also found in high amounts in leaves oil. Hydrodistillation of the flowers also afforded pale yellow oil (yield 0.1% (v/w)). GC/MS analysis of the obtained essential oil resulted in identification of fifteen compounds, of which ar-curcumene (20.5%), caryophyllene oxide (10.9%), espathulenol (10.2%) and bicyclogermacrene (8.8%) were the most abundant components (Table 4). Neophytadiene with the relative percentage of 4.2% was also identified as a diterpenoid present in the essential oil of plant flowers.

Table 1. NMR spectroscopic data of compound 1

Position	δ_C	δ_H (J)	Position	δ_C	δ_H (J)
2	165.47	-	1"	100.79	5.07,(d,8.4)
3	106.82	6.59, s	2"	83.22	*
4	183.37	-	3"	74.69	*
5	152.93	-	4"	70.46	*
6	116.02	-	5"	76.45	*
7	172.08	-	6"	64.03	*
8	102.80	6.70, s	1'''	103.55	4.54
8a	150.78	-	2'''	72.03	*
4a	101.57	-	3'''	67.33	*
9 prenyl	22.76	overlapped	4'''	71.55	*
10	122.90	5.36, br t	5'''	72.41	*
11	128.68	-	6'''	63.77	*
12	19.95	1.34, s	-	-	-
13	25.01	1.29, s	-	-	-
1'	122.13	-	-	-	-
2'	128.86	7.89,(d,8.4)	-	-	-
3'	116.02	6.94,(d,8.4)	-	-	-
4'	161.87	-	-	-	-
5'	116.02	6.94,(d,8.4)	-	-	-
6'	128.86	7.89,(d,8.4)	-	-	-
OCO-CH3	20.01	2.19, s	-	-	-
OCO-CH3	176.82	-	-	-	-

^{1}H (200MHz) and ^{13}C (50MHz) in CD$_3$OD, δ in ppm, J in Hz) ; * overlapping signals in 3.5-4.5ppm.

Table 2. NMR spectroscopic data of compound 2

Position	δ_C	δ_H (J)	Position	δ_C	δ_H (J)
2	156.99	-	1"	102.67	5.34,(d,6)
3	134.17	-	2"	71.79	*
4	177.83	-	3"	73.61	*
4a	104.24	-	4"	70.08	*
5	161.49	-	5"	76.54	*
6	98.68	6.22, (d, 2)	6"	67.32	*
7	164.96	-	-	-	-
8	93.61	6.43, (d, 2)	-	-	-
8a	161.49	-	-	-	-
1'	121.48	-	-	-	-
2'	112.92	8.04, (d, 2)	-	-	-
3'	146.99	-	-	-	--
4'	149.55	-	-	-	-
5'	114.69	6.95, (d, 8)	-	-	-
6'	122.37	7.66,(dd,8.2)	-	-	-
OCH$_3$	55.44	3.99, s	-	-	-

^{1}H (200MHz) and ^{13}C (50MHz) in CD$_3$OD, δ in ppm, J in Hz) ; * overlapping signals in 3.5-4.5ppm.

Table 3. Chemical composition of the leaves essential oil of Z. fabago.

No.	Compound	%	RI
1	β-Damascenone	12.6	1383
2	β-Ionone	15.9	1487
3	Megastigmatrienone	1.6	1585
4	Hexahydroxyfarnesyl acetone (Phytone)	5.1	1857
5	Phytol	62.1	1942
	Oxygenated sesquiterpenes	5.1	-
	Diterpenes	62.1	-
	Non-terpenes	28.5	-
	Total identified	95.7	-

RI: Relative retention indices to C8-C24 n-alkanes on HP-5MS column.

Table 4. Chemical composition of the flowers essential oil of Z. fabago.

No.	Compound	%	RI
1	α-Citral	2.3	1338
2	β-Damascenone	1.4	1383
3	E-Caryophyllene	7.3	1417
4	Alloaromadendrene	0.9	1462
5	ar-Curcumene	20.5	1479
6	β-Ionone	4.6	1487
7	α-Zingiberene	2.9	1493
8	Bicyclogermacrene	8.8	1500
9	δ-Cadinene	1.5	1522
10	Espatulenol	10.2	1577
11	Caryophyllene oxide	10.9	1582
12	Bicyclo[4.4.0]dec-1-ene, 2-isopropyl-5-methyl-9-methylene-	3.8	1653
13	Hexadecanoic acid	7.7	1959
14	Neophytadiene	4.2	2014
15	Pentacosane	4.6	2500
	Oxygenated monoterpenes	2.3	-
	Sesquiterpene hydrocarbons	50.7	-
	Oxygenated sesquiterpenes	21.1	-
	Diterpenes	4.2	-
	Non-terpenes	8.2	-
	Total identified	86.5	-

RI: Relative retention indices to C$_8$-C$_{24}$ n-alkanes on HP-5MS column.

Antioxidant activity

The reduction in the absorption intensity of methanol solutions of DPPH radical in the presence of antioxidants at 517 nm is usually used asa measure of antioxidant activity. The ability of a sample to scavenge DPPH radical was determined on the base of its concentrations providing 50% inhibition (IC$_{50}$). In this experiment, IC$_{50}$ values of the total methanolic extracts of leaves, flowers and roots were obtained 0.24, 0.20 and 0.39 mg/ml, respectively. The IC$_{50}$ value of Butylated HydroxyToluene (BHT) was 0.02 mg/ml. In comparison to BHT (as a powerful antioxidant), the extracts of leaves and flowers of Z. fabago showed the remarkable results in free radical-scavenging activity.

Cytotoxic activity of aerial parts of plant

The results of cytotoxic activity of extracts of leaves and flowers are shown in Table 5.

Based on these results, it is indicated that both of leaves and flowers extracts had low cytotoxic activities (IC$_{50}$>100 µg/ml) on cancerous cell lines in comparison to the literature data for IC$_{50}$ values of cytotoxic materials.

Table 5. The IC$_{50}$ values (µg/ml) obtained from MTT assay

-	MDBK	A-549	MCF-7	HT-29
Leaves extract	>100	>100	99.0	>100
Flowers extract	>100	>100	>100	>100

Discussion

The preparative HPLC of fraction C (40% and 60% MeOH-H$_2$O Sep-pak fraction) resulted in the isolation of two flavonoid glycoside. The structure of isolated compounds was studied by UV, ^{1}H-NMR and ^{13}C-NMR spectral analyses.

The UV spectrum of compound 1 showed a series of peaks at 260, 264, 268, 278(sh) and 310 nm characteristic for a flavone derivative. ^{1}H-NMR spectrum revealed two symmetrical doublet resonance at δ 7.89 and 6.94 (J= 8.4 Hz) representing para-substituted B ring (AA'BB' system). A singlet resonance at δ 6.59 was also assigned for H-3. Three aliphatic resonances at δ 5.36 (1H, br t), 1.29 (3H, s) and 1.34 (3H, s) suggested the presence of a prenyl group which was supported by the ^{13}C-NMR spectrum of compound. The expected doublet resonance of two protons of prenyl group at δ 3.4 (2H, overlapped) was obscured by sugar protons signals. The downfield shift of C-8 from δ 93.4 to 102.8 indicated the connection of sugar moiety to OH-7 of flavone. Prenyl group to C-6 of flavone derivative was proved by a downfield shift of C-6 from 99.40 to 116.02 ppm.[14] Inspection of ^{13}C-NMR spectrum displayed two glucopyranosyl units from anomeric resonances at δ 100.79 and 103.55 as well as other ten resonances at δ 63.77-83.22 ppm. Assignment of two anomeric resonances at δ 5.07 (1H, d, 8.0) and 4.55 (1H, d) and twelve multiple resonances at 3.1-4.4 ppm in ^{1}H-NMR spectrum also confirmed the presence of two glucopyranosyl units in the structure of isolated compound. Comparison of the ^{1}H- and ^{13}C-NMR data with those reported in literature resulted to identification of β -D-glucopyranosyl-(1→2)-β-D-glucopyranosyl as a disaccharide moiety of the isolated flavone glycoside.[15-17]One methyl singlet at δ 2.19 with a carbonyl resonance in δ 176.82 was assigned for one acetyl moiety in ^{1}H and ^{13}C-NMR spectra of the isolated compound. Comparison of the ^{13}C-NMR spectral data of disaccharide moiety with those reported in literature revealed the downfield shifts of C-4''', and upfield shifts for C-3''' and C-5'''. On the basis of this evidence, the acetyl group is located at C-4''' of the sugar moiety.

Consequently, the structure of isolated compound was elucidated as 6-C-prenyl-7-O-[β -D-4'''-O-acetyl-glucopyranosyl-(1'''→2'')-β-D-glucopyranosyl] apigenin, a new compound which was named as Zygocaperoside (Figure 1).

^{1}H-NMR spectrum of compound 2, revealed a doublet resonance at δ 8.04 (1H, *d*, 2.0) was specified for H-2'. The doublets at 6.95 (*J*= 8 Hz) and 7.66 (*J*= 8 Hz) indicated ortho-coupled aromatic H-atoms assignable to H (5') and H (6'), respectively. In addition, doublet resonances at δ 6.22 (1H, 2.0) and δ 6.43 (1H, 2.0) for the H (6) and H (8), indicated the meta coupled connection. Furthermore, some peaks at δ 3-4 ppm showed the presence of glucose at C-3. The assignment of all ^{13}C-NMR signals were confirmed by comparing with the published data.[18-21] Among the volatile compounds diterpenoids and Sesquiterpene hydrocarbons were high amounts in leaves and flowers respectively. In the other words, the amounts of Oxygenated sesquiterpenes in the leaves and the flowers considerably are different. Furthermore, free-radical-scavenging activity of the corresponding extracts was evaluated *in vitro* by the DPPH assay. The DPPH-scavenging capacity of the extracts was compared with known antioxidants, BHT as a positive control. Among the extracts, the MeOH extract showed the most potent free-radical-scavenging activity with a RC$_{50}$ value of 0.39 mg/mL which could be attributed to the presence of the isolated flavones exhibited potent antioxidant activities in the various studies.[22,23] Both DCM and n-Hexane extracts showed low potency in this assay; this may be explained by deficiency of hydrogen donating components. The anti-proliferative property of the aerial parts of extracts has been evaluated by the MTT assay.[24] None of the extracts showed significant effect against cancerous cells. It is also indicated that there was no obvious cytotoxic effect on non-cancerous cell lines (MDBK). It seems that aerial parts of Z. fabago are not the first choices for further evaluations in cancer researches but it is suggested to isolate and purify the compounds from the aerial parts of the plant which would be have cytotoxic effects on cancerous cell lines without cytotoxicity on non-cancerous cell line.

Conclusion

Flavonoids have considered for their various health benefits such as antioxidant, hepatoprotective, anti-inflammatory, anticancer, antibacterial and antiviral activities. It has also been reported that prenylation enhances the antibacterial, anti-inflammatory, antioxidant, cytotoxicity, larvicidal and estrogenic activity of the flavonoids.[16,17] The result of present study on isolation and identification of a prenylated flavon-O- glucoside (compound 1) and Isorhamnetin-3-O glucoside (compound 2) from Z. fabago roots is indicative of more medicinal potentials of this species and suggests it as an appropriate candidate for further biological and pharmacological studies.

Ethical Issues
Not applicable.

Conflict of Interest
The authors have no conflicts of interest to declare.

References
1. Akhyani V. Flora of Iran, No.7: Zygophyllaceae. Tehran: Research Institute of Forests and Rangelands;1992.
2. Khan SS, Khan A, Khan A, Wadood A, Farooq U, Ahmed A, et al. Urease inhibitory activity of ursane type sulfated saponins from the aerial parts of zygophyllum fabago linn. *Phytomedicine* 2014;21(3):379-82. doi: 10.1016/j.phymed.2013.09.009
3. Zargari A. Medicinal herbs. Vol. 2 and 4. Tehran: University of Tehran Press; 1995.
4. Orhan I, Sener B, Choudhary MI, Khalid A. Acetylcholinesterase and butyrylcholinesterase inhibitory activity of some turkish medicinal plants. *J Ethnopharmacol* 2004;91(1):57-60. doi: 10.1016/j.jep.2003.11.016
5. Zaidi MA, Crow SA, Jr. Biologically active traditional medicinal herbs from balochistan, pakistan. *J Ethnopharmacol* 2005;96(1-2):331-4. doi: 10.1016/j.jep.2004.07.023
6. Belchi-Hernandez J, Moreno-Grau S, Bayo J, Rosique C, Bartolome B, Moreno JM. Zygophyllum fabago l: A new source of allergenic pollen. *J Allergy Clin Immunol* 1997;99(4):493-6.
7. Belchi-Hernandez J, Moreno-Grau S, Sanchez-Gascon F, Bayo J, Elvira Rendueles B, Bartolome B, et al. Sensitization to zygophyllum fabago pollen. A clinical and immunologic study. *Allergy* 1998;53(3):241-8.
8. Castells T, Arcalis E, Moreno-Grau S, Bayo J, Elvira-Rendueles B, Belchi J, et al. Immunocytochemical localization of allergenic proteins from mature to activated zygophyllum fabago l. (zygophyllaceae) pollen grains. *Eur J Cell Biol* 2002;81(2):107-15. doi: 10.1078/0171-9335-00223

9. Feng YL, Li HR, Xu LZ, Yang SL. 27-nor-triterpenoid glycosides from the barks of zygophyllum fabago l. *J Asian Nat Prod Res* 2007;9(6-8):505-10. doi: 10.1080/10286020600782157

10. Feng YL, Wu B, Li HR, Li YQ, Xu LZ, Yang SL, et al. Triterpenoidal saponins from the barks of zygophyllum fabago l. *Chem Pharm Bull (Tokyo)* 2008;56(6):858-60.

11. Feng YL, Li HR, Rao Y, Luo XJ, Xu LZ, Wang YS, et al. Two sulfated triterpenoidal saponins from the barks of zygophyllum fabago l. *Chem Pharm Bull (Tokyo)* 2009;57(6):612-4.

12. Feng YL, Xie B, Li HR, Xu QM, Zhang XJ, Wang YS, et al. A new sulfated triterpenoid from the bark of *Zygophyllum fabago* L. *Chinese Chem Lett* 2010;21(9):1100-2. doi:10.1016/j.cclet.2010.04.015

13. Khan SS, Khan A, Ahmed A, Ahmad VU, Farooq U, Arshad S, et al. Two new disulfated triterpenoids from *Zygophyllum fabago*. *Helv Chim Acta* 2010;93(10):2070-4.

14. Abegaz BM, Ngadjui BT, Dongo E, Tamboue H. Prenylated chalcones and flavones from the leaves of dorstenia kameruniana. *Phytochemistry* 1998;49(4):1147-50. doi: 10.1016/S0031-9422(98)00061-2

15. Watjen W, Weber N, Lou YJ, Wang ZQ, Chovolou Y, Kampkotter A, et al. Prenylation enhances cytotoxicity of apigenin and liquiritigenin in rat h4iie hepatoma and c6 glioma cells. *Food Chem Toxicol* 2007;45(1):119-24. doi: 10.1016/j.fct.2006.08.008

16. Kumar S, Pandey AK. Chemistry and biological activities of flavonoids: An overview. *ScientificWorldJournal* 2013;2013:162750. doi: 10.1155/2013/162750

17. Chen X, Mukwaya E, Wong MS, Zhang Y. A systematic review on biological activities of prenylated flavonoids. *Pharm Biol* 2014;52(5):655-60. doi: 10.3109/13880209.2013.853809

18. Agrawal PK. Carbon-13 NMR of Flavonoids. India: Central Institute of Medicinal and aromatic plants, Luck now; 1989.

19. Markham KR. Techniques of flavonoid identification. London: Academic Press, 1982.

20. Harborne JB, Mabry TJ. The flavonoids: advances in research. London: Chapman and Hall; 1982.

21. Mabry TJ, Markham KR, Thomas MB. The systematic identification of flavonoids. New York: Springer; 1970.

22. Choudhary MI, Begum A, Abbaskhan A, Musharraf SG, Ejaz A, Atta ur R. Two new antioxidant phenylpropanoids from lindelofia stylosa. *Chem Biodivers* 2008;5(12):2676-83. doi: 10.1002/cbdv.200890221

23. Asgharian P, Heshmati Afshar F, Asnaashari S, Bamdad Moghaddam S, Ebrahimi A, Delazar A. Characterization of terpenoids in the essential oil extracted from the aerial parts of scrophularia subaphylla growing in Iran. *Adv Pharm Bull* 2015;5(4):557-61. doi: 10.15171/apb.2015.075

24. Tofighi Z, Asgharian P, Goodarzi S, Hadjiakhoondi A, Ostad SN, Yassa N. Potent cytotoxic flavonoids from Iranian *Securigera securidaca*. *Med Chem Res* 2014;23(4):1718-24. doi: 10.1007/s00044-013-0773-3

The Cytotoxic and Apoptotic Effects of *Scrophularia Atropatana* Extracts on Human Breast Cancer Cells

Elham Safarzadeh[1], Abbas Delazar[2], Tohid Kazemi[1], Mona Orangi[1], Dariush Shanehbandi[1], Solmaz Esnaashari[3], Leila Mohammadnejad[1], Saeed Sadigh-Eteghad[4], Ali mohammadi[1], Mehrdad Ghavifekr Fakhr[1], Behzad Baradaran[1]*

[1] Immunology Research Center, Tabriz University of Medical Sciences ,Tabriz, Iran.
[2] Department of Pharmacognosy, Faculty of Pharmacy, Tabriz University of Medical Sciences, Tabriz, Iran.
[3] Drug Applied Research Center, Tabriz University of Medical Sciences, Tabriz, Iran.
[4] Neurosciences Research Center (NSRC), Tabriz University of Medical Sciences ,Tabriz, Iran.

Keywords:
· Scrophularia atropatana
· Breast cancer
· Extract
· Apoptosis
· MCF-7
· Cytotoxic

Abstract

Purpose: Breast cancer is the most frequent malignancy diagnosed in women both in developed and developing countries. Natural products especially those from herbal origin have high potential in producing drug components with a source of novel structures. The present study was designed to explore the cytotoxic effects and the cell death mechanism of *Scrophularia atropatana* extracts.

Methods: MTT assay was employed to evaluate the cytotoxic activity of the extracts of *S. atropatana* on the MCF-7 as well as non-malignant cells. Furthermore, induction of apoptosis was evaluated by TUNEL assay, cell death detection ELISA, DNA fragmentation test, western blotting and Real Time PCR.

Results: In vitro exposures of the MCF-7 cells with different concentration of *S. atropatana* extract significantly inhibited their growth and viability and induced apoptosis in the MCF-7 cells. Cleavage PARP protein, decrease in the mRNA expression levels of bcl-2 and increase expression of Caspase-3 and Caspase-9 mRNA, highlights that the induction of apoptosis was the main mechanism of cell death. Moreover the expression study of Caspase-9 mRNA showed that, the extracts have induced apoptosis via intrinsic mitochondrial pathway.

Conclusion: Our results demonstrated that dichloromethane extract of Scrophularia atropatana has an apoptotic effects and it can be developed as anticancer agents.

Introduction

Cancer is one of the most common causes of death worldwide. It is estimated that by 2030, there will be 21.4 million new cases of cancer and 13.2 million cancer deaths annually in the world.[1-3] The most conventional strategies for cancer therapy involve surgery, radiotherapy and chemotherapy.[4,5] Among these methods, chemotherapy is widely used for treatment of cancer. However, this therapy has serious side effects and complications.[2,3] Hence, seeking for new therapeutic agents and effective therapies to prevent or control the complications and side effects of routine drugs is of a central importance.[1] Natural compounds especially herbal medicines have a long history of use as medication for various diseases such as cancer.[3,6,7] Many conventional drugs have been derived from herbal resources.[8,9] According to the World Health Organization (WHO), herbal medicines account for approximately 80% of therapeutics in the developing countries.[10,11] Herbal medicines are increasingly being investigated to overcome the side effects of conventional cancer treatments.[12,13] Herbal therapies are more accepted among public and are believed to be safe and natural.[14,15]

Several studies suggest that, herbal medicines may halt the tumor promotion and progression and show an acceptable range of cytotoxic activities on cancerous cells without causing excessive damages to normal cells.[16,17] Some of the compounds with natural origin such as taxol (from *Taxus brevifolia*), camptothecin (from *Camptotheca acuminate*), Decne, vinca alkaloids from Catharanthus roseus G. Don and podophyllotoxin from Podophyllum peltuturn L. are often used in oncology and act as antitumor agents.[3,18,19] The most prominent marker of anticancer agents is induction of apoptosis.[20-22] Hence, apoptosis is considered as an impotent key event in cancer chemotherapy.[18,23] Therefore, the identification of medicinal plants which induce apoptosis is of central importance.[24-27] *Scrophularia*, an important herbal medicine, is a genus of the family Scrophulariaceae which includes about 3000 species and 220 genera throughout the world.[28,29] Since ancient times, some species of *Scrophularia* genus are being used for treatment of several ailments such as fever, erythema, eczema, skin inflammation, different types of dermatosis and also for cancer and wound healing.[30] Herein, we report the cytotoxic and apoptotic effects of *Scrophularia atropatana* extracts on MCF-7 (breast carcinoma cell line) for the first time.

Materials and Methods
Preparation of extracts

Scrophularia atropatana was collected from Eastern Azerbaijan province, Iran. The herbarium voucher specimens (8962) were identified and deposited by the Herbarium of the Faculty of Pharmacy, Tabriz University of Medical Sciences. The aerial parts of the *S. atropatana* (leaves and stems) were washed thoroughly with distilled water and air-dried at room temperature for 2 weeks. Then, the samples were ground using a blender and stored in an airtight container. Extracts from the ground samples were obtained by Soxhlet apparatus using n-hexane, dichloromethane and methanol. *S. atropatana* extracts were concentrated by rotary evaporator (Heildolph, Germany) at 45 °C dried under reduced pressure. Then, 20 mg of each extract was separately re-suspended in 100 µL of Dimethyl Sulfoxide (DMSO) (Merck, Germany) and diluted with serum-free culture medium, RPMI-1640. Finally, the plant extracts were sterilized with 0.22 µm syringe filters (Nunc, Denmark) and stored at 4 °C as a stock solution for further biological assays.

Cell Culture

The Human breast carcinoma cell line (MCF-7) and a normal control cell line (L929) were purchased from Pasteur Institute of Iran (National Cell Bank). The cells were grown in RPMI-1640 medium (Sigma, Germany) supplemented with 10% heat inactivated fetal calf serum (FCS) (Sigma, Germany), 100 Units/ml penicillin and 100 µg/ml streptomycin (Sigma, Germany) and maintained at 37 °C in a humidified atmosphere of 5% CO_2. MCF-7 cells were maintained in their growing phase at 80% confluence with routine passage using 0.025% Trypsin-EDTA treatment. According to the aims of the study, the cells sub cultured into $75cm^2$ flasks, 6-well Plates or 96-well plates (Nunc, Denmark).

Cell Cytotoxicity Assay

The effect of n-hexane, dichloromethane and methanol extracts of *S. atropatana* on cell growth was analyzed by the MTT method based on the ability of live cells to convert 3-(4,5-dimethylthiazolyl-2-yl)-2,5-diphenyltetrazolium Bromide (MTT) into Purple formazan by mitochondrial dehydrogenases. Briefly, cells in early log phase were trypsinized and cultured in 96-well plates with concentration of 10^4 cells/well/200 µl and incubated overnight at 37°C and 5% CO2. Twenty-four hours later, the existing medium was replaced with fresh medium containing different concentrations of extracts (0, 100, 150, 200, 300, 400, 500 and 600 µg/mL). Furthermore, 0.2 % (v/v) DMSO (Merck, Germany) as a negative control and Taxol (Paclitaxel) as a positive control were considered for this assay. After 24, 36 and 48 h of treatments, 10 µl MTT (5 mg/mL) was added to each well

and incubated for 4h in a humidified atmosphere at 37°C following the manufacturer's instructions. These incubation times in the present study were calculated according to the previous study of Iloki Assanga et al and doubling time of the cell lines.[31-33] The formazan crystals were solubilized with DMSO and 25µL of Sorenson buffer. Then the absorbance at a wavelength of 570nm was measured using ELISA plate reader (Bio Teck, Germany). All experiments were performed in triplicates. The dose-response curve was plotted and IC50 value (the concentration that caused 50% of cell growth inhibition) was calculated. Data were normalized by setting the DMSO control to one.

Trypan blue dye exclusion assay

10^4 MCF-7 cells as well as L929 cell (as a normal control cell) were seeded in 96-plate and treated with 0, 100, 200 and 300 µg/mL concentration of dichloromethane and methanol extracts of *S. atropatana* in 0.2 % (v/v) DMSO for 24, 36, 48 and 72 hours. Subsequently, the cells were detached by adding 50 µl of 0.5 % trypsin/EDTA. Then 50 µl of the suspended cells was mixed with an equal volume of trypan blue and incubated for 3 min. Finally, 20 µl of this solution transferred to a hemocytometer and the numbers of viable and non-viable cells were counted under an inverted microscope. The viability was calculated as follows: viability (%) = (live cell count/total cell count) ×100

Cell Death Detection

Cell death detection ELISA (Roche Applied Science, Germany), determinates the mono- and oligonucleosomes in the cytoplasmic fraction of cell lysates after induced cell death using mouse monoclonal antibodies against DNA and histones.[34] Briefly, cells were incubated with the IC50 concentrations of methanolic and dichloromethane extract *S. atropatana*. DMSO and Taxol were used as negative and positive controls respectively. After 24 hours of incubation at 37°C, the culture supernatants were utilized for quantification of necrosis and cell lysates for apoptosis. The assay was performed according to the manufacturer's instructions. The absorbance was measured using an ELISA plate reader at 405 nm and the percentage of apoptosis and necrosis obtained from the ratio of absorbance in the treated samples to that of the untreated controls.

TUNEL assay

TUNEL assay (Terminal deoxynucleotidyl transferase dUTP nick end labeling) was carried out for detection of apoptosis in the treated cells. The *in situ* cell death detection kit (Roche Diagnostics GmbH, Germany) was employed for this purpose. This method is based on the presence of a multitude of DNA strand breakages during programmed cell death. Terminal deoxynucleotidyl transferase enzyme (TdT) adds secondarily conjugated dUTPs to the end nicks.[35,36] Concisely, MCF-7 cells and L929 cell were seeded on chamber slides. After 24 h, the medium was replaced with fresh one. The cells were treated with IC50 concentration of *S. atropatana* dichloromethane extract. Following incubation, cells were washed with PBS and fixed in freshly prepared 4% (w/v) paraformaldehyde (pH 7.4) for 60 min at room temperature. Subsequently, cells were incubated with blocking solution (3% H_2O_2 in methanol) (Merck, Germany) at room temperature for 10 min to inactivate the endogenous peroxidases. The cells were washed once with PBS and permeabilized in 0.1% Triton X-100 in 0.1% sodium citrate for 2 min on ice. Then the fixed and permeabilized cells were incubated in TUNEL reaction mixture (containing TdT-enzyme and Biotinated-dUTP) for 60 min at 37°C in the dark. For negative control, label solution (without TDT) was used instead of reaction mixture. Cells incubated with DNase I (to induce DNA strand nicks) served as positive control. All cells were washed twice with PBS and incubated with streptavidin-HRP conjugate (50μL per specimen) for 30 min and then rewashed. The cells were incubated with diaminobenzidine solution (DAB) for 10 min in the dark place. Afterward, the stained cells (dark brown cells) were analyzed under inverted biological microscope.

DNA Fragmentation
A key event during apoptosis is DNA laddering in which, DNA is degraded by caspase-activated DNase (CAD). Genomic DNA at inter-nucleosomal linkers is cleaved by CADs into nucleosomal units, which are multiples of about 180-bp fragments.[37,38] To perform this experiment, 4 × 10⁵ cells/well were cultured in 6-well plates and treated with 300 and 600 μg/mL concentrations of dichloromethane extracts of *S. atropatana* for 24 hours. DMSO 0.2 % (v/v) was exploited as a negative control. After trypsinizing, the cells were harvested by centrifugation (1000 g, 5 min, 4°C) and washed with 1X PBS. Then the cells were lysed with 1 ml lysis buffer (5 mM Tris [pH 8.0] 20 mM EDTA, 0.5% Triton X-100) and incubated overnight at 56 °C (proteinase K, Thermo scientific). After 24 h, NaCl (5M) was added and the procedure was followed by phenol chloroform method. DNA was precipitated by ethanol (100%) and the pellet was air-dried at room temperature. Finally the DNA pellet was washed once with ethanol (70%) and dissolved in nuclease free distilled water. The extracted DNA was treated with 1 μl of RNase A (DNase free, Fermentas) and incubated for 30 min at 37 °C. Electrophoresis was carried out utilizing agarose gel (1.8%) and the results were subsequently visualized under UV light.

Quantitative Real Time-PCR
Cells were seeded in 6-well plates and exposed to dichloromethane extract of *S. atropatana* in concentration of 300 and 600μg/mL for 12 h at 37°C. Following incubation cells were washed and were added RNX™ – PLUS. Then the sample incubated with chloroform for 5 min on the ice and centrifuged. Transfer the aqueous phase to a fresh tube RNase free and were added isopropanol and incubate for 15 min at 4°C. Washed RNA pellet with 70% EtOH, dissolved the pellet in DEPC water and quantified

extracted RNA by spectrometric assay. Then cDNA were synthesized using Revert Aid ™ first strand synthesis kit (Fermentase, Canada). Synthesized cDNA was measured on a Corbett Rotor Gene 6000 real-time PCR detection system using a SYBR Green I PCR Master Mix (ABI, Foster City, USA). PCR cycling conditions were 95°C for 10 min as hold step, followed by 45 cycles of 95°C for 20 s, 60°C for 30s. β- actin was used as an internal reference. The sequence of primers were: β-actin: Forward: 5′TCCCTGGAGAAGAGCTACG 3′, Reverse: 5′ GTAGTTTCGTGGATGCCACA 3′, bcl-2: Forward: 5′ CCTGTGGATGACTGAGTACC 3′, Reverse: 5′ GAGACAGCCAGGAGAAATCA 3′, caspase 3: Forward: 5′ TGTCATCTCGCTCTGGTACG 3′Reverse:5′AAATGACCCCTTCATCACCA 3′. Caspase-9: forward: GCAGGCTCTGGATCTCGGC and reverse: GCTGCTTGCCTGTTAGTTCGC.

Western blotting for assessment of Poly (ADP-ribose) polymerase (PARP) protein cleavage
MCF-7 cells were grown in 6-well plates and treated with dichloromethane extracts of *S. atropatana* and DMSO, as a control for 24h. After treatment, cells were lysed in RIPA Extraction Buffer (Thermo Scientific, Canada) and equal amounts of proteins (100 μg) from cell lysates were subjected to sodium dodecyl sulfate– polyacrylamide gel electrophoresis (SDS- PAGE). Subsequently, blotting onto polyvinyl-difluoride (PVDF) membrane (Roche Diagnostics GmbH, Germany) was performed in 150 mA for one hour. The membrane was subsequently blocked with 4% skim milk, washed and incubated with specific primary antibodies of a mouse anti-PARP monoclonal antibody and anti-β-actin as a normalizing control (Roche Diagnostics GmbH, Germany) for overnight. Then the membrane was probed with horseradish peroxidase-conjugated secondary antibody. Protein detection was carried out by exposing the membrane to ECL western blotting detection system (Amersham Phamacia Biotech Inc, USA).

Statistical analysis
All statistical analyses were carried out using Graph Pad Prism 6.01 software (Graph Pad Software Inc., San Diego, CA, USA) and statistical significance of differences were analyzed using two-way ANOVA test. Each experiment was performed in triplicates (n = 3) and Data are presented as the means ± S.D. The criterion for statistical significance between groups were considered as $P<0.05$.

Results
S.atropatana treatment inhibited MCF-7 cells viability and proliferation
To evaluate the cytotoxic effects of *S. atropatana* n-hexane, dichloromethane and methanol extracts on the growth of MCF-7 breast cancer cell line and L929, the cells were treated with different concentration of the extracts and then analyzed by MTT and trypan blue assay. As shown in Figure1, compared with untreated cells, dichloromethane and methanol extracts of *S. atropatana*

significantly suppressed MCF-7 cell growth in a time and dose dependent manner, whereas the cytotoxic effects was not observed in the cells treated with n-hexane extract. Based on MTT results, the IC50 (50% growth inhibition) values of dichloromethane and methanolic extracts are shown in Table 1. According to the outcomes, dichloromethane extract exhibited a higher cytotoxic activity on MCF-7 cells than methanolic extract. Moreover, interestingly the cytotoxic effects of dichloromethane and methanol extracts of *S. atropatana* on the MCF-7 cells were significantly higher than on the L929 cells (p<0.05). In addition, dye exclusion assay was utilized for assessment of viability in MCF-7 and L929 cells treated with dichloromethane and methanol extract of *S.atropatana*. Taxol (paclitaxel) was employed as a positive control at the same concentration. Microscopic cell count using a hemacytometer indicated a significant decrease in the number of viable MCF-7 cells in the treated cells compared to untreated ones. As a result, the dichloromethane extract was more cytotoxic compared with methanolic extract (p<0.05) Figure 2.

Table 1. The IC50 values of dichloromethane and methanolic extracts in MCF-7 and L929cells.

	IC50 µg/ml					
	24 h		36 h		48 h	
Cell line	MCF-7	L929	MCF-7	L929	MCF-7	L929
Dichloromethane	223.0	557.0	153.9	303.8	114.7	264.3
Methanol	289.9	543.3	226.6	370.2	197.9	321.0

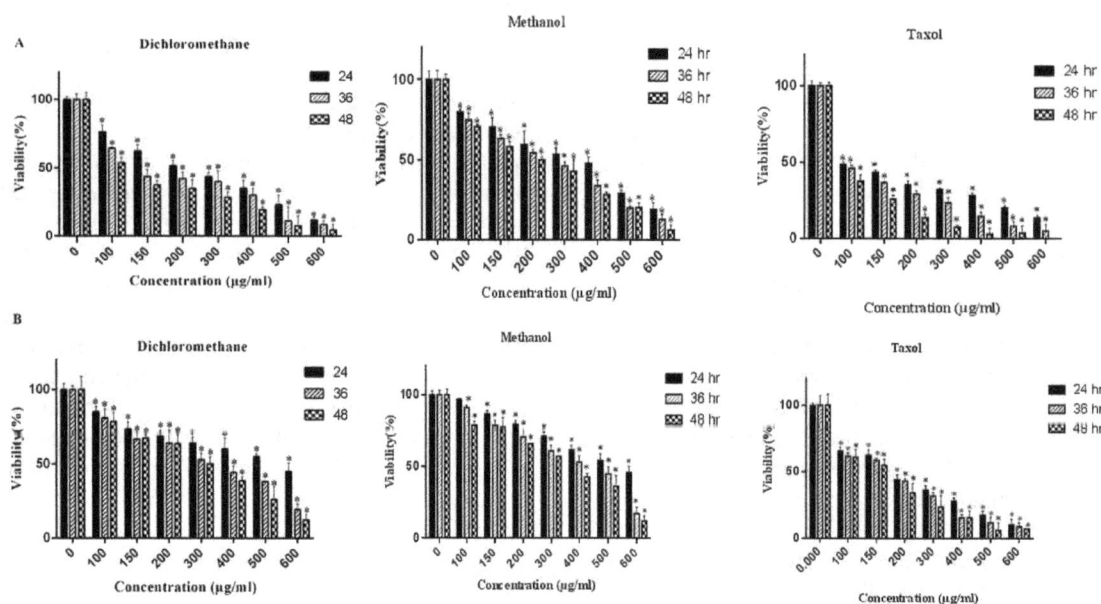

Figure 1. Cytotoxic effect of *S. atropatana* extract in **A**.MCF-7 cells, **B**.L929 cells Experiment was carried out in triplicates (n=3) and values are presented as the mean ± SEM.

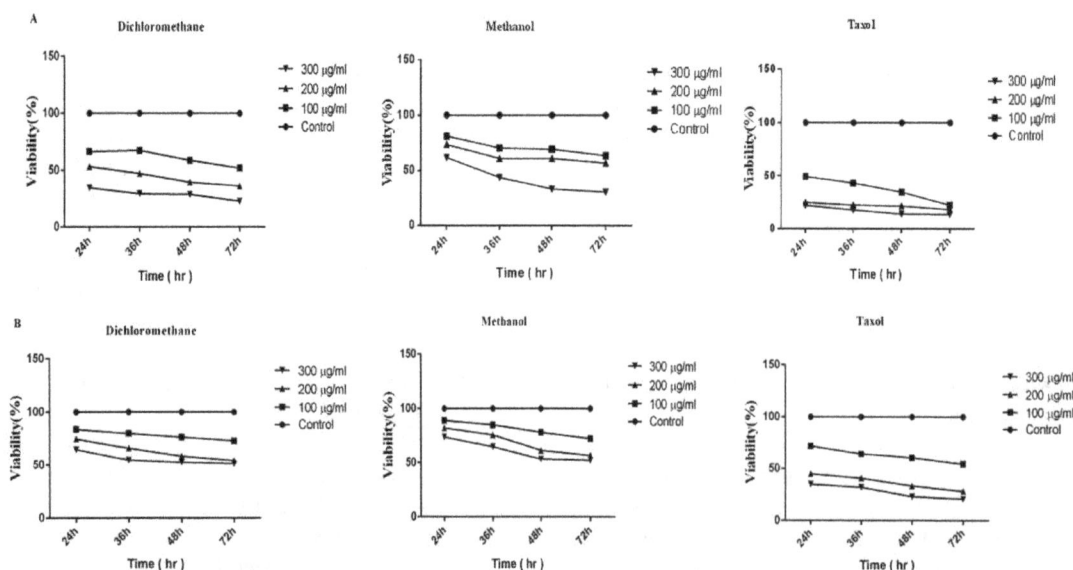

Figure 2. Viability of **A**.MCF-7 cells, **B**.L929 cells treated with various concentrations of *S. atropatana* (100, 200 and 300 µg/ml) for 24, 36, 48, and 72 hours.

S. atropatana treatment induced apoptosis in MCF-7 cells
Cell death ELISA kit, was used to assess apoptosis or necrosis occurrence in cells treated with dichloromethane and methanol extracts. Taxol was used as positive control for induction of apoptosis. After 24 h of treatment with IC50 concentrations of S. atropatana extracts, apoptosis values for dichloromethane extract and methanol extract in MCF-7 cells were 51.21% and 30.72% respectively (Figure 3). The acquired data indicated that, dichloromethane extract exhibits more apoptotic activity than methanol extract on the studied cells. Therefore, the next experiments were performed relying on dichloromethane extract. In addition, TUNEL test was performed to identify presence of DNA strand breaks and confirm the induction of apoptosis in MCF-7 cells exposed to dichloromethane extract S. atropatana. As shown in Figure 4, following 24 h of exposure to

IC50 concentrations of the extracts despite the normal cells, apoptotic cells developed brown precipitates.

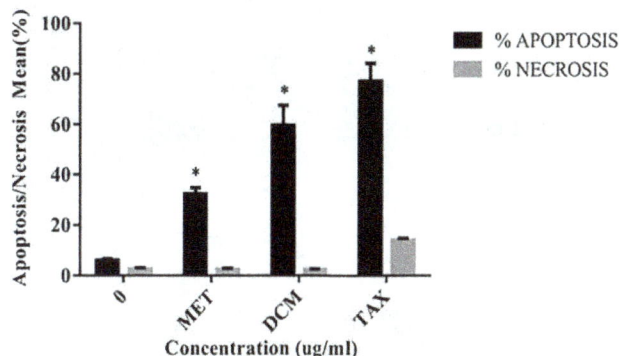

Figure 3. The percentages of apoptosis and necrosis by Cell Death assay in MCF-7 cells.
Data are presented as means ± S.E. *: $p < 0.05$ was considered as significant statistical difference.

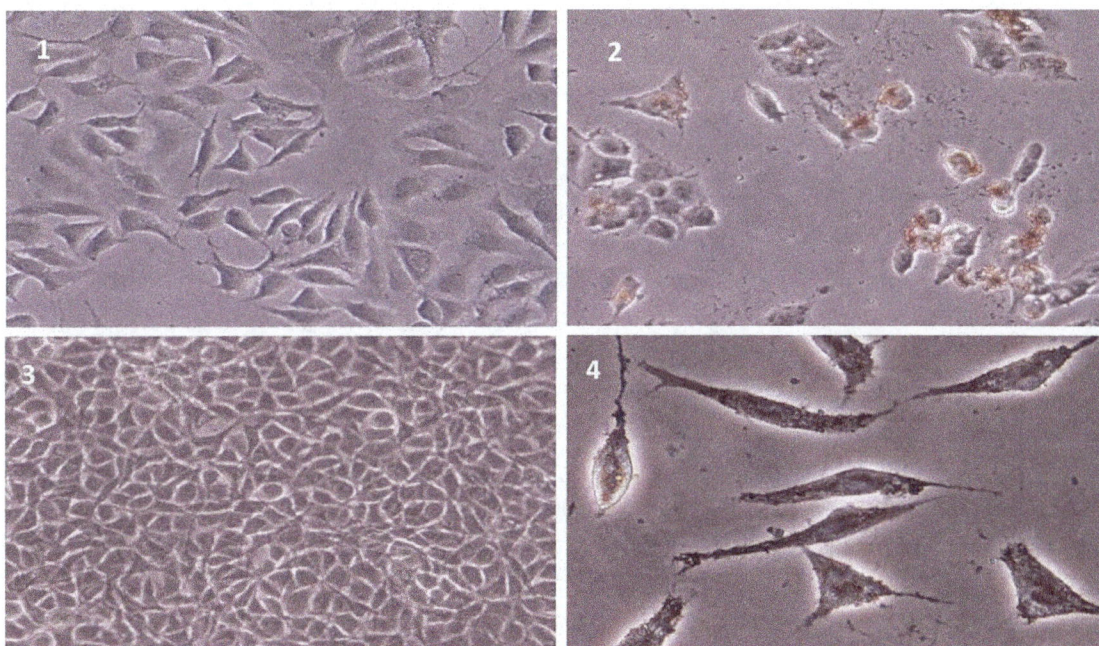

Figure 4. Apoptotic effects of S. atropatana on MCF-7 cells observed by TUNEL assay. (1) MCF-7 control, (2) treated MCF-7 (3) L929 control and (3) treated L929. Arrows indicate apoptotic cells.

S. atropatana treatment of MCF-7 cells induced DNA fragmentation
A key feature of apoptosis is DNA fragmentation via nuclease activity of caspase-3 protein. Dichloromethane extract of S. atropatana was able to form apoptotic DNA ladders in MCF-7 cells after 24 h of treatment with the concentration of 300 and 600μg/mL (Figure 5). Moreover, DNA fragmentation was not observed in L929 cells. The results further confirmed that, S. atropatana extract could induce apoptosis on tumor cells.

S. atropatana treatment of MCF-7 cells changed the expression of apoptotic genes
Changes in the expression level of apoptosis-related genes, bcl-2 (anti apoptotic gene), caspase 3 (pro-

apoptotic gene) and caspase 9 following the treatment with dichloromethane extract of S. atropatana was investigated using real time PCR. According to the data, bcl-2 expression was decreased by 6.25 and 22.22 fold in 300 and 600 μg/ml concentrations respectively compared to the untreated control cells, whereas a noticeable increase was detected in caspase 3 expression. The rate of this increase was 3.02 and 4.58 fold in 300 and 600 μg/ml groups respectively. Caspase 9 also indicated a 5.3 and 7.3 fold increases in 300 and 600 μg/ml groups respectively (Figure 6).

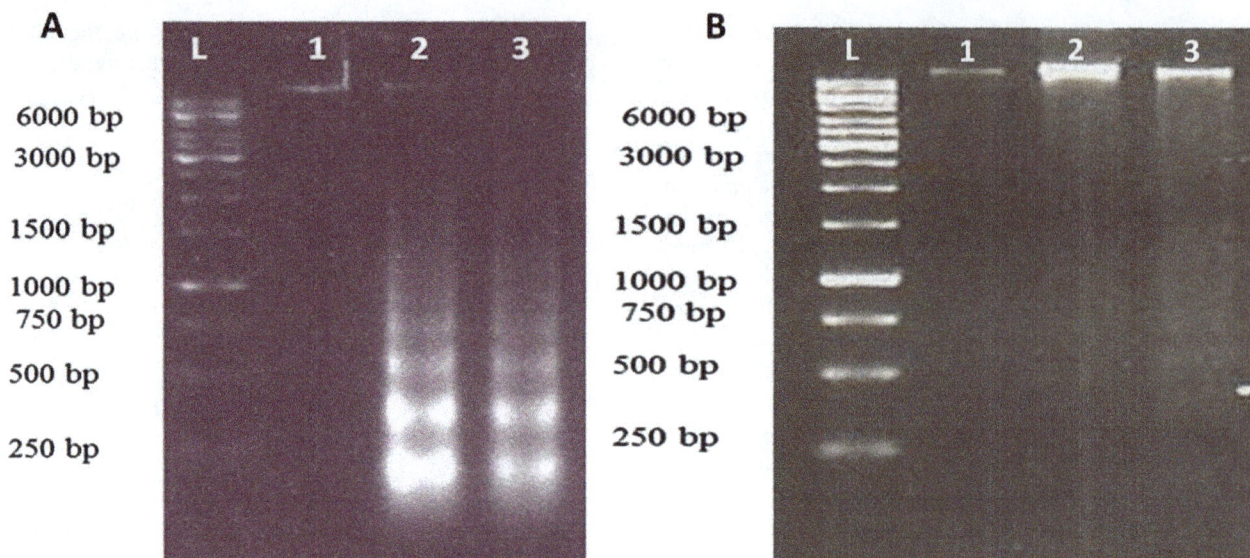

Figure 5. DNA fragmentation assay in MCF-7 cells(A) and L929 cells (B) treated with S. atropatana for 24 hr. (1) control,(2) 300 µg/mL, (3) 600 µg/mL and L= size Ladder. DNA fragments were separated on 1.8% agarose gel electrophoresis.

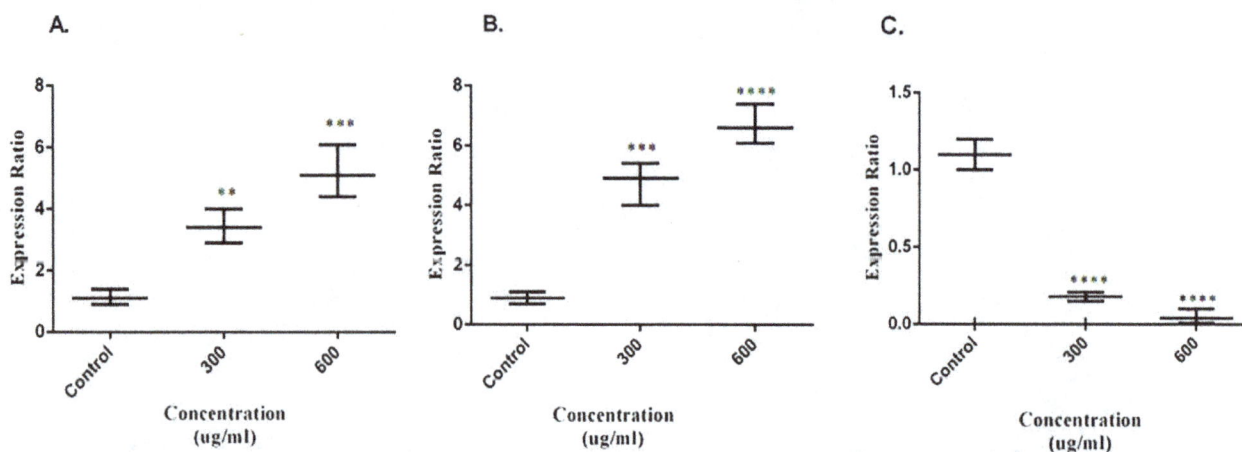

Figure 6. Effects of dichloromethane extract of S. atropatana on **A.** Caspase-3, **B.** Caspase-9 and **C.** Bcl-2 mRNA expression in MCF-7 cells at 24 h. Relative expression was acquired by qRT-PCR using 2(-ΔΔCt) method. The results are presented as mean ± SD (n = 3); ****p<0.00001 versus control ***p<0.0001 versus control.

S.atropatana treatment of MCF-7 cells induced PARP cleavage

During programmed cell death, the intact PARP molecule (116 kDa) is cleaved into 89 kDa and 24 kDa fragments by activated caspase-3.[39] After 24 h of treatment with *S. atropatana* dichloromethane extract, the PARP molecule cleavage was detected in MCF-7 cells by western blot analysis. However, no cleavage of PARP molecule was observed in untreated control cells (Figure 7).

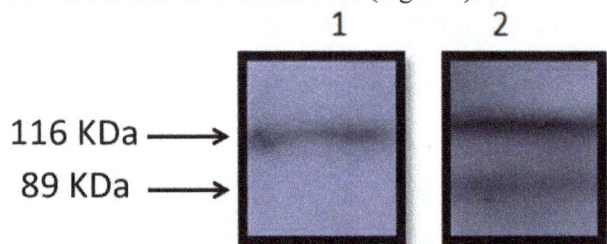

Figure 7. PARP molecule (116 kDa) cleavage to 89 kDa and 24 kDa fragments by activated caspase-3. (1) Control, (2) treated

Discussion

High prevalence of cancer makes it the second mortality cause following cardiovascular diseases. Nowadays, because of the priority and importance of neoplasia, numerous studies have focused on the introduction of safe and effective compounds for the treatment of various types of cancer. In this regard, the mechanisms involved in carcinogenesis has a critical role in developing the methods for neoplasm treatment.[3,40] Among these compounds, drugs with herbal origin are the most popular. Because, these products are more cost effective, available and exert fewer side effects.[41] Consequently, targeting the mechanisms which cause tolerance to death stimuli and apoptosis could be a suitable strategy in cancer treatment.[20] Different studies have shown that, herbal medicines have different functional mechanisms, but inducing apoptosis is a common feature among them.[3] Most synthesized anti carcinogenic drugs such as; taxol which used in treatment of breast and ovarian cancers have herbal origin.[3]

Numerous studies have shown the cytotoxic and anti-tumor effects of different species of Scrophularia genus. A study has shown that *Scrophularia lucida* has remarkable cytotoxic and apoptotic effects on HL-60 leukemic cells. It has been reported that methanolic extract of *S. lucida* leads to cell cycle blockage in G2-M phase, inhibiting activation of caspase-3 and breaking down PARP protein into 89 kDa compartments.[42] In another study, the cytotoxic effects of *Scrophularia striata* on astrocytes (1321) has been assessed and shown that it had significant suppressing effects on the growth and replication of these cell types.[28] Another study showed that methanolic and dichloromethanolic extracts of *Scrophularia oxysepala* suppresses the growth of MCF-7 cells by apoptosis induction.[43] In the present study, the cytotoxic effect of n-hexane, dichloromethanolic and methanolic extracts of *S. atropatana* on MCF-7 and L929 cells has been assessed. The ability of elimination of tumor cells is one of the chemotherapeutic drug characteristics. The results of this study showed that dichloromethanolic and methanolic extracts of *S. atropatana* had significant cytotoxic effect on tumor cells but there was no significant activity in L929 normal cells. Nontoxic properties of these extracts on normal cells, makes them as suitable candidates for future in vivo studies. Moreover, N hexane extract did not indicate noticeable impacts on cancerous and normal cells. As shown in Figure1, the toxicity of the extracts is comparable with that of Taxol chemotherapeutic drug. Furthermore, the cytotoxic effect of dichloromethanolic and methanolic extracts was time and concentration dependent. It means that, by enhancing the concentration of extract and time of exposure, the cytotoxic effect on MCF-7 cells was increased. Also the comparison of IC50 showed that dichloromethanolic extract had greater effect on MCF-7 tumor cells than methanolic extract, suggesting that dichloromethanolic extract contain high level of active cytotoxic components. Cytotoxic effects are not solely enough for herbal extracts to be considered as antitumor agent. Beside this feature, chemotherapeutic extracts should also induce apoptosis. Microscopic observations showed that, the exposure of MCF-7 cells to dichloromethanolic and methanolic extracts led to morphological alteration and apoptotic bodies' formation. For evaluating the apoptosis induction, ELISA cell death assay was utilized. According to the results, dichloromethanolic and methanolic extracts exert apoptotic characteristics. Data analysis suggested that, these extracts had substantial apoptotic effects on MCF-7 cells compared to taxol. DNA fragmentation as one of the hallmarks of apoptosis could be demonstrated by TUNEL and DNA fragmentation test. The results of these tests were in conformity with earlier tests. In order to detect antitumor mechanism(s) of *S. atropatana*, the expression rate of genes involved in apoptosis such as caspase 3, caspase 9 and BCL-2 were assessed by real time PCR. CASP 3 and CASP 9 genes belong to

cysteine- aspartic acid protease family play a central role in the induction of apoptosis. BCL-2 is a regulatory protein that as an oncogene has anti apoptotic effects. The increased expression of CASP 9 gene in the treated cells could be regarded as an indicator of intrinsic (mitochondrial) apoptosis. Data analysis showed that following the treatment of MCF-7 cells, the expression of caspase 3 and caspase 9 mRNAs were increased significantly and expression of bcl-2 gene decreased in contrast to the untreated controls. On the other hand Caspase-3 activity could result in the breakdown of different proteins including PARP. According to western blot results, PARP protein was fragmented to 89 kDa and 24kDaproteins in size demonstrating the occurrence of apoptosis in treated cells. Consequently, the aforementioned features prove the occurrence of apoptosis in the cells exposed to *S. atropatana* extracts.

Conclusion

The treatment of MCF-7 cells with dichloromethanolic and methanolic extracts of *S. atropatana* resulted in morphological changes, cytotoxic and apoptotic effect on this tumor cells while there was no significant inhibitory effect on normal cells. Induced cytotoxic effects were related to exposure time and concentration of the extract, so that by enhancing the time and concentration the viability of cells declined. These findings suggested that dichloromethanolic extracts of *S. atropatana* may contained more bioactive components compare to methanolic and n hexane extracts. According to these results, dichloromethanolic extract of *S. atropatana* can be a proper candidate for extraction of antitumor component.

Acknowledgments
The authors wish to thank the Immunology Research Center of Tabriz University of Medical Sciences, for supporting the research (Grant#91/61).

Ethical Issues
Not applicable.

Conflict of Interest
The authors declare no conflict of interests.

References
1. Wang Z, Wang N, Chen J, Shen J. Emerging glycolysis targeting and drug discovery from chinese medicine in cancer therapy. *Evid Based Complement Alternat Med* 2012;2012:873175. doi: 10.1155/2012/873175
2. Taraphdar AK, Roy M, Bhattacharya R. Natural products as inducers of apoptosis: Implication for cancer therapy and prevention. *Curr Sci* 2001;80(11):1387-96.
3. Hemalswarya S, Doble M. Potential synergism of natural products in the treatment of cancer. *Phytother Res* 2006;20(4):239-49. doi: 10.1002/ptr.1841
4. Qi F, Li A, Inagaki Y, Gao J, Li J, Kokudo N, et al. Chinese herbal medicines as adjuvant treatment during

chemo- or radio-therapy for cancer. *Biosci Trends* 2010;4(6):297-307.

5. Sahranavard S, Naghibi F, Mosaddegh M, Esmaeili S, Sarkhail P, Taghvaei M, et al. Cytotoxic activities of selected medicinal plants from iran and phytochemical evaluation of the most potent extract. *Res Pharm Sci* 2009;4(2):133-7.

6. Nho KJ, Chun JM, Kim HK. Ethanol extract of dianthus chinensis l. Induces apoptosis in human hepatocellular carcinoma hepg2 cells in vitro. *Evid Based Complement Alternat Med* 2012;2012:573527. doi: 10.1155/2012/573527

7. Koehn FE, Carter GT. The evolving role of natural products in drug discovery. *Nat Rev Drug Discov* 2005;4(3):206-20. doi: 10.1038/nrd1657

8. Vickers A, Zollman C, Lee R. Herbal medicine. *West J Med* 2001;175(2):125-8.

9. Mansoori B, Mohammadi A, Hashemzadeh S, Shirjang S, Baradaran A, Asadi M, et al. Urtica dioica extract suppresses mir-21 and metastasis-related genes in breast cancer. *Biomed Pharmacother* 2017;93:95-102. doi: 10.1016/j.biopha.2017.06.021

10. Bent S, Ko R. Commonly used herbal medicines in the united states: A review. *Am J Med* 2004;116(7):478-85. doi: 10.1016/j.amjmed.2003.10.036

11. Treasure J. Herbal medicine and cancer: An introductory overview. *Semin Oncol Nurs* 2005;21(3):177-83. doi: 10.1016/j.soncn.2005.04.006

12. Ekor M. The growing use of herbal medicines: issues relating to adverse reactions and challenges in monitoring safety. *Front Pharmacol* 2013;4:177. doi: 10.3389/fphar.2013.00177

13. Mohammadi A, Mansoori B, Baradaran PC, Khaze V, Aghapour M, Farhadi M, et al. Urtica dioica extract inhibits proliferation and induces apoptosis and related gene expression of breast cancer cells in vitro and in vivo. *Clin Breast Cancer* 2017. doi: 10.1016/j.clbc.2017.04.008

14. Olaku O, White JD. Herbal therapy use by cancer patients: A literature review on case reports. *Eur J Cancer* 2011;47(4):508-14. doi: 10.1016/j.ejca.2010.11.018

15. Hosseini BA, Pasdaran A, Kazemi T, Shanehbandi D, Karami H, Orangi M, et al. Dichloromethane fractions of scrophularia oxysepala extract induce apoptosis in mcf-7 human breast cancer cells. *Bosn J Basic Med Sci* 2015;15(1):26-32. doi: 10.17305/bjbms.2015.1.226

16. Hsieh MJ, Yang SF, Hsieh YS, Chen TY, Chiou HL. Autophagy inhibition enhances apoptosis induced by dioscin in huh7 cells. *Evid Based Complement Alternat Med* 2012;2012:134512. doi: 10.1155/2012/134512

17. Mohammadi A, Mansoori B, Baradaran B. Cytotoxic effects of anacyclus pyrethrum plant extract in oral cancer cell (kb cell line). *J Urmia Univ Med Sci* 2016;27(4):257-65.

18. Naveen Kumar DR, Cijo George V, Suresh PK, Ashok Kumar R. Cytotoxicity, apoptosis induction and anti-metastatic potential of oroxylum indicum in human breast cancer cells. *Asian Pac J Cancer Prev* 2012;13(6):2729-34.

19. Safarzadeh E, Sandoghchian Shotorbani S, Baradaran B. Herbal medicine as inducers of apoptosis in cancer treatment. *Adv Pharm Bull* 2014;4(Suppl 1):421-7. doi: 10.5681/apb.2014.062

20. Ait-Mohamed O, Battisti V, Joliot V, Fritsch L, Pontis J, Medjkane S, et al. Acetonic extract of buxus sempervirens induces cell cycle arrest, apoptosis and autophagy in breast cancer cells. *PLoS One* 2011;6(9):e24537. doi: 10.1371/journal.pone.0024537

21. Asadi H, Orangi M, Shanehbandi D, Babaloo Z, Delazar A, Mohammadnejad L, et al. Methanolic fractions of ornithogalum cuspidatum induce apoptosis in pc-3 prostate cancer cell line and wehi-164 fibrosarcoma cancer cell line. Adv Pharm Bull 2014;4(Suppl 1):455-8. doi: 10.5681/apb.2014.067

22. Mohammadi A, Mansoori B, Aghapour M, Baradaran B. Urtica dioica dichloromethane extract induce apoptosis from intrinsic pathway on human prostate cancer cells (pc3). *Cell Mol Biol (Noisy-le-grand)* 2016;62(3):78-83.

23. Mohammadi A, Mansoori B, Aghapour M, Shirjang S, Nami S, Baradaran B. The urtica dioica extract enhances sensitivity of paclitaxel drug to mda-mb-468 breast cancer cells. *Biomed Pharmacother* 2016;83:835-42. doi: 10.1016/j.biopha.2016.07.056

24. Valiyari S, Jahanban-Esfahlan R, Zare Shahneh F, Yaripour S, Baradaran B, Delazar A. Cytotoxic and apoptotic activity of Scrophularia oxysepala in MCF-7 human breast cancer cells. *Toxicol Environ Chem* 2013;95(7):1208-20. doi: 10.1080/02772248.2013.854362

25. Mohammadi A, Mansoori B, Goldar S, Shanehbandi D, Khaze V, Mohammadnejad L, et al. Effects of urtica dioica dichloromethane extract on cell apoptosis and related gene expression in human breast cancer cell line (mda-mb-468). *Cell Mol Biol (Noisy-le-grand)* 2016;62(2):62-7.

26. Mohammadi A, Mansoori B, Aghapour M, Baradaran PC, Shajari N, Davudian S, et al. The herbal medicine utrica dioica inhibits proliferation of colorectal cancer cell line by inducing apoptosis and arrest at the g2/m phase. *J Gastrointest Cancer* 2016;47(2):187-95. doi: 10.1007/s12029-016-9819-3

27. Mohammadi A, Mansoori B, Baradaran PC, Baradaran SC, Baradaran B. Anacyclus pyrethrum extract exerts anticancer activities on the human colorectal cancer cell line (hct) by targeting apoptosis, metastasis and cell cycle arrest. *J Gastrointest Cancer* 2016. doi: 10.1007/s12029-016-9884-7

28. Ardeshiry Lajimi A, Rezaie-Tavirani M, Mortazavi SA, Barzegar M, Moghadamnia SH, Rezaee MB. Study of anti cancer property of scrophularia striata extract on the human astrocytoma cell line (1321). *Iran J Pharm Res* 2010;9(4):403-10.

29. Goldar S, Baradaran B, Shekari Khaniani M, Azadmehr A, Derakhshan SM, Mohammadi A, et al. Extracts of scrophularia frigida boiss display potent

antitumor effects in human breast cancer cells by inducing apoptosis and inhibition of expression of the human epidermal growth factor receptor 2. *Cell Mol Biol (Noisy-le-grand)* 2016;62(9):83-9.

30. Stevenson PC, Simmonds MS, Sampson J, Houghton PJ, Grice P. Wound healing activity of acylated iridoid glycosides from scrophularia nodosa. *Phytother Res* 2002;16(1):33-5.

31. Iloki Assanga SB, Gil-Salido AA, Lewis Luján LM, Rosas-Durazo A, Acosta-Silva AL, Rivera-Castañeda EG, et al. Cell growth curves for different cell lines and their relationship with biological activities. *Int J Biotechnol Mol Biol Res* 2013;4(4):60-70. doi: 10.5897/IJBMBR2013.0154

32. Sutherland RL, Hall RE, Taylor IW. Cell proliferation kinetics of mcf-7 human mammary carcinoma cells in culture and effects of tamoxifen on exponentially growing and plateau-phase cells. *Cancer Res* 1983;43(9):3998-4006.

33. Osborne CK, Hobbs K, Trent JM. Biological differences among mcf-7 human breast cancer cell lines from different laboratories. *Breast Cancer Res Treat* 1987;9(2):111-21.

34. Frankfurt OS, Krishan A. Enzyme-linked immunosorbent assay (elisa) for the specific detection of apoptotic cells and its application to rapid drug screening. *J Immunol Methods* 2001;253(1-2):133-44.

35. Darzynkiewicz Z, Galkowski D, Zhao H. Analysis of apoptosis by cytometry using tunel assay. *Methods* 2008;44(3):250-4. doi: 10.1016/j.ymeth.2007.11.008

36. Loo DT. In situ detection of apoptosis by the tunel assay: An overview of techniques. *Methods Mol Biol* 2011;682:3-13. doi: 10.1007/978-1-60327-409-8_1

37. Matassov D, Kagan T, Leblanc J, Sikorska M, Zakeri Z. Measurement of apoptosis by DNA fragmentation. *Methods Mol Biol* 2004;282:1-17. doi: 10.1385/1-59259-812-9:001

38. Rahbar Saadat Y, Saeidi N, Zununi Vahed S, Barzegari A, Barar J. An update to DNA ladder assay for apoptosis detection. *Bioimpacts* 2015;5(1):25-8. doi: 10.15171/bi.2015.01

39. Morales P, Haza AI. Selective apoptotic effects of piceatannol and myricetin in human cancer cells. *J Appl Toxicol* 2012;32(12):986-93. doi: 10.1002/jat.1725

40. Shukla Y, Singh R. Resveratrol and cellular mechanisms of cancer prevention. *Ann N Y Acad Sci* 2011;1215:1-8. doi: 10.1111/j.1749-6632.2010.05870.x

41. Pal SK, Shukla Y. Herbal medicine: Current status and the future. *Asian Pac J Cancer Prev* 2003;4(4):281-8.

42. Giessrigl B, Yazici G, Teichmann M, Kopf S, Ghassemi S, Atanasov AG, et al. Effects of scrophularia extracts on tumor cell proliferation, death and intravasation through lymphoendothelial cell barriers. *Int J Oncol* 2012;40(6):2063-74. doi: 10.3892/ijo.2012.1388

43. Valiyari S, Baradaran B, Delazar A, Pasdaran A, Zare F. Dichloromethane and methanol extracts of scrophularia oxysepala induces apoptosis in mcf-7 human breast cancer cells. *Adv Pharm Bull* 2012;2(2):223-31. doi: 10.5681/apb.2012.034

16

Antimicrobial Activity of Two Garlic Species (*Allium Sativum* and *A. Tuberosum*) Against Staphylococci Infection. *In Vivo* Study in Rats

Paulo César Venâncio[1], Sidney Raimundo Figueroba[2]*, Bruno Dias Nani[2], Luiz Eduardo Nunes Ferreira[2], Bruno Vilela Muniz[2], Fernando de Sá Del Fiol[3], Adilson Sartoratto[4], Edvaldo Antonio Ribeiro Rosa[5], Francisco Carlos Groppo[2]

[1] *Department of Exact Sciences, Technical School of Limeira, Cotil, UNICAMP, Limeira, São Paulo, Brazil.*
[2] *Department of Physiological Sciences, Piracicaba Dental School, UNICAMP, Piracicaba, São Paulo, Brazil.*
[3] *Department of Pharmacological Sciences, School of Pharmacy of Sorocaba, UNISO, Sorocaba São Paulo, Brazil.*
[4] *Research Center for Chemistry, Biology and Agriculture, CPQBA, UNICAMP, Paulínia, São Paulo, Brazil.*
[5] *Xenobiotics Research Unit, PUC-Paraná, Curitiba, Paraná, Brazil.*

Keywords:
· Garlic
· Chinese chive
· Amoxicillin
· *Staphylococcus aureus*
· Infection

Abstract

Purpose: This study observed the effect of garlic extracts and amoxicillin against an induced staphylococcal infection model. MIC and MBC were also obtained for aqueous extracts of *Allium sativum* (*Asa*) and *Allium tuberosum* (*Atu*) against *Staphylococcus aureus* penicillin-sensitive (PSSA - ATCC 25923) and MRSA (ATCC 33592).

Methods: Granulation tissues were induced in the back of 205 rats. After 14 days, 0.5 mL of 10^8 CFU/mL of PSSA or MRSA were injected inside tissues. After 24h, animals were divided: G1 (Control) – 0.5 mL of NaCl 0.9%; G2 – *Asa* 100 mg/kg or 400mg/kg; G3 – *Atu* 100 mg/kg or 400 mg/kg; G4 – amoxicillin suspension 50 mg/kg, considering PSSA infection; and G5 (Control) - 0.5 mL of NaCl 0.9%; G6 – *Asa* 400mg/kg; G7 – amoxicillin 50 mg/kg; and G8 - *Asa* 400 mg/kg + amoxicillin 50 mg/kg for MRSA. All treatments were administered P.O. every 6h. Animals were killed at 0, 6, 12 and 24h. Samples were spread on salt-mannitol agar. Colonies were counted after 18 h at 37 °C. *Atu* was not able to inhibit or kill PSSA and MRSA. Considering *Asa*, MIC and MBC against PSSA were 2 mg/mL and 4 mg/mL, respectively; and 16 mg/mL and 64 mg/mL against MRSA.

Results: No effect was observed *in vivo* for control, *Asa* 100 mg/kg and *Atu* 100 mg/kg, while amoxicillin, *Atu* 400 mg/kg and *Asa* 400 mg/kg decreased PSSA counts in all-time points. No effect of any group against MRSA was observed at any time.

Conclusion: Thus, *A. sativum* and *A. tuberosum* were able to reduce PSSA infection, but not MRSA infection.

Introduction

Among all staphylococci, *Staphylococcus aureus* is the most important cause of infectious diseases in humans. This microorganism is part of the commensal microbiota, causing opportunistic infections under appropriate conditions.[1] Besides, intrinsic virulence factors, life-threatening staphylococcal infections occur due to its ability to develop antibiotic resistance.[2] The antimicrobial resistance against penicillins is remarkable in the most known *S. aureus* strains. The minimum inhibitory concentration (MIC) of amoxicillin against penicillin-sensitive *S. aureus* strains is usually below to 0.5 µg/mL.[3] The beta-lactams' MIC against resistant strains could be hundred times higher than the usual MIC of sensitive strains. Thus, there is a clear need for novel antimicrobials or new methods to improve the efficacy of old antibiotics.

Natural products are the most important source of innovative contributions to antimicrobial therapeutic.[4]

The genus *Allium* is often used and studied in medicine as antibacterial and anti-viral agents among many other properties.[5] There are over 600 species of *Allium* found throughout the world, most of them in Asia. Most species have characteristic aroma and odor; some are used as ornamentals or spices. Garlic is often used in many forms (oils, powder, etc.), being also present in many pre-packaged foods, soups and bread used in a daily diet.[6]

Among the species of *Allium* spp., *A. tuberosum* ("Chinese chive") is an important ingredient in Asian cuisine, being used as a medicinal herb for many disorders and diseases.[7] Both pressed juice and essential oil showed inhibition properties against a broad range of gram-positive and gram-negative microorganisms as well as many fungi.[8]

Allium sativum contains several biologically active chemical constituents, such as alliin, allicin, alliinase,

---

*Corresponding author: Sidney Raimundo Figueroba, Email: sfigueroba@uol.com.br

S-allylcysteine and other organosulfur compounds.[9] Alliin is a natural sulfoxide constituent of fresh garlic. It is derivate from the amino acid cysteine, being converted to allicin by the enzyme aliinase when bulbs are mashed. Allicin is a precursor of sulphur compounds, responsible for the odor and some of the pharmacological properties of garlic. Once exposed to the atmospheric air, allicin is converted into diallydissulphinate, which has antimicrobial activity.[10,11]

Garlic extract and some of its products, such as diallyl sulphide and diallyl disulphide showed protective action against MRSA infection in mice.[12] The additive or complimentary effect of garlic or its products on some antibiotics against bacterial infections was previously demonstrated *in vitro*[13] and *in vivo*.[14]

The aim of this study was to observe the effect of garlic extracts alone or in combination with amoxicillin on the staphylococcal infection, which was induced with penicillin-sensitive or penicillin-resistant strains, in rats.

Materials and Methods
Preparation of garlic extracts
Garlic bulbs (*Allium sativum*) and Chinese chive (*Allium tuberosum*) were supplied by Research Center for Chemistry, Biology and Agriculture – CPQBA-UNICAMP (Campinas, SP, Brazil). The dry peel around the bulbs was removed and they were used to prepare *A. sativum* extract. *A. tuberosum* extract were prepared using only the plant leaves. Bulbs are the most common part of *A. sativum* used by population and in most of studies. Considering *A. tuberosum* the few studies in literature used its leaves as a primary source for extracts. Both aqueous extracts were prepared by using 100 g of fresh rootless bulbs of *A. sativum* or 100 g of *A. tuberosum* leaves and 100 mL of distilled/deionized water. Both plants were ground in a blender for 10 min and the resulting extracts were filtered in qualitative paper filters, and sterilized through 0.2 μm membrane filters by using a vacuum pump. All residues were weighed, and the concentration of the final solution of both extracts was considered 25% (w/v) or 250 mg/mL, as previously described.[15,16]

Analysis of extracts compounds
The extracts were analyzed using a gas chromatograph (Hewlett-Packard – HP-5890) with a mass-selective detector (Hewlett-Packard – HP-5971), equipped with DB-1 capillary column (25 m x 0.2 mm x 0.33 μm). Carrier gas was helium at a flow rate of 1.0 mL/min. The injection temperature was 240 °C and the detector was set at 300 °C. The column temperature program was 60 °C (2 min) to 300 °C at 4 °C/min.

The injection volume was 1.0 μL and the detector was a quadropole system with ionization energy of 70 eV. Both extracts were assayed under the same conditions, using the NIST98 electronic library for GC/MS.

Bacteria
Both *Staphylococcus aureus* ATCC 25923 (penicillin sensitive - PSSA) and ATCC 33592 (methicillin resistant - MRSA) were used in the *in vitro* and *in vivo* models. Both strains were kept in TSA medium.

In vitro study
Minimal inhibitory (MIC) and bactericidal (MBC) concentrations
Eleven culture tubes containing 5 mL of Mueller–Hinton broth were used for each strain. Two-fold progressive concentrations of both extracts were added in the first 10 tubes. The last tube had microorganisms only (positive control). An extra tube was used as negative control (without microorganisms or extracts). The extracts' concentrations were 1, 2, 4, 8, 16, 32, 64, 128, 256 and 512 mg/mL. Amoxicillin was used in concentrations of 0.5, 1, 2, 4, 8, 16, 32, 64, 128 and 256 μg/mL for PSSA and 32, 64, 128 and 256, 512, 1024, 2048, 4096 and 8192 μg/mL for MRSA.

All tubes received 250 μL of 10^6 CFU/mL of either PSSA or MRSA. Tubes were incubated in aerobic conditions at 37 °C. Bacterial concentration was adjusted by using a spectrophotometer. After 18 h, the culture medium was observed and the turbidity of medium was measured and compared with the negative-control tubes. The first tube without bacterial growth was considered as MIC. Amounts of 5 μL from the tubes without bacterial growth were spread on Petri dishes containing BHI agar. The first concentration without any bacterial growth on agar was considered as MBC.

In vivo study
This study was approved by the Ethical Committee of Animal Experimentation of Biology Institute-UNICAMP (protocol # 1457-1).

Two assays were carried out. The first one was designed to compare both garlic extracts against the PSSA infection. The second one was designed to compare the effect of *A. sativum*, which was the most efficient formulation in assay 1, and amoxicillin against MRSA infection.

First assay
140 adult-male Wistar rats (*Rattus norvegicus*-albinus), 60 days of age and weighing 175 g ± 25 g, were obtained from CEMIB-UNICAMP (Centro de Bioterismo – ICLAS Monitoring/Reference Centre, Campinas, Brazil).

Granulation tissue was induced by insertion of four sterilized polyurethane sponge discs (density = 35 kg/m³) subcutaneously in the back of each animal, according to a method previously described.[17] These sponge discs (Proespuma Com. & Ind. Ltd., Sao Paulo, Brazil) were 12 mm in diameter and 5 mm thick, weighing 12 ± 1 mg, being all of them were previously sterilized.

Animals were anesthetized by an injection of ketamine (40-87 mg/kg/I.P.) and xylasine (5-13 mg/kg/I.P.). After careful antisepsis with povidone-iodine, the back skin was incised and the sponge discs were carefully distributed considering a distance of approximately 2 cm among them, two in tail direction and two in head direction. Meperidine chlorhydrate (2 mg/kg/I.M.) was used to control post-operative pain. After 14 days of sponge insertion, a well-delimited granulation tissue was formed around and inside the sponge disks. This tissue was used as a scaffold for the staphylococcal infection.

In order to establish the staphylococcal infection, a careful antisepsis was carried out in the back of all animals and 0.5 mL of a suspension of PSSA (10^8 CFU/mL) was injected into the four granulation tissues. After 24 hours of infection, the animals were submitted to the following treatments:

1) Control – 20 animals received 0.5 mL of 0.9% NaCl. These animals were killed (n = 5 per group) right after the administration (t=0) and after 6, 12 and 24 hours after saline administration.
2) *Allium sativum* - 15 animals received 100 mg/kg of an *A. sativum* aqueous extract and 15 animals received 400 mg/kg of an *A. sativum* aqueous extract.
3) *Allium tuberosum* – 15 animals received 100 mg/kg of an *A. tuberosum* aqueous extract and 15 animals received 400 mg/kg of an *A. tuberosum* aqueous extract.
4) Amoxicillin – 15 animals received amoxicillin suspension 50 mg/kg/P.O. every 6 hours.

Treatments were administered P.O. every 6 hours. Animals of groups 2, 3, and 4 were killed after 6, 12 and 24 hours after drugs administration.

Second assay

After 14 days of sponge implants and careful antisepsis, 65 animals received 0.5 mL of a suspension of 10^8 CFU/mL MRSA strain (*S. aureus* ATCC 33592) into the granulation tissue. After 24 hours of the infection procedure, the animals were divided into the following groups:

1. Control – 20 animals received 0.5 mL of NaCl 0.9% P.O. every 6 hours. These animals were killed (n = 5 per group) right after the administration (t = 0) and after 6, 12 and 24 hours after saline administration.
2. *Allium sativum* - 15 animals received *A. sativum* aqueous extract 400 mg/kg. Both extracts were administered P.O. every 6 hours and the animals were killed after 6, 12 and 24 hours after the first administration.
3. Amoxicillin– 15 animals received amoxicillin suspension 50 mg/kg/P.O. every 6 hours. These animals were killed after 6, 12 and 24 hours after amoxicillin administration.
4. *A. sativum* + amoxicillin - 15 animals received both *A. sativum* extract 400 mg/kg and amoxicillin

suspension 50 mg/kg. Both extract and amoxicillin suspension were administered P.O. every 6 hours. Animals were killed after 6, 12 and 24 hours after the first administration.

Granulation tissue removal

All infected granulation tissues were surgically removed after general anesthesia and blood removal by cutting carotid plexus. Tissue samples were individually disposed into assay tubes with 10 mL of 0.9% NaCl. Tubes were weighed before and after the tissue insertion. Samples were dispersed using an ultrasonic system (Vibra Cell 400W, Sonics & Materials Inc, Danbury, CT, USA) and 10 µL of the resulting suspension was spread on salt mannitol agar and incubated at 37 °C. Eighteen hours after incubation, the colonies were counted by using a manual colony counter.

Statistical analysis

Results were submitted to the Bartlett's test to assess variance homogeneity, and the Kolmogorov & Smirnov test to observe data distribution. Data of the first assay were transformed and analyzed by two-way ANOVA and Tukey's test adjusted for multiple comparisons (*post hoc*). Second assay data were submitted to Kruskal-Wallis' and Dunn's tests. GraphPad Prism 6.0 was used to analyze all data, considering 5% of a significant level.

Results
Gas chromatography profile

Figure 1 and (Table 1) show respectively the gas chromatography profile and the probable chemical composition of both *A. tuberosum* and *A. sativum* aqueous and hydroalcoholic extracts.

The most abundant compound of the *A. tuberosum* aqueous extract was not identified by gas chromatography, being only 8% of its compounds identified. However, *A. tuberosum* hydroalcoholic extract had phytol as the most abundant compound (48.4%) followed by other acyclic compounds (23.4%) and only 1.8% of sulphides. *A. sativum* aqueous extract showed 82% of sulphur compounds, being disulphides the most prevalent ones. The hydroalcoholic extract of *A. sativum* showed trisulphides (31%) as the most abundant compound.

MIC and MBC

A. tuberosum was not able to inhibit or kill both resistant and sensitive staphylococci strains in MIC and MBC tests. *A. sativum* and amoxicillin inhibited (MIC) the penicillin-sensitive strain respectively at 2 mg/mL and 0.1 µg/mL. They killed (MBC) this strain at 4 mg/mL and 2 µg/mL, respectively. However, it was necessary 2048 µg/mL of amoxicillin to inhibit the MRSA strain and 8192 µg/mL to kill it. *A. sativum* was able to inhibit MRSA at 16 mg/mL, being able to kill it at 64 mg/mL.

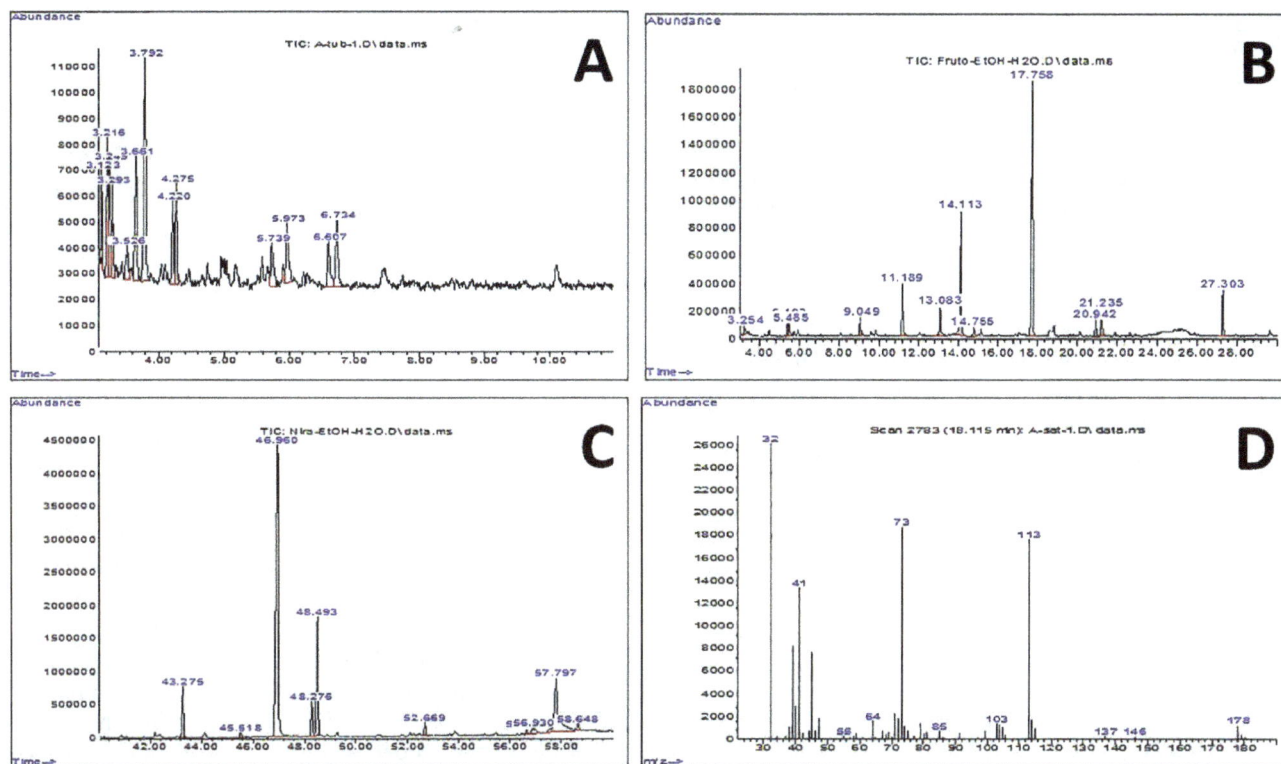

Figure 1. GC-Chromatograms of both *A. tuberosum* (A and C) and *A. sativum* (B and D) extracts. Aqueous extracts are presented in A and B and the hydroalcoholic ones in C and D.

Table 1. Probable chemical composition of both aqueous and hydroalcoholic extracts of *A. tuberosum* and *A. sativum*.

	Allium	Retention time (min)	Kovats index	Probable identification	Class	Relative %
Aqueous extracts	tuberosum	3.22	---	2,5-dimethyl-heptane	Alkane	1.0
		3.25	---	ethylcyclohexane	Alkane	0.7
		3.61	---	1-propene,3,3'-thiobis or diallyl sulfide	**Monosulfides**	0.6
		3.79	---	p-xylene	Aromatic	2.3
		4.23	---	o-xylene	Aromatic	0.8
		4.28	900	nonane	Alkane	1.0
		6.61	994	1,2,4-trimethylbenzene	Aromatic	0.8
		6.74	999	decane	Alkane	1.0
	sativum	3.21	---	2,5-dimethyl-heptane	Alkane	1.0
		3.77	---	p-xylene	Aromatic	2.3
		4.26	900	nonane	Alkane	1.0
		6.61	994	1,2,4-trimethylbenzene	Aromatic	0.8
		13.45	1183	3-vinyl-1,2-dithiacyclohex-4-ene	**Disulfides**	21.7
		14.50	1209	3-vinyl-1,2-dithiacyclohex-5-ene	**Disulfides**	57.3
		18.12	1296	di-2-propenyl trisulfide	**Trisulfides**	3.0
Hydroalcoholic extracts	tuberosum	5.73	958	Dimethyl trisulfide	**Trisulfides**	0.5
		8.55	1053	S-methyl methanethiosulfonate	**Disulfides**	1.3
		43.28	1981	palmitic acid ethyl ester	Ester	5.2
		46.96	---	phytol	Alcohol	48.4
		48.27	---	linoleic acid ethyl ester	Ester	3.7
		48.50	---	linolenic acid ethyl ester	Ester	13.0
		52.67	---	ethyl 3-(4-hydroxy-3-methoxyphenyl)propanoate	Ester	1.4
	sativum	13.08	1174	3-vinyl-1,2-dithiacyclohex-4-ene	**Disulfides**	3.5
		14.11	1200	3-vinyl-1,2-dithiacyclohex-5-ene	**Disulfides**	13.9
		17.76	1288	di-2-propenyl trisulfide or diallyl trisulfide	**Trisulfides**	31.2
		27.30	1523	di-2-propenyl tetrasulfide or diallyl tetrasulfide	**Tetrasulfides**	5.1
		42.20	1948	dibutyl-o-phthalate	Ester	2.2
		48.26	---	linoleic acid ethyl ester	Ester	1.8

First in vivo assay

Figure 2 shows the effect of treatments in the number of bacteria in all-time points. There are no significant differences ($p > 0.05$) among periods for control, *A. sativum* 100 mg/kg and *A. tuberosum* 100 mg/kg. Amoxicillin decreased the CFU counts after 6 and 12 hours, but no differences were found between 24 hours and 6 or 12 hours. *A. tuberosum* 400 mg/kg decreased the bacterial counts starting from 6 to 24 hours and *A. sativum* showed a decrease after 6 and 24 hours.

Comparison among groups in each period showed no significant differences among control, *A. sativum* 100 mg/kg and *A. tuberosum* 100 mg/kg, except for 6 hours period, when both aqueous solutions significantly decreased the CFU in comparison with control. Amoxicillin and *A. sativum* 400 mg/kg decreased CFU in comparison with control, *A. sativum* 100 mg/kg and *A. tuberosum* 100 mg/kg in each period, but they did not differ from *A. tuberosum* 400 mg/kg. This formulation also decreases CFU in comparison with control, *A. sativum* 100 mg/kg and *A. tuberosum* 100 mg/kg in all periods, except for 6 hours.

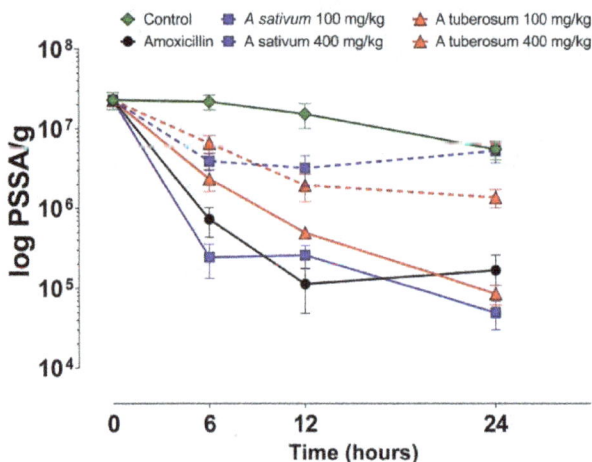

Figure 2. Effect of the treatments on the concentration (mean±SD) of PSSA per gram of tissue in all-time points.

Second in vivo assay

Figure 3 shows the effect of treatments against the resistant bacteria in all-time points. CFU increased after 12 h for control and amoxicillin + *A. sativum*, and after 6 hours for *A. sativum* 400 mg/kg and amoxicillin. Comparison among groups in the 6 hours period showed greater number of CFU for the amoxicillin group than the others groups, which did not differ one from each other. After 12 hours, control showed bigger number of CFU than amoxicillin alone or combined with *A. sativum*. No significant differences were observed in this period among *A. sativum* and the other groups. No significant differences were observed at the 24 hours period.

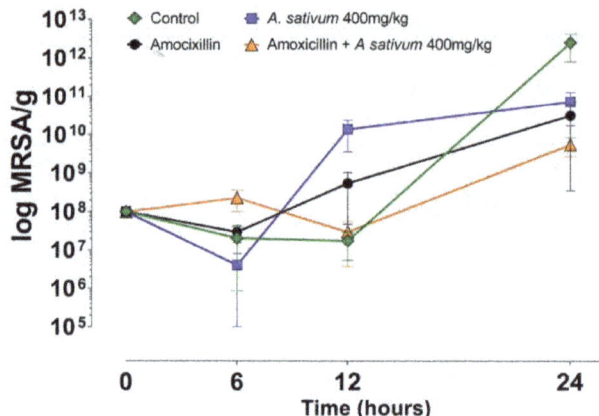

Figure 3. Effect of the treatments on the concentration (mean±SD) of MRSA per gram of tissue in all-time points.

Discussion

Among many other models, the use of PVC or polyurethane sponges to induce a well-delimited infection was previously described for research on anti-staphylococci substances. This model allowed a well-delimited staphylococcal infection development, since one of the most important phenomena for the infection establishment is bacterial surface adherence. The validity of the model was previously demonstrated for acute staphylococcal infection.[17]

Most of the important infections results from bacterial adherence on some tissue surface, and the first line of the host defense against the bacterial invasion also request a surface to exert its defensive function.[18] Thus, the surface provided by the granulomatous tissue was suitable to both staphylococcal infection development and host defensive events.

It is remarkable that amoxicillin was not able to kill all the PSSA microorganisms, and, thus, it did not eradicate the staphylococcal infection. This result is similar to the ones previously obtained using the same model. The main reason for this phenomenon is probably due to the penicillin mechanism of action. It is well stablished that bacteria growing in tissues surrounded by immune cells show slow reproduction, which decreases the penicillin activity.[17]

As anticipated, the chemical composition differed between the two garlic species. The main chemical composition of *A. tuberosum* is thiosulphinates,[19] and various steroidal saponins,[20] which were observed in both *A. tuberosum* hydroalcoholic and aqueous extracts in the present study.

A. sativum chemical composition was similar to the one previously described by others.[9,21,22] Discrepancies on chemical composition of *A. sativum* can occur due to the method to obtain the plant extract. In the present study, *A. sativum* extract was obtained as previously described,[15,23] and it provided antimicrobial activity in both *in vivo* and *in vitro* assays. In addition, we used raw garlic extracts since these extracts showed higher antimicrobial activity than some isolated compounds, such as allicin.[12,24] Besides, progressive concentrations of a raw extract of *A. sativum* (100 to 1000 μg/mL) strongly inhibited many microorganisms.[25]

The MIC observed for *A. sativum* in the present study (2 mg/mL) against PSSA was lower than MIC observed by,[26] which observed 11.25 mg/mL against the same strain. Probably, the difference occurred because those authors used agar dilution techniques in spite of liquid medium as used in the present study.

Very few information regarding the antimicrobial activity of *A. tuberosum*, especially against bacteria, was found in literature. The *in vitro* antifungal activity was previously demonstrated for *A. tuberosum* raw extracts against *C. albicans*,[27] and for the essential oil against Aspergillus species,[8] observed both antibacterial and antifungal activity of *A. tuberosum* in disk diffusion tests. The aqueous extract was able to inhibit many bacterial species, such as *Bacillus subtilis*, *Escherichia coli*, *Pseudomonas aeruginosa*, and *Salmonella typhimurium*, but not *Staphylococcus aureus*.

In the present study, the *in vitro* anti-staphylococcal activity of *A. tuberosum* was not observed against both PSSA and MRSA strains. However, it was able to decrease the PSSA strain counts in the *in vivo* model. Thus, it is possible that the anti-staphylococcal activity of *A. tuberosum* was indirect. As observed in many antimicrobial models, *in vitro* assays do not provide the variability observed in the *in vivo* assays, especially considering immunological aspects.[28] Differences between *in vitro* and *in vivo* models in antimicrobial research are well recognized and future studies are necessary to address the effects of *A. tuberosum* on host immune response.

A. sativum is a well-recognized anti-staphylococcal agent against the biofilm formation in burn wounds,[29] and against both PSSA and MRSA in an *in vitro* MIC model,[30] as observed in the present study. In addition, diallyl sulphide and diallyl disulphide from a raw *A. sativum* extract showed protective action against MRSA-infection in both diabetic,[31] and non-diabetic mice.[12]

Raw garlic extracts (100% and 50% concentrations) administered orally, exhibited comparable effect with both diallyl sulphide and diallyl disulphide, being safer than the two sulphides.[12] However, in the present study *A. sativum* did not show antibacterial activity against the MRSA strain, despite of the activity against the PSSA strain. The animal model and the garlic concentration used in the present study could have affected the results.

Conclusion

We concluded that both garlic species showed constitution comparable to other similar strains and they have molecules related to antimicrobial properties. Both species were able to reduce staphylococcal infection, despite only *A. sativum* showed in vitro anti-staphylococci activity. No additive or complementary effect was observed by adding *A. sativum* extract with amoxicillin against the strains studied.

Acknowledgments

Part of this work was presented at the International Dental Research Association - IADR, Barcelona, Spain, 2010 (poster presentation #1876). This study was supported by FAPESP (foundation for Research Support of the state of São Paulo, grants #2007/08076-5, #08/01021-3).

Ethical Issues

This study was approved by the Ethical Committee of Animal Experimentation of Biology Institute-UNICAMP (protocol # 1457-1).

Conflict of Interest

The authors declare no competing interests exist.

References

1. Tohidpour A, Sattari M, Omidbaigi R, Yadegar A, Nazemi J. Antibacterial effect of essential oils from two medicinal plants against methicillin-resistant staphylococcus aureus (mrsa). *Phytomedicine* 2010;17(2):142-5. doi: 10.1016/j.phymed.2009.05.007

2. Tanaka H, Sato M, Oh-Uchi T, Yamaguchi R, Etoh H, Shimizu H, et al. Antibacterial properties of a new isoflavonoid from erythrina poeppigiana against methicillin-resistant staphylococcus aureus. *Phytomedicine* 2004;11(4):331-7. doi: 10.1078/0944711041495137

3. Moroni P, Pisoni G, Antonini M, Villa R, Boettcher P, Carli S. Short communication: Antimicrobial drug susceptibility of staphylococcus aureus from subclinical bovine mastitis in italy. *J Dairy Sci* 2006;89(8):2973-6. doi: 10.3168/jds.S0022-0302(06)72569-3

4. Groppo FC, Bergamaschi Cde C, Cogo K, Franz-Montan M, Motta RH, de Andrade ED. Use of phytotherapy in dentistry. *Phytother Res* 2008;22(8):993-8. doi: 10.1002/ptr.2471

5. Shouk R, Abdou A, Shetty K, Sarkar D, Eid AH. Mechanisms underlying the antihypertensive effects of garlic bioactives. *Nutr Res* 2014;34(2):106-15. doi: 10.1016/j.nutres.2013.12.005

6. Filocamo A, Nueno-Palop C, Bisignano C, Mandalari G, Narbad A. Effect of garlic powder on the growth of commensal bacteria from the gastrointestinal tract. *Phytomedicine* 2012;19(8-9):707-11. doi: 10.1016/j.phymed.2012.02.018

7. Fang YS, Cai L, Li Y, Wang JP, Xiao H, Ding ZT. Spirostanol steroids from the roots of allium tuberosum. *Steroids* 2015;100:1-4. doi: 10.1016/j.steroids.2015.03.015

8. Kocevski D, Du M, Kan J, Jing C, Lacanin I, Pavlovic H. Antifungal effect of allium tuberosum, cinnamomum cassia, and pogostemon cablin essential oils and their components against population of aspergillus species. *J Food Sci* 2013;78(5):M731-7. doi: 10.1111/1750-3841.12118

9. Sendl A. Allium sativum and allium ursinum: Part 1 chemistry, analysis, history, botany. *Phytomedicine* 1995;1(4):323-39. doi: 10.1016/S0944-7113(11)80011-5

10. Wang J, Cao Y, Wang C, Sun B. Low-frequency and low-intensity ultrasound accelerates alliinase-catalysed synthesis of allicin in freshly crushed garlic. *J Sci Food Agric* 2011;91(10):1766-72. doi: 10.1002/jsfa.4377

11. Khodavandi A, Harmal NS, Alizadeh F, Scully OJ, Sidik SM, Othman F, et al. Comparison between allicin and fluconazole in candida albicans biofilm inhibition and in suppression of hwp1 gene expression. *Phytomedicine* 2011;19(1):56-63. doi: 10.1016/j.phymed.2011.08.060

12. Tsao SM, Hsu CC, Yin MC. Garlic extract and two diallyl sulphides inhibit methicillin-resistant staphylococcus aureus infection in balb/ca mice. *J Antimicrob Chemother* 2003;52(6):974-80. doi: 10.1093/jac/dkg476

13. Reuter HD. Allium sativum and allium ursinum: Part 2 pharmacology and medicinal application. *Phytomedicine* 1995;2(1):73-91. doi: 10.1016/S0944-7113(11)80052-8

14. Sohn DW, Han CH, Jung YS, Kim SI, Kim SW, Cho YH. Anti-inflammatory and antimicrobial effects of garlic and synergistic effect between garlic and ciprofloxacin in a chronic bacterial prostatitis rat model. *Int J Antimicrob Agents* 2009;34(3).215-9. doi: 10.1016/j.ijantimicag.2009.02.012

15. Elnima EI, Ahmed SA, Mekkawi AG, Mossa JS. The antimicrobial activity of garlic and onion extracts. *Pharmazie* 1983;38(11):747-8.

16. Groppo FC, Ramacciato JC, Simoes RP, Florio FM, Sartoratto A. Antimicrobial activity of garlic, tea tree oil, and chlorhexidine against oral microorganisms. *Int Dent J* 2002;52(6):433-7.

17. Groppo FC, Simoes RP, Ramacciato JC, Rehder V, de Andrade ED, Mattos-Filho TR. Effect of sodium diclofenac on serum and tissue concentration of amoxicillin and on staphylococcal infection. *Biol Pharm Bull* 2004;27(1):52-5.

18. Lorian V. In vitro simulation of in vivo conditions: Physical state of the culture medium. *J Clin Microbiol* 1989;27(11):2403-6.

19. Seo KI, Moon YH, Choi SU, Park KH. Antibacterial activity of s-methyl methanethiosulfinate and s-methyl 2-propene-1-thiosulfinate from chinese chive toward escherichia coli o157:H7. *Biosci Biotechnol Biochem* 2001;65(4):966-8.

20. Zou ZM, Yu DQ, Cong PZ. A steroidal saponin from the seeds of allium tuberosum. *Phytochemistry* 2001;57(8):1219-22.

21. Banerjee SK, Mukherjee PK, Maulik SK. Garlic as an antioxidant: The good, the bad and the ugly. *Phytother Res* 2003;17(2):97-106. doi: 10.1002/ptr.1281

22. Lemar KM, Turner MP, Lloyd D. Garlic (allium sativum) as an anti-candida agent: A comparison of the efficacy of fresh garlic and freeze-dried extracts. *J Appl Microbiol* 2002;93(3):398-405.

23. Groppo FC, Ramacciato JC, Motta RH, Ferraresi PM, Sartoratto A. Antimicrobial activity of garlic against oral streptococci. *Int J Dent Hyg* 2007;5(2):109-15. doi: 10.1111/j.1601-5037.2007.00230.x

24. Fujisawa H, Watanabe K, Suma K, Origuchi K, Matsufuji H, Seki T, et al. Antibacterial potential of garlic-derived allicin and its cancellation by sulfhydryl compounds. *Biosci Biotechnol Biochem* 2009;73(9):1948-55. doi: 10.1271/bbb.90096

25. Gomaa NF, Hashish MH. The inhibitory effect of garlic (allium sativum) on growth of some microorganisms. *J Egypt Public Health Assoc* 2003;78(5-6):361-72.

26. Tessema B, Mulu A, Kassu A, Yismaw G. An in vitro assessment of the antibacterial effect of garlic (allium sativum) on bacterial isolates from wound infections. *Ethiop Med J* 2006;44(4):385-9.

27. Furletti VF, Teixeira IP, Obando-Pereda G, Mardegan RC, Sartoratto A, Figueira GM, et al. Action of coriandrum sativum l. Essential oil upon oral candida albicans biofilm formation. *Evid Based Complement Alternat Med* 2011;2011:985832. doi: 10.1155/2011/985832

28. Henry-Stanley MJ, Hess DJ, Wells CL. Aminoglycoside inhibition of staphylococcus aureus biofilm formation is nutrient dependent. *J Med Microbiol* 2014;63(Pt 6):861-9. doi: 10.1099/jmm.0.068130-0

29. Nidadavolu P, Amor W, Tran PL, Dertien J, Colmer-Hamood JA, Hamood AN. Garlic ointment inhibits biofilm formation by bacterial pathogens from burn wounds. *J Med Microbiol* 2012;61(Pt 5):662-71. doi: 10.1099/jmm.0.038638-0

30. Tsao SM, Yin MC. In-vitro antimicrobial activity of four diallyl sulphides occurring naturally in garlic and chinese leek oils. *J Med Microbiol* 2001;50(7):646-9. doi: 10.1099/0022-1317-50-7-646

31. Tsao SM, Liu WH, Yin MC. Two diallyl sulphides derived from garlic inhibit meticillin-resistant staphylococcus aureus infection in diabetic mice. *J Med Microbiol* 2007;56(Pt 6):803-8. doi: 10.1099/jmm.0.46998-0

17

Preparation of the Potential Ocular Inserts by Electrospinning Method to Achieve the Prolong Release Profile of Triamcinolone Acetonide

Shahla Mirzaeei[1,2*], Kaveh Berenjian[3], Rasol Khazaei[3]

[1] *Pharmaceutical Sciences Research Center, School of Pharmacy, Kermanshah University of Medical Sciences, Kermanshah, Iran.*
[2] *Nano Drug Delivery Research Center, School of Pharmacy, Kermanshah University of Medical Sciences, Kermanshah, Iran.*
[3]*Student Research Committee, School of Pharmacy, Kermanshah University of Medical Sciences, Kermanshah, Iran.*

Keywords:
· Ocular
· Insert
· Electrospinning
· Nanofiber
· Chitosan
· Triamcinolone acetonide

Abstract

Purpose: The poor bioavailability of drugs in the ocular delivery systems is an important issue and development of delivery systems with prolonged release profile could be in a major importance. This study aims to develop an ocular delivery system using electrospun nanofibers to be a candidate insert for delivery of triamcinolone acetonide.

Methods: For this purpose, three different chitosan-based formulations were prepared by electrospinning method, and electrospun nanofibers were compared to a formulation comprising hydrophobic polymers (Eudragit S100 and Zein). The electrospun nanofibers were characterized by SEM and FTIR analyses. The release profile and release kinetic models of all the formulations were also examined.

Results: The SEM photographs of electrospun nanofibers revealed that among the four designed formulations, formulation obtained by electrospinning of chitosan and PVP possessed the best quality and the minimum size (120 ±30 nm) , which resulted the most uniform and bead-free nanofibers. This formulation also possessed the prolonged release profile of triamcinolone acetonide and was the only electrospun nanofiber following the zero-order kinetic profile. Due to the small diameter and uniformity of this formulation, the prolonged and well controlled release profile, it could be taken into account as a candidate to overcome the drawbacks of the commonly used ocular delivery systems and be used as ocular insert.

Conclusion: This study confirmed the ability of electrospun nanofibers to be used as ocular inserts for delivery of ophthalmic drugs.

Introduction

Topical formulations of corticosteroids, including drops and ointments, are the most prescribed formulations for treatment of different ocular disorders. Eye drops are the most frequently used ophthalmic drugs, due to the ease of instill and topical administration.[1] This type of administration of ophthalmic drugs affects the anterior segment of the eye and is associated by significant drawbacks; the poor bioavailability of drug (due to nasolacrimal drainage and dilution of drug by tear turnover), requirement of frequent administration, unpredictable and uncontrolled doses, blurred vision, messy and difficult dosing, and short residence time are some of these drawbacks.[2-4]

Several efforts have been conducted to attain an effective formulation, with a desired concentration of drug at the intended site of action, for a programmed period of treatment.[5] The therapeutic efficacy of an ocular drug can be greatly improved by prolonging its contact with the corneal surface.[6]

Ocular inserts are the solid and semi-solid drug-impregnated formulations which could be placed into cul-de-sac or conjunctiva sac.[6] These inserts have been used frequently for reducing the frequency of administration, attaining the extended release duration, predictable and controlled release profile, and desired efficacy in treatment of eye infections such as conjunctivitis, keratitis, corneal ulcers.[3,7-10]

The main objective of this study is to produce the electrospun formulations which could be used as ophthalmic inserts and to incorporate triamcinolone acetonide into these formulations. These formulations hoped to be able to increase the contact time between the drug and conjunctival tissue, decrease the number of administration, achieve a controlled and prolonged release suited for topical treatment of infection, and improve the therapeutic efficacy of drug at the site of action.

Electrospinning is prevailing as a remarkably simple, well-established method which provides a versatile technique for generating various nanofibers with controlled surface morphology from different sources (polymers, ceramics, and composite).[11] Electrospun fibers with different characteristics are promising scaffolds for drug encapsulation and cell incorporation and also can offer the cells an environment for mimicking the native extracellular matrix (ECM). These nano-scale scaffolds have been studied for adhesion, proliferation, and differentiation of different types of cells.[12] Incorporation of bioactive agents into nanofibers can be occurred in one-step process with almost no loss of the agents. The high surface area to volume ratio of nanofibers, flexibility in surface functionalities,[13] porous structure, and good mechanical strength make them promising candidates for many biomedical applications,[14-16] such as controlling delivery of antibiotics and other antibacterial compounds.[17,18] Natural polymers have been implicated as the opportunistic biomedical applications because of their biocompatibility, biodegradability and similarity to the ECM. The most frequently used natural polymers attracting much attention for the biomedical applications are the polysaccharides and proteins.[19] Chitosan is a hydrophobic linear polysaccharide obtained from deacetylated chitin.[20] Chitosan was chosen as the main polymer in this study because it is a water insoluble mucoadhesive polymer which can provide the prolong release of drugs and improve the ocular bioavailability of triamcinolone acetonide.[21,22] Chitosan can interact chemically with the negatively charged mucus layer or the eye tissues and enhance the residence time of drug. [3] Based on the literature review, in spite of overwhelming popularity of electrospinning, no study has been devoted to the application of electrospinning in preparation of ocular inserts for delivery of ophthalmic therapeutics. Just besides of this study, one study investigated the application of electrospun PLA/PVA nanofibers as inserts in ocular delivery of dexamethasone.[23] To the best of our knowledge, this is the first attempt towards preparing ocular inserts by chitosan-based electrospun nanofibers, to be used as the ocular inserts capable of controlling and prolonging the delivery of triamcinolone acetonide. In this study, electrospun chitosan-based nanofibers were fabricated to be used as ocular inserts. Furthermore, a formulation comprising two hydrophobic components (Eudragit/ Zein) was prepared and the results were compared to the chitosan-based nanofibers. Eudragit was chosen because it is suitable for loading the anionic drugs and also can attach to the negatively charged cells.[24]

Materials and Methods
Chitosan and Zein were purchased from Sigma Aldrich (St. Louis, Missouri, USA). Eudragit S100 was procured from Evonik Industries, Parsippany, NJ, USA. Poly vinyl alcohol (PVA 13-23 kDa, 98% hydrolysis), poly vinyl pirolidine (PVP), and ethanol were procured from Merck (Germany). Triamcinolone acetonide was purchased from Crystal Pharma (Spain). All the other compounds were in analytical grade and were performed without further purification.

Preparation of electrospinning solutions
In this study, four formulations were performed for producing triamcinolone acetonide-loaded nanofibers (Table 1). Chitosan-based electrospun nanofibers were obtained from the solution of chitosan in acetic acid. In order to prepare formulation T_2, chitosan was dissolved in 1% acetic acid to obtain the concentration of 6% (w/v) and stirred for 4h at 300 rpm and PVA (12% w/v) was added to the solution. Formulation T_3 comprised of chitosan, PVP, and PVA dissolving in water with concentrations of 6, 3, and 9%, respectively. The formulation T_3 was obtained by co-dissolving chitosan (6% w/v) in acetic acid and addition of PVP (12% w/v) under stirring conditions at 300 rpm. The electrospinning solution of formulation T_1 was prepared by dissolving Eudragit S100 in ethanol and Zein in isopropyl alcohol the solution was stirred for 5h. A drug solution with concentration of 1% w/v in acetic acid was added to each formulation.

Table 1. Different formulations prepared for electrospinning process, the arithmetic mean size and standard deviation of nanofibers.

Formulation	PVA%	PVP%	Zein%	Eudragit%	Chitosan%	Mean* size(nm)	Standard Deviation(nm)	Viscosity (cps)
T_1	-	-	12.5	5	-	169	36	925
T_2	-	12	-	-	6	120	30	1850
T_3	9	3	-	-	6	260	73	1948
T_4	12	-	-	-	6	172	48	1172

* Arithmetic mean size of nanofibers

Electrospinning
After preparation of electrospinning solutions, the solutions were placed in a 5 mL syringe connected with a metallic needle, with inner and outer diameters of 0.6 and 0.9 mm, at the nozzle. The solutions were pumped at the flow rate of 0.7 mL/h using a syringe pump (SP1000, fanavaran Nano-meghyas, Iran). The positive electrode of the Fanavaran Nano-meghyashigh-voltage power supply (D04X-05TH, Fanavaran Nano-meghyas, Iran) was clamped to the tip of the needle and the electrospun nanofibers were collected on a grounded rotating cylindrical collector covered by aluminum foil. The needle tip to collector distance was fixed at 8 cm and the solutions were electrospun at a fixed voltage of 22 kV. The electrospinning of solutions were carried out at constant temperature of 40°C by controlling the temperature in a metallic box enclosing the electrospinning apparatus.

Characterization of electrospun nanofibers
The diameter and morphology of electrospun nanofibers were analyzed by Scanning Electron Microscope (SEM,

Hitachi, HT-4160-02, Japan). The nanofiber samples were placed on the aluminum stub and were gold coated prior to SEM imaging. The mean diameter of nanofibers was determined using ImageJ software. The diameter of at least 100 samples was measured and the arithmetic average diameter was obtained. The viscosity of electrospinning solutions was determined using BROOKFIELD ULTRA DV III Rheometer .

The structural change during electrospinning and the interaction of different chemical groups were observed by Fourier Transform Infrared (FTIR) spectroscopy using potassium bromide tabs. The range of spectra was in 400-4000 cm^{-1} with the accuracy of 4cm^{-1}.

Release study

The *in-vitro* release profile of triamcinolone acetonide from different formulations was determined to obtain the best formulation which is close to the aim of this study. The specified pieces of drug loaded electrospun nanofibers were placed in a dialysis bag (Mw cut-off= 12,000–14,000 Daltons; Delchimica Scientific Glassware, Milan, Italy), containing PBS (pH=7.4). The dialysis bag was sunk in PBS (pH=7.4) as release medium. The system was stirred continuously at 100 rpm and maintained at 37°C.At predetermined time intervals, a specified amount of release medium was replenished by fresh medium. The

concentration of triamcinolone acetonide in withdrawn samples at different times was determined using UV spectrophotometer at 238 nm. This study was carried out in triplicate and the release curve of triamcinolone acetonide from each electrospun nanofiber was prepared.

Results and Discussion
Size and morphology of electrospun nanofibers

The SEM photographs of the four electrospun nanofibers with different formulations are demonstrated in Figure 1 (a-d). The size and standard deviation of electrospun nanofibers were determined using ImageJ software, and the results were tabulated in Table 1. The SEM photographs indicated that formulations T_1, T_2, and T_4 resulted in bead-free electrospun nanofibers with a smooth surface and uniform diameters, but in the formulation T_3, some scattered droplets were formed on the nanofiber and its beaded structure made formulation T_3 unsuitable for medical applications. A glance at figure indicated that adding PVP to the structure of chitosan/PVA nanofibers caused bead formation and a decrease in the uniformity of nanofiber. The size of nanofibers was also compared and among the prepared formulations the best one with smallest diameter and standard deviation was formulation T_2 (chitosan/ PVP) with the mean diameter of 120±30 nm. The viscosity of electrospinning solutions is also indexed in Table 1.

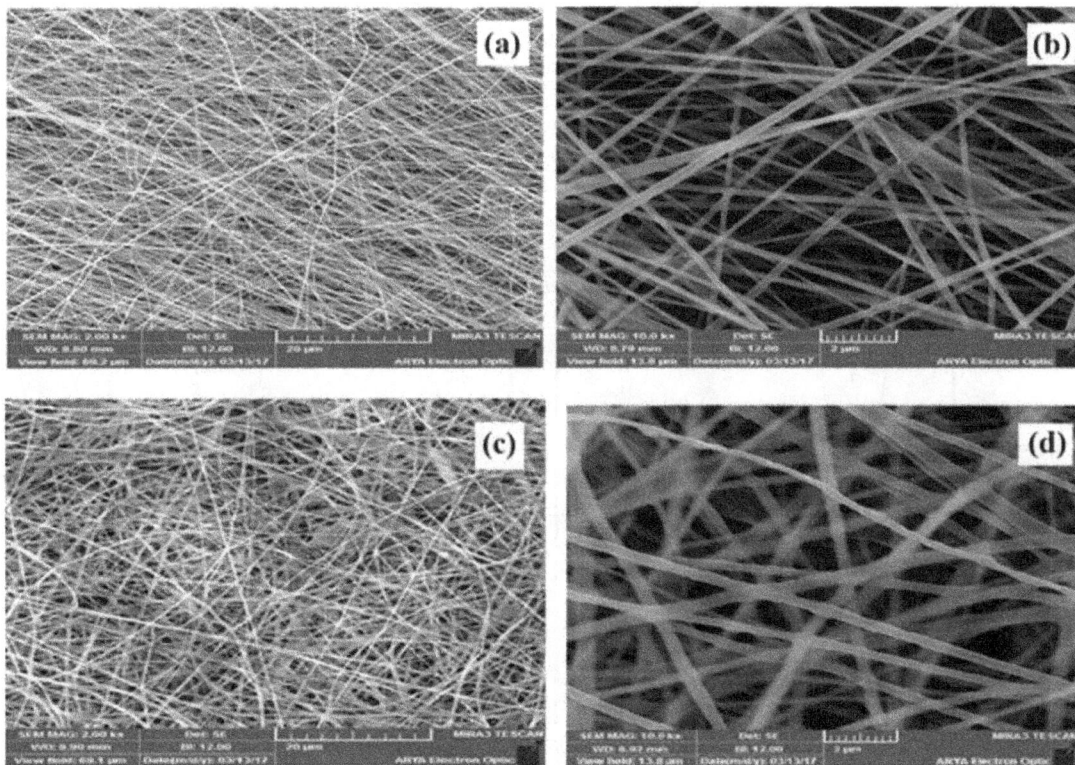

Figure 1. The SEM photographs of formulations (a) T_1, (b) T_2, (c) T_3, and (d) T_4.

FTIR results

In drug delivery systems, it could be an important issue to find out the possible interactions of drug and polymer. The FTIR analysis could help the identification of these interactions based on the alteration of the spectra of the

samples. In the present study, the FTIR spectra of pure polymers (Eudrsgit S100, Zein, chitosan, PVA, and PVA) and free drug were compared with the spectra of the four formulations. The FTIR spectrum of triamcinolone acetonide is demonstrated in Figure 2. FTIR spectrum of triamcinolone acetonide included the hydroxyl group stretching vibration at 3392 cm^{-1}, the carbonyl group (C=O) band at 1708 cm^{-1}, C=C stretching vibration band at 1662 cm^{-1}, and C-O stretching vibration at 1207cm^{-1}. In the spectrum of Eudragit S100, the characteristic peak at 1724 cm^{-1}could be attributed to the esterified carbonyl group. Two peaks were observed at 1150, 1245cm^{-1} corresponding to the ester vibration. The broad peak from 3224 to 3452cm^{-1} could be assigned to the absorption band of the hydroxyl group. The spectrum of Zein revealed characteristic peaks of amide I and amide II at 1651 and 1523 cm^{-1}, which were respectively due to C=O stretching vibrations, N-H bending, and C-N stretching vibrations. The FTIR spectra of formulation T_1 clarified that no significant interaction could be observed between the components of this formulation and drug because of the presence of major bands of components and drug, as well as the absence of new characteristic peaks. The typical infrared bands corresponding to the OH group of chitosan at 3410 cm^{-1}, the NH_2 group of chitosan at 1641 cm^{-1}, and stretching band of the C-O functional group at

1365 cm^{-1} could be observed in the spectra of formulations T_2, T_3, and T_4, while there were no significant shifting and alteration in the position of these peaks. The characteristic peaks of triamcinolone acetonide were identified in the spectra of these three formulations, at the same wavelengths (3292, 1708, 1600-1690, and 1234cm^{-1}), compare to those of pure drug.

In the spectra of the formulation T_2 andT_3, the characteristic peaks of PVP (1716 cm^{-1} for C=O vibration, 1238 cm^{-1} corresponding to C-N vibration, and 3066-3522 cm^{-1}corresponding to OH functional group) and those corresponding to PVA (at 3296 cm^{-1} attributing to the OH vibration, the range of 2850-3000 representing the alkyl vibration) were observed without any alteration in the wavelength of the peaks.

The characteristic peaks of these three formulations seem to be the superposition of their components (polymers and drug) and the FTIR results of these formulations exhibited that drug has been physically dispersed into the polymeric chain, without the presence of detectable chemical interactions.

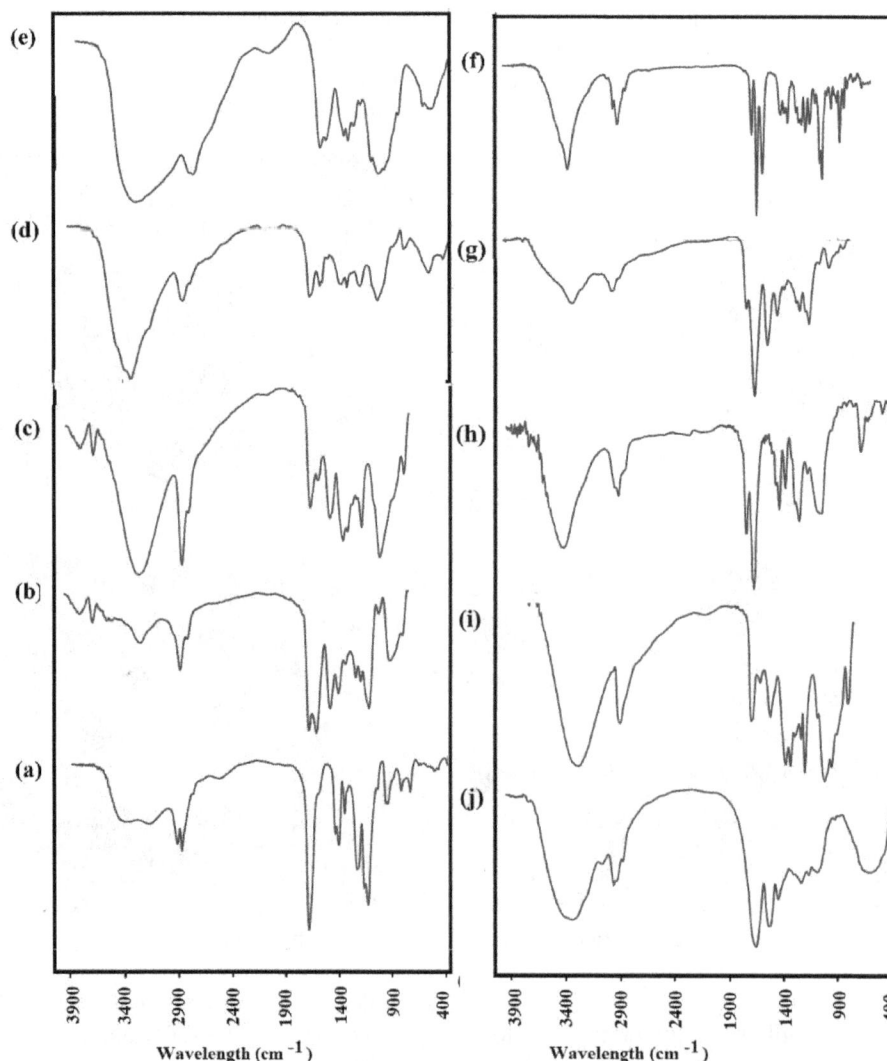

Figure 2. The FTIR spectra of pure Eudragit S100 (a), Zein (b), PVP (c), PVA (d), chitosan (e), triamcinolone acetonide (f), and electrospun nanofibers T_1 (g), T_2 (h), T_3 (i) and T_4 (k).

Release study and release kinetic

In order to study the release pattern of triamcinolone acetonide from different electrospun nanofibers, the concentration of drug in release medium at specified time intervals were determined using a UV-Vis spectrophotometer. The absorbance band of solutions was recorded and the concentration of drug was calculated using the standard calibration curve, which correlated the concentration of triamcinolone acetonide to the absorbance intensity. The calibration curve followed the below equation:

$$y=0.035x+0.0038 \quad R^2 = 0.9998$$

Where y is the absorbance intensity at 238 nm and x is the concentration of triamcinolone acetonide in release medium.

The release pattern of different electrospun nanofibers is represented in Figure 3.

A glance at figure indicated that triamcinolone acetonide released from these electrospun nanofibers T_1, T_2, and T_3 without inducing burst release, but the formulation T_4 released up to 30% of the loaded drug within the first hour. The absence of the burst release in the release profile of these nanofibers showed the potential of these formulations to control the release and delivery of triamcinolone acetonide. These formulations could be advantageous over the other forms of chitosan-based inserts because the release profile of drug contained burst release and those inserts were not able in controlling the release rate and delivery of drugs. According to the figure, the release profile of these formulated electrospun nanofibers was prolonged and these insert candidates released the drug for up to 4 days, while the release profile of free triamcinolone acetonide has been reported more than 70% within 8h.[24] The slowest release rate was achieved for formulation T_1, in which the EudragitS100 and Zein were performed in the electrospinning solution, following the formulation T_2 (chitosan/PVP nanofiber). In order to compare the release rate of these formulations the time corresponding to 80% release of triamcinolone acetonide ($t_{80\%}$) was recorded. The $t_{80\%}$ was found up to 23, 25, and 44.8 h for formulations T_4, T_3, and T_2 respectively, while formulation T_1 did not release 80% of the loaded drug within the study period. The completed release of drug (about 99% release) was achieved for electrospun nanofiber T_2 within 4 days, while the nanofiber T_1 released about 77% of the loaded drug within this period. The slow release pattern of formulation T_1 could be due to the hydrophobic nature of the polymers (Eudragit and Zein) and lower the dissolution rate of these polymers in release medium. The release profile of triamcinolone acetonide from Eudragit RS100 nanofibers with 20% polymer concentration showed a burst release within the first hour following the plateau release and 65% of drug released the nanofiber within 8h,[24] while in the present study the release of 65% of loaded triamcinolone acetonide from Eudragit/Zein nanofibers took more than 70 h.

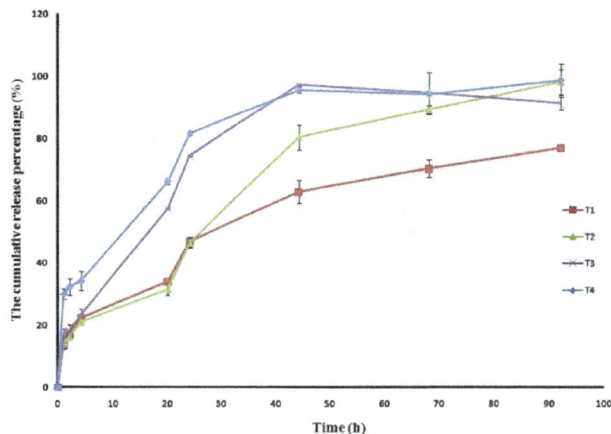

Figure 3. The release profile of triamcinolone acetonide from different electrospun nanofibers.

In order to perform a further comparison the triamcinolone acetonide release from different electrospun nanofibers, the kinetic study was conducted to find the best model correlating the release percentage to the time. The release data of each formulation were fitted to three commonly used empirical models (Higuchi, Zero-order, and First-order) and the amount of R^2 corresponding to each model was compared (Table 2). The kinetic study suggested that the Higuchi was the best fitting model for formulations T_1, T_3, and T_4, while formulation T_2 fitted to the Zero-order kinetic model. Zero-order kinetic with constant release rate and independent drug concentration was known as the ultimate goal of controlled-release delivery systems. The zero-order release profile of formulation T_2, the small size, and size distribution of nanofibers suggested that this formulation is the closest one to the aim of this study.

Table 2. The R-squared of the fitted kinetic models for different formulations.

Formulation	Higuchi	Zero-order	First-order
T_1	**0.9443**	0.8546	0.8861
T_2	0.9074	**0.9461**	0.9060
T_3	**0.9863**	0.9514	0.9337
T_4	**0.9550**	0.8725	0.9313

The well-controlled and monotonic release profile of this formulation could be attributed to the monodispersity of the size of nanofibers. The nanofibers with different sizes released the drug with different rates, but the monodisperse nanofibers with homogenous sizes released the drug more predictably. This formulation was selected as the best electrospun nanofiber to be used as an ophthalmic insert. The release study also revealed the promising ability of Eudragit and Zein to prolong the release time of triamcinolone acetonide and achieve the sustained release, but based on the hydrophobic nature of the polymers, the swelling ability of this formulation in the cul-de-sac must be further investigated. It should be noted that although the release rate of the drug from hydrophobic formulation T_1 was slower than formulation T_2, the formulation T_2 could be advantageous over T_1. Based on the water solubility (and consequently the high swelling ability) of polymers and muco-adhesive nature of chitosan, the formulation T_2 could be swelled in neutral pH of the lacrimal fluid and the solid inserts could be converted to a gel phase and could interact with mucus within muco-adhesion process.[3] Therefore, the controlled drug lixiviation for a prolonged period could be achieved. While the hydrophobic nature of formulation T_1 could possibly cause the degradation and erosion of the insert and dispersion into cul-de-sac, which might cause the problems such as blurred vision within the treatment period. Therefore the formulation T_2 could be suggested for further investigations as a desired candidate for alternating the typical ocular delivery systems with ophthalmic inserts. This formulation also could be advantageous over the other ocular inserts suggested in the previous study, according to the monotonic, well-controlled, and well-prolonged release profile of triamcinolone acetonide.

The previous studies showed the lack of control over the release profile of ocular therapeutics from chitosan-based inserts (prepared by different methods), attributing the accumulation of drug on the surface of inserts and existence of burst release in their profile.[25-27] Jahangiri et al.[28] used the electrospray method to prepare the triamcinolone acetonide-loaded PLGA nanobeads and nanofibers as the alternative delivery system for ophthalmic drops. In spite of the advantages of the prepared formulations as the ophthalmic inserts, the release profile included the initial burst release following the plateau release. Beside, the release period was much shorter than that of the electrospun formulations in this study. Prajapati et al. used the PVA/chitosan films as the ocular insert for prolonging the delivery of ofloxacin. The release of ofloxacin from the films was completed within the first 6h.[29]

The facility of the electrospun nanofibers administration on the ocular surface could be another important advantage of the suggested formulation. Furthermore, the other advantage of these inserts over the conventional ophthalmic delivery systems such as drops was that the multiple-dose typical ophthalmic delivery systems (such as drops) required and contained preservatives (such as benzalkonium chloride) in the formulation for protecting the therapeutics against the contamination by microorganisms.[3] The presence of preservatives could mediate inflammation and corneal and conjunctival cell death,[29] while these solid-state inserts did not require the addition of any preservative and could overcome the side effects corresponding to the presence of preservatives.

Conclusion

For the first time in the present study, hydrophilic chitosan-based ocular inserts were developed for delivery of triamcinolone acetonide by electrospinning method and the results were compared with a hydrophobic (Eudragit/Zein) electrospun insert candidate. The prepared ophthalmic delivery system could achieve prolonged therapeutic drug concentrations and could be promising candidates as ocular inserts and it could be used in a single dose at longer time intervals. The Zero-order release profile indicated the prolonged, monotonic, and well-controlled release of drug from the suggested formulation, and consequently, limited systemic exposure and side effects and the possibility to improve the patient adherence to therapy could be taken into account as some of the advantages of the suggested formulation. The suggested formulation could be converted from solid to gel form after exposition into the ocular pH, and the muco-adhesive nature of the suggested formulation caused the longer period for control of lixiviation than other similar formulations. Based on the advantages of the suggested formulation, it could be performed for ocular delivery of other similar drugs.

Acknowledgments
The authors would like to acknowledge the Research Council of Kermanshah University of Medical Sciences (Grant number: 95416) for financial support of this work. Also faithfully thanks to Mr Komail Sadrjavadi and Miss Marziyeh Hajialyani for their assistances and valuable ideas.

Ethical Issues
Not applicable.

Conflict of Interests
The authors declared no conflict of interest for this study.

References
1. Kumar BP, Harish G, Bhowmik D. Ocular inserts: A novel controlled drug delivery system. *Pharm Innov* 2013;1(12).
2. Tanwar Y, Patel D, Sisodia S. In vitro and in vivo evaluation of ocular inserts of ofloxacin. *DARU* 2007;15(3):139-45.
3. De Souza JF, Maia KN, Patrício PSDO, Fernandes-Cunha GM, Da Silva MG, Jensen CEDM, et al. Ocular inserts based on chitosan and brimonidine tartrate: Development, characterization and biocompatibility. *J Drug Deliv Sci Tec* 2016;32:21-30. doi: 10.1016/j.jddst.2016.01.008
4. Vaishya RD, Khurana V, Patel S, Mitra AK. Controlled ocular drug delivery with nanomicelles. *Wiley Interdiscip Rev Nanomed Nanobiotechnol* 2014;6(5):422-37. doi: 10.1002/wnan.1272
5. Ananthula HK, Vaishya RD, Barot M, Mitra AK. Duane's Ophthalmology. In: Tasman W, Jaeger EA, editors. *Bioavailability*. Philadelphia: Lippincott Williams & Wilkins; 2009.
6. Madhuri B, Gawali Vikas B, Mahesh B. Ocular inserts: A rate controlled drug delivery system–a review. *Int J Pharmaceut* 2012; 2(1): 49-63.
7. Di Colo G, Zambito Y, Burgalassi S, Serafini A, Saettone MF. Effect of chitosan on in vitro release and ocular delivery of ofloxacin from erodible inserts

based on poly(ethylene oxide). *Int J Pharm* 2002;248(1-2):115-22.

8. Sreenivas S, Hiremath S, Godbole A. Ofloxacin ocular inserts: Design, formulation and evaluation. *Iran J Pharmacol Therapeut (IJPT)* 2006;5(2):159-62.

9. Reddy ES. Design and characterization of ofloxacin and dexamethasone ocular inserts using combination of hydrophobic and hydrophilic polymers. *Asian J Pharm* 2017;11(01). doi: 10.22377/ajp.v11i01.1089

10. Reshu S, Laxmi G, Preeti K. Formulation and evaluation of ocular inserts of acyclovir. *Int J Drug Res Tech* 2013;3(4):88-95.

11. Manea LR, Hristian L, Leon AL, Popa A. Recent advances of basic materials to obtain electrospun polymeric nanofibers for medical applications. *IOP Conf Ser: Mat Sci Eng* 2016;45(3):032006. doi:10.1088/1757-899X/145/3/032006

12. Da Silva GR, Lima TH, Orefice RL, Fernandes-Cunha GM, Silva-Cunha A, Zhao M, et al. In vitro and in vivo ocular biocompatibility of electrospun poly(varepsilon-caprolactone) nanofibers. *Eur J Pharm Sci* 2015;73:9-19. doi: 10.1016/j.ejps.2015.03.003

13. Kataria K, Sharma A, Garg T, K Goyal A, Rath G. Novel technology to improve drug loading in polymeric nanofibers. *Drug Deliv Lett* 2014;4(1):79-86.

14. Villarreal-Gomez LJ, Cornejo-Bravo JM, Vera-Graziano R, Grande D. Electrospinning as a powerful technique for biomedical applications: A critically selected survey. *J Biomater Sci Polym Ed* 2016;27(2):157-76. doi: 10.1080/09205063.2015.1116885

15. Eatemadi A, Daraee H, Zarghami N, Melat Yar H, Akbarzadeh A. Nanofiber: Synthesis and biomedical applications. *Artif Cells Nanomed Biotechnol* 2016;44(1):111-21. doi: 10.3109/21691401.2014.922568

16. Duque Sanchez L, Brack N, Postma A, Pigram PJ, Meagher L. Surface modification of electrospun fibres for biomedical applications: A focus on radical polymerization methods. *Biomaterials* 2016;106:24-45. doi: 10.1016/j.biomaterials.2016.08.011

17. Chen J, Liu Z, Chen M, Zhang H, Li X. Electrospun gelatin fibers with a multiple release of antibiotics accelerate dermal regeneration in infected deep burns. *Macromol Biosci* 2016;16(9):1368-80. doi: 10.1002/mabi.201600108

18. Nagarajan S, Soussan L, Bechelany M, Teyssier C, Cavaillès V, Pochat-Bohatier C, et al. Novel biocompatible electrospun gelatin fiber mats with antibiotic drug delivery properties. *J Mater Chem B* 2016;4(6):1134-41. doi: 10.1039/C5TB01897H

19. Malafaya PB, Silva GA, Reis RL. Natural-origin polymers as carriers and scaffolds for biomolecules and cell delivery in tissue engineering applications. *Adv Drug Deliv Rev* 2007;59(4-5):207-33. doi: 10.1016/j.addr.2007.03.012

20. Alves NM, Mano JF. Chitosan derivatives obtained by chemical modifications for biomedical and environmental applications. *Int J Biol Macromol* 2008;43(5):401-14. doi: 10.1016/j.ijbiomac.2008.09.007

21. Scherliess R, Buske S, Young K, Weber B, Rades T, Hook S. In vivo evaluation of chitosan as an adjuvant in subcutaneous vaccine formulations. *Vaccine* 2013;31(42):4812-9. doi: 10.1016/j.vaccine.2013.07.081

22. Laurienzo P. Marine polysaccharides in pharmaceutical applications: An overview. *Mar Drugs* 2010;8(9):2435-65. doi: 10.3390/md8092435

23. Bhattarai RS, Das A, Alzhrani RM, Kang D, Bhaduri SB, Boddu SHS. Comparison of electrospun and solvent cast polylactic acid (pla)/poly(vinyl alcohol) (pva) inserts as potential ocular drug delivery vehicles. *Mater Sci Eng C Mater Biol Appl* 2017;77:895-903. doi: 10.1016/j.msec.2017.03.305

24. Payab S, Davaran S, Tanhaei A, Fayyazi B, Jahangiri A, Farzaneh A, et al. Triamcinolone acetonide-eudragit((r)) rs100 nanofibers and nanobeads: Morphological and physicochemical characterization. *Artif Cells Nanomed Biotechnol* 2016;44(1):362-9. doi: 10.3109/21691401.2014.953250

25. Fulgencio Gde O, Viana FA, Ribeiro RR, Yoshida MI, Faraco AG, Cunha-Junior Ada S. New mucoadhesive chitosan film for ophthalmic drug delivery of timolol maleate: In vivo evaluation. *J Ocul Pharmacol Ther* 2012;28(4):350-8. doi: 10.1089/jop.2011.0174

26. Foureaux G, Franca JR, Nogueira JC, Fulgencio Gde O, Ribeiro TG, Castilho RO, et al. Ocular inserts for sustained release of the angiotensin-converting enzyme 2 activator, diminazene aceturate, to treat glaucoma in rats. *PLoS One* 2015;10(7):e0133149. doi: 10.1371/journal.pone.0133149

27. Verestiuc L, Nastasescu O, Barbu E, Sarvaiya I, Green KL, Tsibouklis J. Functionalized chitosan/nipam (hema) hybrid polymer networks as inserts for ocular drug delivery: Synthesis, in vitro assessment, and in vivo evaluation. *J Biomed Mater Res A* 2006;77(4):726-35. doi: 10.1002/jbm.a.30668

28. Jahangiri A, Davaran S, Fayyazi B, Tanhaei A, Payab S, Adibkia K. Application of electrospraying as a one-step method for the fabrication of triamcinolone acetonide-plga nanofibers and nanobeads. *Colloids Surf B Biointerfaces* 2014;123:219-24. doi: 10.1016/j.colsurfb.2014.09.019

29. Ammar DA, Kahook MY. Effects of glaucoma medications and preservatives on cultured human trabecular meshwork and non-pigmented ciliary epithelial cell lines. *Br J Ophthalmol* 2011;95(10):1466-9. doi: 10.1136/bjophthalmol-2011-300012

18

Phytochemical Synthesis of Silver Nanoparticles by Two Techniques Using *Saturaja rechengri* Jamzad Extract: Identifying and Comparing *in Vitro* Anti-Proliferative Activities

Fataneh Narchin[1], Kambiz Larijani[1]*, Abdolhossein Rustaiyan[1], Samad Nejad Ebrahimi[2], Farzaneh Tafvizi[3]

[1] Department of Chemistry, Science and Research Branch, Islamic Azad University, Tehran, Iran.
[2] Department of Phytochemistry, Medicinal Plants and Drugs Research Institute, Shahid Beheshti University, Evin Tehran, Iran.
[3] Department of Biology, Parand Branch, Islamic Azad University, Parand, Iran.

Keywords:
· Satureja
· Nanoparticle
· Green chemistry
· Silver
· Phytochemical
· Cytotoxicity

Abstract

Purpose: A lot of plants are available which can produce nanoparticles used in medicine, life sciences, and the pharmaceutical industry. The present study aims to introduce safe biological and eco-friendly methods for synthesizing silver nanoparticles (AgNPs) by using *Saturaja rechengri* Jamzad extract, which can replace traditional chemical methods. In addition, the chemical nature and antimicrobial activities were identified and accordingly the anticancer effects of AgNPs was successfully reported on colon cancer cells (HT-29).

Methods: Light and ultrasound, as two green chemistry techniques were first used for AgNPs synthesis. Then, morphological and crystalline structure of AgNPs was evaluated by scanning electron microscopy (SEM) and X-ray diffraction (XRD) analysis, respectively. In addition, functional groups were determined by using the Fourier transform infrared spectroscopy (FTIR) spectrum. Further, a maximum adsorption of AgNPs was observed in UV-visible spectrum. In the next stage, antibacterial activity of green synthesized AgNPs was evaluated against two pathogenic bacteria including Escherichia coli and Staphylococcus aureus. Finally, the cytotoxicity of AgNPs on HT-29 at different concentrations and times of AgNPs was determined by MTT assay.

Results: The findings indicated that the synthesis of AgNPs by ultrasonic technique leads to smaller particle size and more distribution. Based on the results of MTT test for calculating the IC50%, the anti-proliferative effects of the light and ultrasound AgNPs were observed on HT-29 cell lines depending on the dose and time. Finally, the AgNPs had the most cytotoxicity HT-29 cell lines at 100 µg/ml concentration although the lowest toxicity effect was reported on HEK-293 cell lines at the same conditions.

Conclusion: The change in the concentration, physical and chemical properties of AgNPs including the form and size of particles, and their type of covering and fields can influence the induction of cytotoxicity and morphological change in the treated cells. The present research opens a new horizon on the development of new biological and cytotoxicity agents.

Introduction

Bio-nanotechnology is regarded as one of the most valuable nanotechnology in the modern era. In addition, it is an interdisciplinary area related to physics, electronic materials, biology, chemistry and medicine, which uses these scientific fields to control matter at the molecular scale.[1] The use of plan biomass to produce nanoparticles is a relatively simple and cost-effective technique. In addition, the biomass derived from live or dead plants is used as a renewable energy source to generate electricity, biogas, fuel, and the like. Further, the use of biomass for producing nanoparticles is exciting.[2,3] Generally, this technique helps to protect the environment and reduce the risk of damage for human beings, nature, air and the ecosystem.[4,5] Nanoparticles used in diagnosing and treating diseases are divided into organic and inorganic category.

Organic nanoparticles include albumin, lipid nanoparticle and chitosan, and the like while inorganic nanoparticles are often found as metal nanoparticles including magnetic, copper, gold and silver, etc.[6] The use of nanoparticles is important since they are comparable with cellular components in human cells in term of size. It seems that the nature has used materials at a nano-scale to construct biological systems. If someone is supposed to accompany the nature in treating the diseases, he should use materials at a scale which is similar to the nature in some areas like correcting defective genes,[7] preventing the proliferation of viral genomes[8] and cancer cell death,[9] and restoring to cellular metabolism.[10] Among different synthesized nanoparticles, AgNPs are considered as one of the most widely used drug-delivery nanotechnologies for treating

*Corresponding author: Kambiz Larijani, Email: klarijani@yahoo.com

diseases. In this regard, a large body of research was conducted on the related anticancer,[11] antibacterial,[12] antifungal,[13] and antiviral effects.[14] The results indicated that AgNPs can damage DNA by destructing the mitochondrial respiratory chain in cancer cells, leading to the cell death.[15,16] However, silver, in itself, can play a minor role or lacks the properties. Compared with macro silver particles, this dual effect of nanoparticles is caused by increasing the areas, along with the reactivity of matter and its compliance with quantum physics and chemistry in nano mode.[17] Based on green chemical compounds, producing AgNPs by using green chemistry includes choosing the solvent environment, a safe operating environment revivalist, and non-toxic materials for the stability of the nanoparticles (Eshleman, 2011). Hera et al. reported the formation of Ag^+ from alfalfa biomass in an aqueous solution in a pH-dependent manner.[18] Mata et al. examined the cytotoxic effects of AgNPs synthesized by the aqueous extract of Abution indicum leaf in the cancer cell line (COLO 205) (human colon cancer) and MDCK (normal) cell *in vitro* conditions and observed that concentration-depend AgNPs, inhibit the growth of this cancer cell line. In addition, it was observed that AgNPs cause morphological changes in chromatin densities and the membranes of treated cells, which ultimately lead to the cell death.[19] Savory with the scientific name (Satureja hortensis) belongs to the Lamiaceae family. Lamiaceae is one the largest plant families with a global distribution. This genus has 15 species in Iran, among which 9 species such as *S. edmondi, S. sahendica, S. kallarica, S. bachtiarica, S. intermedia, S. isophylla, S.atropatana, S. khuzestanica. S. Rechingeri* are exclusive to Iran. Some studies reported carvacrol and flavonoids as the main components of Satureja species[20,21] including antioxidant properties.[22] During recent years, a number of studies reported anti-viral properties,[23] analgesic and anti-inflammatory,[24] antibacterial and antifungal,[25-27] antispasmodic and anti-diarrhea,[28] vasodilatory properties[29] for different species of this plant, among which we can refer to Satureja rechingeri as one of the endemic species of this plant. In this study, the green synthesized AgNPs extracted from *S.rechengeri* were used to determine the antimicrobial and anti-cancer effects on colon cancer cell lines. However, no study has yet addressed different AgNPs synthesis methods of *S.rechingeri* by using light and ultrasonic techniques. Based on the review of the literature, this is the first study addressing the quick and simple synthesis of AgNPs by using *S.rechingeri* extract as a reducing and stable agent to determine its effect on colon cancer cells. It seems that the introduction of drugs used in traditional medicine, especially medicinal herbs, represents a good starting point for the development of research projects to produce new drugs for the treatment of cancer.[30]

Materials and Methods
Plant Extract Preparation
The aerial parts of the plant were collected at the flowering stage from a farm owned by Khoraman Company in Lorestan Province (Iran) in July 2016 with the Herbarium code MPH-1348. The fresh plants of *S.rechengri* were dried in the shade for 10 days and then were powdered. In order to prepare aqueous solution of the plant extract, 20 g of plant powder was weighed and was kept for 24 hours in the laboratory conditions after being ionized into 80 ml water. In the next stage, the solution was placed in water bath with 80°C for 45 min and was filtered by Watman Filter Paper No. 2. Accordingly, the extract was treated by vacuum rotary evaporation (Rv10 digital, Germany) and was kept at 4°C for use and identification by various techniques in order to remove the extra solvent and obtain a good concentration.

AgNPs Synthesis
In order to synthesize AgNPs, the two following methods as green chemistry were used. The solution of silver nitrate salt ($AgNO_3$) (Merck, Germany) 0.001 M was prepared in both methods.

A) Light: Silver nitrate solution and the extract were mixed with a ratio of 1:4 for the synthesis of AgNPs. The sample was exposed to direct sunlight for 5 min at pH=7. The rapid color change from pale yellow to reddish-brown indicated a reduction of Ag^+ to Ag^0 and the formation of AgNPs. Then, the sample was placed at room temperature for 24 hours.

B) Ultrasound: One part of $AgNO_3$ solution 0.001M was mixed with four parts of the extract (a mix ratio of 1:4) and the same was exposed at ultrasound irradiation of 40 Hz in the dark for three times, each time for 30 min, at 40°C and pH= 7 Changes in color from pale yellow to reddish-brown indicated the formation of AgNPs.

Charactization of AgNPs
Spectroscopy (UV-visible) to identify AgNPs
The color change was observed under light and ultrasound conditions, which was very fast and clear in light conditions. The absorption spectra were measured by using a spectrophotometer (JASCO V-670 Spectrophotometer) in the range of 300-600 as silver absorption occurs in this range.

XRD diffraction analysis
X-ray diffraction analysis XRD was used to identify the phase and determine the crystalline structure of AgNPs in the range of $5 > 2\emptyset > 90$. Sharp peaks indicated the crystallization properties of the produced sample. The precipitation from the interaction of the aqueous extract of the plant and silver ion was centrifuged three times at 1200 rpm and washed with deionized water. Then, it was dried at 45°C for 24 hours and accordingly used for its identification.

Infrared Fourier transform spectrum analysis (FTIR)
In the next stage, the functional groups of AgNPs were determined by ultrasound and light techniques by using Fourier transform spectrometer. This technique involves the identification of functional groups AgNPs in the range of 500-4000 cm^{-1}.

Scanning electron microscopy
Scanning electron microscopy SEM is a considered as a technique used for direct observation of AgNPs and estimating their size and surface morphology. This technique is appropriate for identifying the particles with smaller particle size and is regarded as a good standard for determining the validity of other techniques. Further, it provides some information about the structure of particles through electron distribution and dimensions of synthesized nanoparticles. In the next procedure, SEM image of AgNPs was photographed to determine the shape and size of the nanoparticles. To this end, a thin layer of sediment was placed on a gold cloth at a low voltage and under vacuum pressure (5-8 Torr) by using Philips XL30 electron microscope. It was found that the particles are mainly spherical in shape and their diameter is in the range of 44.2 and 65.3 nm, which are stacked together in some areas.

Antimicrobial test
MIC and MBC evaluation
The Minimum inhibitory concentration (MIC) of synthesized AgNPs light and ultrasound for *Escherichia coli* and *Staphylococcus aureus* was determined by the Mueller-Hinton broth (Merck, Germany) micro dilution method (CLSI, 2010) on 96-well plates with incubation at 37°C for 24 hours. Further, MIC and higher concentrations were cultured on nutrient agar (Merck, Germany) plates and incubated at 37°C for 24 hours in order to evaluate the minimum bactericidal concentration (MBC) of AgNPs light and ultrasound. Then, the MIC value was determined for the least dose of synthesized AgNPs, which prevented the growth of tested bacteria. In order to achieve a better result, the test was repeated twice.

Cytotoxicity effect
Preparation of cell lines and culture
The HT-29 cells (Human colorectal adenocarcinoma, IBRC C10097) and Normal HEK-293 (IBRC C10139) were purchased from National Cell Bank in Iranian Biological Resource Center (Cell Bank of Pasteur Institute Tehran-Iran). Then, they were defrozen and cultured in the IMPR environment enriched with 10% SBF and bovine serum and 1% penicillin –streptomycin. After the cell lines were grown sufficiently, they were counted and a total number of 10^4 cell lines were cultured in a 96-well plate and incubated within incubators (Binder) at 37°C and 5% CO_2.

MTT Assay
MTT assay is a colorimetric method based on the revival and break of yellow crystals with chemical formula 3- [4, 5-dimethylthiazol-2-yl] -2, 5-diphenyl-] which are regenerated by tetrazolium bromide enzyme succinate dehydrogenase in the active cellular mitochondria and the formation of insoluble blue crystals. The color is proportional to the cellular activity and the number of living cells.[31] After 24 hours, 100 ml of the cultured cells was covered with 100 ml of AgNPs of salt with a concentration of 0.5 mg ml for 4 hours by using a foil. Then, the cell cytotoxicity was estimated through colorimetric method (MTT) on colon cancer cells HT-29 and healthy cells HEK-293 by measuring the light and ultrasound absorbance based on the concentration of AgNPs. In the next stage, the results were compared with the rate of cell survival. In addition, the cells were cultured in a 96-well plate with a density of 10^4 cells per plant and were incubated in a CO_2 incubator (37°C) for 24 h. Further, HT-29 cancer cells were treated with different concentration of AgNPs synthesized from the aqueous extract of the plant for 24 and 48 h, respectively. After treating the samples, 10 µl of MTT solution (5 mg/ml) was added to each plate containing AgNPs-treated cells and incubated at 37°C and 5% CO_2 for 5 h. Finally, DMSO (0.5 µl) was added to each well until dissolving the purple crystals, and the light absorbance was read by a spectrophotometer at 570 nm after 20 min at room temperature.[32] In addition, the inhibitory concentration ($IC_{50\%}$) for the samples was determined as follows:

$$Percentage\ of\ cell\ viability\ \% = \frac{Average\ absorbance\ by\ the\ treatment\ sample}{Average\ absorbance\ by\ the\ control\ sample} \times 100$$

Statistical analysis
The quantitative data was evaluated using SPSS software (Version 16) (SPSS Inc., Chicago, IL) and the results were analyzed by ANOVA at a software using statistical tests at significant level. The data were determined as mean ± SD and $p < 0.05$ was considered statistically significant.

Results and Discussion
Synthesis Charactization of AgNPs
This study was designed to synthesize AgNPs by using *S.rechengri* extract based on light and ultrasonic

techniques, which are economical and ecofriendly. In addition, the enormous potentials of the nature can be employed for synthesizing nanoparticles in these two techniques, without damaging the environment. Recently, a lot of plant extracts have been studied for AgNPs synthesis. However, in the present study, aqueous extracts were extracted from the aerial parts of dried *S.rechengri* for AgNPs synthesis and the extracts prepared by using a solution of AgNO$_3$ 0.001 M (from Merck Company, Germany) with a purity of 99/99% were mixed. In order to synthesize the AgNPs from the obtained solution, both light and ultrasound techniques (absence of light) were used. The results showed a change in color of the extract from pale yellow to dark brown at room temperature and the formation of a colloidal mix of AgNPs. The observation of the color change due to the interaction of herbal extracts and silver salt solution was similar to the results of the study by Reddy and Gandhi (2012) and is considered as the first microscopic signs of the production of AgNPs.[33] The speed of the reaction reducing Ag[+] in the aqueous extract of *S.rechengri* by using the light technique was found to be higher than that of ultrasound technique. Further, the color change in the light technique was considerably clearer than of the ultrasound technique. In the ultrasound techniques, the silver nitrate solution and the extracts were exposed to ultrasonic irradiation with intensity (40 Hz) at 40°C for 30 minutes while the solution was exposed to direct sunlight (visible waves) for 5 min in the optical techniques. The completion of the synthesis of AgNPs at higher speeds is regarded as one of the benefits of these methods. Furthermore, UV-visible absorption occurred in the 300-600 nm region for both methods. The observation of absorption in the region of x nm confirms the synthesis of AgNPs. In the present study, the presence of AgNPs peak at a wavelength of 430 nm is consistent with the observations made by Song and Kim (2009) and Sathyavathi et al (2010).[34] Todays, there are many plants which are used for synthesizing metal nanoparticles such as Ag.[35,36] However, only one of these species, *S.rechengri* is used for AgNPs synthesis although Satureja has many species. Biological organisms are significant at both capping and oxidant agents in the synthesis of AgNPs. A large body of research indicates that the synthesis of AgNPs by using bioorganic compounds is successful. In addition, the reduction of Ag[+] by biomolecules including the cell extract such as enzymes, proteins, vitamins, amino acids, and polysaccharides are compatible with the nature.

Dehghanizade et al. (2017) investigated the synthesis of AgNPs using Anthemis atropatana extract and its antimicrobial and anticancer effects, and showed that biosynthesis of AgNPs by green chemistry is easily affordable and there is no require any reducing agents.[37] Extensive studies have shown that a combination of phenolic acids and amine acids, flavonoids, enzymes and proteins present in the plant extract may be the main cause for rapid and easy reduction of metallic silver ions,[38] which play an important role in the synthesis of AgNPs.[39,40] However, the chemical synthesis of such nanoparticles brings about many environmental disadvantages and problems, which is not environment-friendly.[41]

UV-Visible

The UV-visible spectrum was used to determine the absorption wavelength of AgNPs, which indicated a high absorption occurred in the wavelength 430 nm. Based on the theory of the effect of quantum restraint, lower wavelength leads to higher energy of the wave and smaller particle size.[42] Thus, this spectrum confirms the formation and fineness of AgNPs (Figure 1).

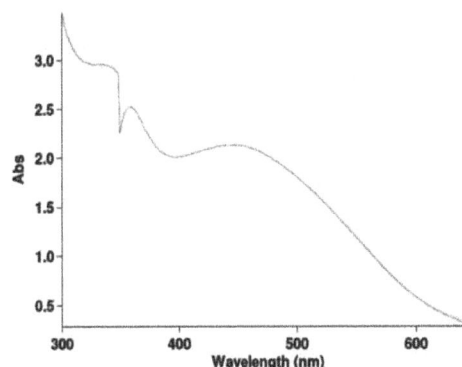

Figure 1. UV-visible spectrum of green synthesized AgNPs

XRD analysis of AgNPs

In addition, XRD diffraction was used to determine the crystalline structure of the synthesized AgNPs. The relative intensity of each peak represents the type of synthesized AgNPs and their phase qualitatively. As observed in Figure 2, the peak intensity in regions 111, (200), (220), (311), and (222) confirms the regular crystal structure of the synthesized AgNPs at angles 5> 2 Ǿ > 90. Further, sharp peaks represent the crystalized nature of the produced samples. Furthermore, the analysis of the diffraction patterns of the irradiation could confirm the cubic crystal structure of the samples.[43]

FTIR spectroscopy

In order to study the tensile and flexural frequency of the bonds in the synthesized AgNPs, the Fourier transform infrared (FTIR) spectrometer was used (Figure 3). In general, the peaks of 3417.79 and 1636.27 cm[-] represent tensile and flexural modes of the absorbed surface water (H-O-H) of this blend, respectively. Additionally, the bending vibration mode of Ag-O in the peak numbers of 521.73 and 472.96 cm[-] confirms the formation of AgNPs. In this spectrum, the peak close to the wave number 600 cm[-] is related to two split peaks. It seems that this splitting is the result of separating energy levels of AgNPs, which are quantized.

SEM and EDX analysis

The analysis of the structure and morphology of nanoparticles, as well as their size and surface morphology, was performed by SEM microscopy. The synthesized AgNPs in the colloidal solution were exposed to irradiation by using light and ultrasound techniques. The comparison of the produced spherical AgNPs indicated that the synthesized AgNPs produced through ultrasonic irradiation technique are smaller in size and more spherical in shape and have a better distribution. The particle size in the ultrasound technique ranges from 44 to 65.3 nm and is 54.75 nm on average

(Figure 4) while the particle size in the light technique ranges from 57.1 to 88.5 nm, with an average of 72.8 nm (Figure 5). Further, the Energy Dispersive X- ray Spectroscopy (EDS) spectrum was determined to indicate that it is coated with 100% silver (Figure 6).

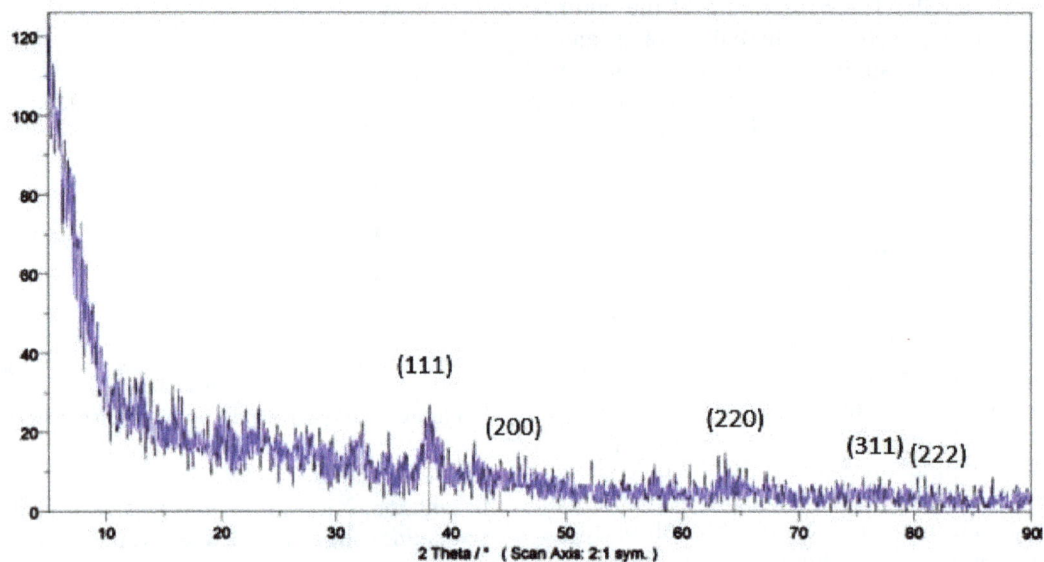

Figure 2. XRD pattern of AgNPs synthesized. Schema of XRD peak related to face-centered cubic (fcc) (111), (200), (220), (311) and (222) in sample silver spectrum. 2θ angles related to silver schema are observed in 38.01, 44.5, 64.78, 77.7 and 82.1.

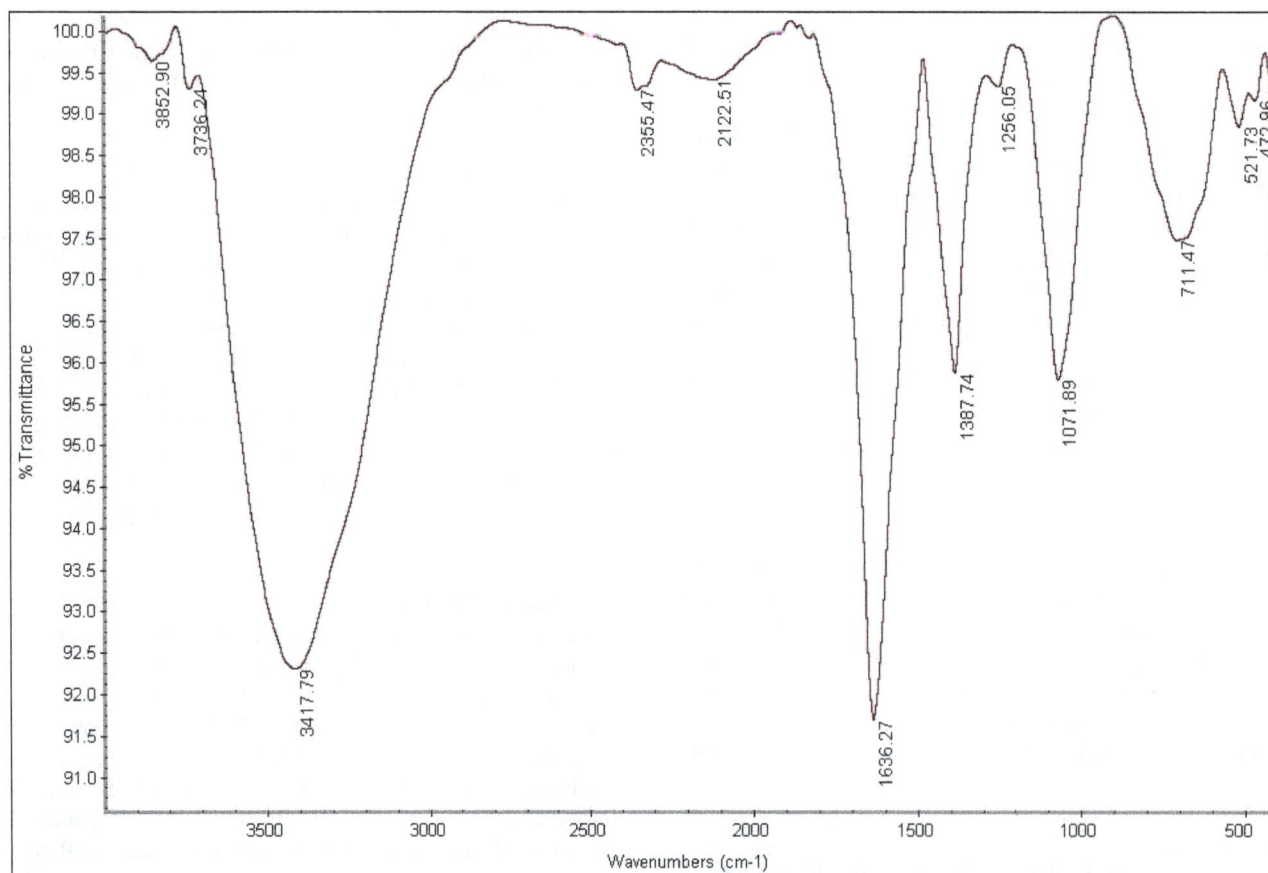

Figure 3. FTIR of AgNPs. The analysis of the AgNPs showed the stretching frequencies in 472.99, 521.73, 711.74, 1071.89, 1387.74,16, 36.27 and 3417.79 cm^{-1}.

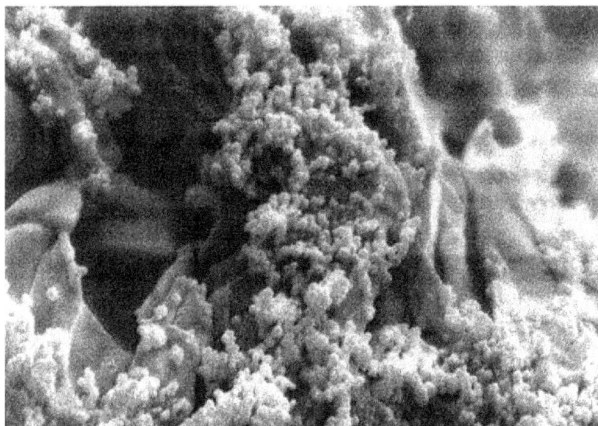

Figure 4. SEM analysis of AgNPs using green chemistry in Ultrasound technique.

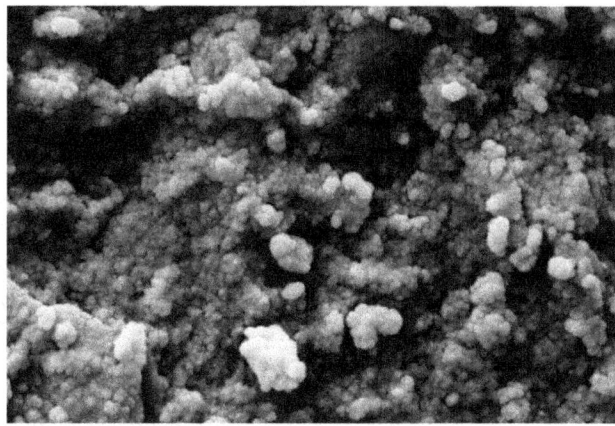

Figure 5. SEM analysis of AgNPs using green chemistry in light technique.

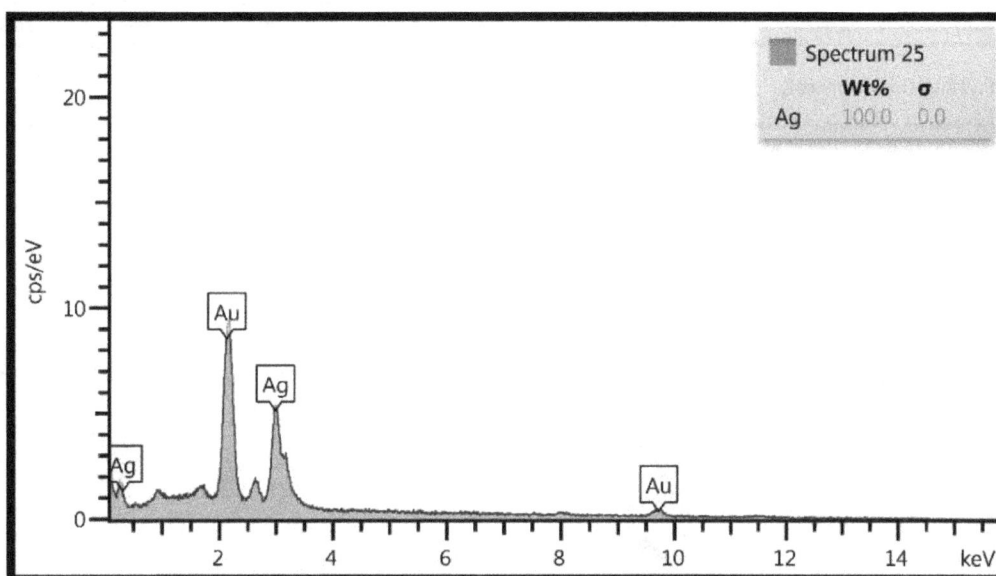

Figure 6. EDS analysis of AgNPs green chemistry

Antibacterial test

The antibacterial activity of the synthesized AgNPs from the aqueous extract of *S.rechengri* was considered based on two bacterial pathogens including *Escherichia coli* and *Staphylococcus aureus*. The results were evaluated for the lowest inhibitory concentration (MIC) of AgNPs in terms of the growth of selected bacteria. The results of some studies indicated that the synthesized AgNPs cause bacterial cell death by destructing the cell membrane of the bacteria such as Staphylococcus and E-coli at a given concentration (Table 1) while bacterial growth are inhibited in other concentrations.[44,45]Another proposed mechanism for the death of bacteria is related to the AgNPs release of Ag^+ which can bind biological macromolecules including oxygen, nitrogen, and sulfur, and disrupt the function of biological molecules, leading to the death of the bacterial cell.[46]

MTT assay

The cytotoxicity of AgNPs was first estimated with colorimetric method (MTT) by measuring the optical density based on the concentrations (3.125-6.5-12.5-25-

50-100 µg/ml) of green synthesized AgNPs through light and ultrasound techniques. Then, the results were compared with cell survival rate. In addition, the effects of synthesized AgNPs on colon cancer cell lines (HT-29) and normal cells (HEK-293) were evaluated. In the next procedure, the survival rate of the treated cells with AgNPs was measured, compared to the survival rate of the untreated (control) cells during 24 and 48 hours after the treatment. Based on the results, the reduction of the cell survival rate was observed with increasing concentrations of AgNPs. In addition, at the highest dose (100 µg /ml), the cell viability for the cells treated by synthesized AgNPs by light and ultrasound techniques were found to be at the lowest rate. Tables 2 and 3 represent the results of biological power of the cells in terms of the color change in salt dimethylthiazol by light and ultrasound AgNPs, respectively. Further, the values were obtained on the mean ± SD and the mean differences were compared at the significance level of P ≤ 0.05 (ANOVA and t-test). Figures 7, 8, 9 and 10 illustrate the dose dependence of anticancer effects of AgNPs on HT-29 cell lines.

Table 1. Minimum inhibitory concentration (MIC µg /ml) against the two bacteria withsynthesized AgNPs by light and ultrasound

Bacteria	Minimum inhibitory concentration (µg/ml)	
	light	ultrasound
Escherichia coli	6.25	-
Staphylococcus aureus	1.56	100

Table 2. The cell viability for HT-29 cells with light AgNPs during 24 and 48 hours by MTT.

Concentrations (µg/ml)	3.125	6.25	12.5	25	50	100
Cell viability (% of control)	[a]42.5 ± 0.36	22.5 ± 0.49	11.75±0.44	7.7±0.34	5.25±0.27	1.27±0.12
	[b]34.25± 0.44	13.7 ± 0.42	9.2 ± 0.37	4.7±0.28	2.5±0.22	1±0.09

* Percentage of cell survival within 24 (a) and 48 (b) hours

Table 3. The cell viability for HT-29 cells with ultrasound AgNPs during 24 and 48 hours by MTT.

Concentrations (µg/ml)	3.125	6.25	12.5	25	50	100
Cell viability (% of control)	[a]63.5± 0.38	37.5 ± 0.88	24.75±0.78	22.25±0.28	11.5±0.58	4.5±0.36
	[b]50.2± 0.57	36.6± 0.52	23.8 ± 0.44	14.7±0.25	10.3±0.15	3.9±0.02

* Percentage of cell survival within 24 (a) and 48 (b) hours

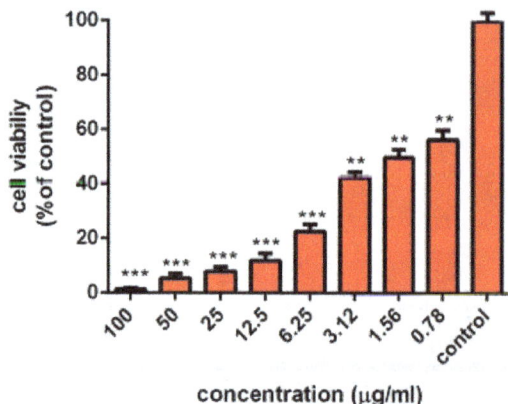

Figure 7. Survival percentage of HT-29 cells against different concentrations of light AgNPs within 24 hours. Results have been reported as survival rate compared with control samples (n=3 P <0.001 ***, P < 0.01**, P <0.05 *).

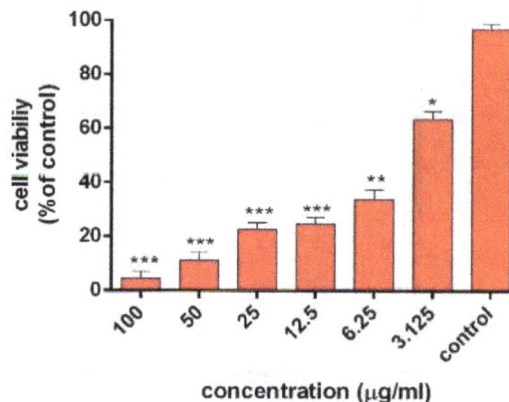

Figure 9. Survival percentage of HT-29 cells against different concentrations of ultrasound AgNPs within 24 hours. Results have been reported as survival rate compared with control samples (n=3 P <0.001 ***, P < 0.01**, P <0.05 *).

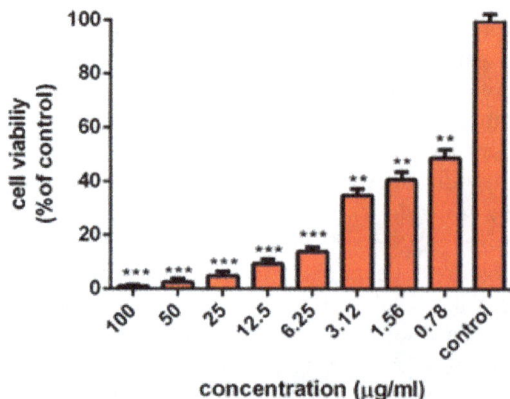

Figure 8. Survival percentage of HT-29 cells against different concentrations of light AgNPs within 48 hours. Results have been reported as survival rate compared with control samples. (n=3 P <0.001 ***, P < 0.01**, P <0.05 *).

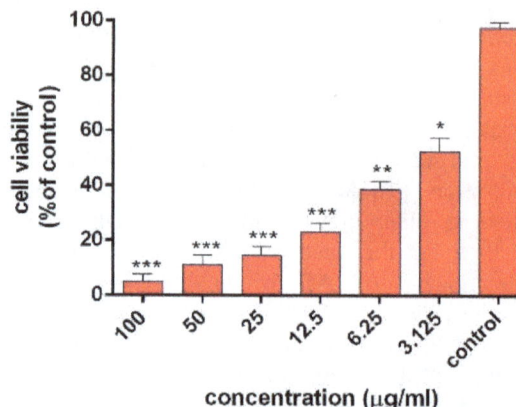

Figure 10. Survival percentage of HT-29 cells against different concentrations of ultrasound AgNPs within 48 hours. Results have been reported as survival rate compared with control samples. (n=3 P <0.001 ***, P < 0.01**, P <0.05 *).

The induction of cytotoxicity of ultrasound AgNPs was observed at higher concentrations and was found to be more intense than that caused by light AgNPs. The results indicated that the effect on cell lines HT-29 relies on their concentration, in addition to the size and shape of AgNPs, Further, the results of calculating the $IC_{50\%}$ for the light AgNPs showed that such nanoparticles can inhibit 50% of the cells during 24 and 48 hours at concentrations of 1.3 and 0.71 µg /ml. Furthermore, light AgNPs within 48 hours with lower doses can prevent the growth of 50% of the cancer cells HT-29, indicating a significant difference during 24 hours. Additionally, the results of ultrasound AgNPs in 24 and 48 hours at the concentrations of 4.7 and 2.6 µg /ml indicated that these AgNPs can inhibit 50% of the cells. In addition, the MTT results of synthesized AgNPs through light and ultrasound technique were performed on a healthy HEK-293 cell line. The values were determined for ultrasound AgNPs 3.125-6.5-12.5-25-50-100 µg/ml for 24 hours (Table 4). Based on the results, both AgNPs had more effective cytotoxicity against HT-29 cells than HEK-293 cell lines. Figure 11 displays the concentration dependence of cytotoxicity effect of AgNPs on HEK-293 cell line.

Table 4. The cell viability for HEK-293 cells with AgNPs during 24 hours by MTT.

Concentrations (µg/ml)	3.125	6.25	12.5	25	50	100
cell viability (% of control)	[a]94.76± 0.43	87.97±0.25	63.56±0.34	25.88±0.25	22.21±0.28	17.76±0.21

* Percentage of cell survival within 24 (a) hours

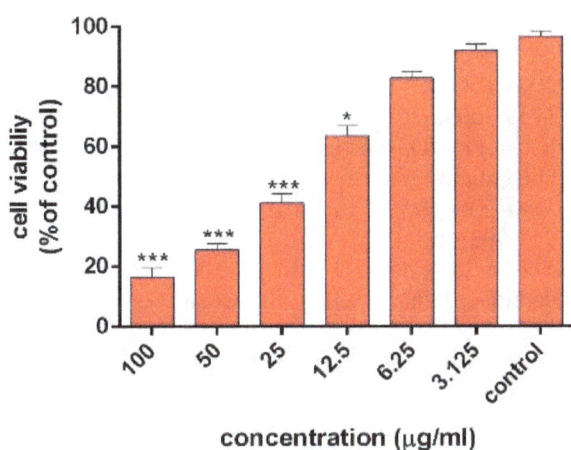

Figure 11. Survival percentage of normal HEK-293 cells against different concentrations of AgNPs within 24 hours. Results have been reported as survival percentages compared with control samples (n=3 P <0.001 ***, P < 0.01**, P <0.05 *).

Conclusion

The present study seek to address the use of nano-synthesis compounds of *S.rechengri* for the preparation of AgNPs. In addition, its chemical properties and effectiveness for treating colon cancer cell lines were taken into consideration. The results indicated that targeted synthesized AgNPs include desired properties, shape, size and useful biological effects. Furthermore, various methods of synthesizing AgNPs by considering biocompatibility as a priority were examined in this study. Therefore, *S.rechengri* has been first used as a living factory for the production of AgNPs. The importance of these techniques is related to their simplicity and speed of AgNPs synthesis, irrespective of the need for using hazardous chemicals. In addition to medicinal properties, *S.rechengri* has a unique feature anticancer, which play a significant role in destructing the cancer cell line HT-29. Finally, it can be used to produce AgNPs for medical and pharmaceutical purposes. It suggested that further researches were performed for AgNPs pharmaceutical effects.

Acknowledgments
We would like to appreciate all colleagues, in particular Dr. Hassan Noorbarzgan and Dr. Rahem Khoshbakht who helped us in analyzing biological data (MIC & MTT) and Dr. Amir Mirzaie for useful guidance. This research was sponsored by Islamic Azad University, Science and Research Branch of Tehran, Iran.

Ethical Issues
This project was conducted in accordance with the principles laid down in the Helsinki Protocol and approved by the Ethics Committee of the Council of Science and Research of the Islamic Azad University.

Conflict of Interest
The authors report no conflicts of interest in this study.

References
1. Sarikaya M, Tamerler C, Jen AK, Schulten K, Baneyx F. Molecular biomimetics: Nanotechnology through biology. *Nat Mater* 2003;2(9):577-85. doi: 10.1038/nmat964
2. Sezik E, Yesilada E, Honda G, Takaishi Y, Takeda Y, Tanaka T. Traditional medicine in Turkey X. Folk medicine in Central Anatolia. *J Ethnopharmacol* 2001;75(2-3):95-115. doi: 10.1016/s0378-8741(00)00399-8
3. Sharma NC, Sahi SV, Nath S, Parsons JG, Gardea-Torresdey JL, Pal T. Synthesis of plant-mediated gold nanoparticles and catalytic role of biomatrix-embedded nanomaterials. *Environ Sci Technol* 2007;41(14):5137-42. doi: 10.1021/es062929a
4. Donaldson K, Tran L, Jimenez LA, Duffin R, Newby DE, Mills N, et al. Combustion-derived nanoparticles: A review of their toxicology following inhalation exposure. *Part Fibre Toxicol* 2005;2:10. doi: 10.1186/1743-8977-2-10
5. Forough M, Farhadi KH. Biological and green synthesis of silver nanoparticles. *Turkish J Eng Env Sci* 2010;34:281-7.

6. Paulus PM, Bönnemann H, Van der Kraan AM, Luis F, Sinzig J, De Jongh LJ. Magnetic properties of nanosized transition metal colloids: the influence of noble metal coating. *Eur Phys J D* 1999;9(1):501-4. doi: 10.1007/s100530050487

7. Chavez A, Scheiman J, Vora S, Pruitt BW, Tuttle M, Iyer E, et al. Highly efficient Cas9-mediated transcriptional programming. *Nat Methods* 2015;12(4):326-8. doi: 10.1038/nmeth.3312

8. Griffin J, Singh AK, Senapati D, Lee E, Gaylor K, Jones-Boone J, et al. Sequence-Specific HCV RNA Quantification Using the Size-Dependent Nonlinear Optical Properties of Gold Nanoparticles. *Small* 2009;5(7):839-45. doi: 10.1002/smll.200801334

9. Han Y, Li S, Cao X, Yuan L, Wang Y, Yin Y, et al. Different inhibitory effect and mechanism of hydroxyapatite nanoparticles on normal cells and cancer cells *in vitro* and *in vivo*. *Sci Rep* 2014;4:7134. doi: 10.1038/srep07134

10. Braydich-Stolle L, Hussain S, Schlager JJ, Hofmann MC. *In vitro* cytotoxicity of nanoparticles in mammalian germline stem cells. *Toxicol Sci* 2005;88(2):412-9. doi: 10.1093/toxsci/kfi256

11. Kennedy DC, Orts-Gil G, Lai CH, Muller L, Haase A, Luch A, et al. Carbohydrate functionalization of silver nanoparticles modulates cytotoxicity and cellular uptake. *J Nanobiotechnology* 2014;12:59. doi: 10.1186/s12951-014-0059-z

12. Satyavani K, Gurudeeban S, Ramanathan T, Balasubramanian T. Toxicity Study of Silver Nanoparticles Synthesized from Suaeda monoica on Hep-2 Cell Line. *Avicenna J Med Biotechnol* 2012;4(1):35-9.

13. Yamasaki K, Nakano M, Kawahata T, Mori H, Otake T, Ueba N, et al. Anti-HIV-1 activity of herbs in Labiatae. *Biol Pharm Bull* 1998;21(8):829-33. doi: 10.1248/bpb.21.829

14. Abad MJ, Bermejo P, Gonzales E, Iglesias I, Irurzun A, Carrasco L. Antiviral activity of Bolivian plant extracts. *Gen Pharmacol* 1999;32(4):499-503. doi: 10.1016/s0306-3623(98)00214-6

15. He Y, Du Z, Ma S, Cheng S, Jiang S, Liu Y, et al. Biosynthesis, Antibacterial Activity and Anticancer Effects Against Prostate Cancer (PC-3) Cells of Silver Nanoparticles Using Dimocarpus Longan Lour. Peel Extract. *Nanoscale Res Lett* 2016;11(1):300. doi: 10.1186/s11671-016-1511-9

16. Nayak D, Pradhan S, Ashe S, Rauta PR, Nayak B. Biologically synthesised silver nanoparticles from three diverse family of plant extracts and their anticancer activity against epidermoid A431 carcinoma. *J Colloid Interface Sci* 2015;457:329-38. doi: 10.1016/j.jcis.2015.07.012

17. Bhainsa KC, D'Souza SF. Development of a preliminary. Biosynthesis of silver nanoparticles using the fungus Aspergillums fumigates. *BI* 2006;47(4):160-4.

18. Herrera I, Gardea-Torresdey JL, Tiemann KJ, Peralta-Videa JR, Armendariz V, Parsons JG. Binding of Silver(I) Ions by Alfalfa Biomass (Medicago Sativa): Batch PH, Time, Temperature, and Ionic Strength Studies. *J Hazard Subst Res* 2003;4:1-16. doi: 10.4148/1090-7025.1026

19. Mata R, Nakkala JR, Sadras SR. Biogenic silver nanoparticles from Abutilon indicum: Their antioxidant, antibacterial and cytotoxic effects in vitro. *Colloids Surf B Biointerfaces* 2015;128:276-86. doi: 10.1016/j.colsurfb.2015.01.052

20. Dai Y, van Spronsen J, Witkamp GJ, Verpoorte R, Choi YH. Natural deep eutectic solvents as new potential media for green technology. *Anal Chim Acta* 2013;766:61-8. doi: 10.1016/j.aca.2012.12.019

21. Dai Y, Witkamp GJ, Verpoorte R, Choi YH. Natural deep eutectic solvents as a new extraction media for phenolic metabolites in carthamus tinctorius L. *Anal Chem* 2013;85(13):6272-8. doi: 10.1021/ac400432p

22. Parker IM, Rodriguez J, Loik ME. An Evolutionary Approach to Understanding the Biology of Invasions: Local Adaptation and General-Purpose Genotypes in the Weed Verbascum thapsus. *Conserv Biol* 2003;17(1):59-72. doi: 10.1046/j.1523-1739.2003.02019.x

23. Esclapez MD, García Pérez JV, Mulet A, Cárcel JA. Ultrasound-assisted extraction of natural products. *Food Eng Rev* 2011;3:108-20. doi: 10.1007/s12393-011-9036-6

24. Mason TJ, Chemat F, Vinatoru M. The extraction of natural products using ultrasound or microwaves. *Curr Org Chem* 2011;15(2):237-47. doi: 10.2174/138527211793979871

25. Chan CH, Yusoff R, Ngoh GC, Kung FW. Microwave-assisted extractions of active ingredients from plants. *J Chromatogr A* 2011;1218(37):6213-25. doi: 10.1016/j.chroma.2011.07.040

26. Tang B, Bi W, Tian M, Row KH. Application of ionic liquid for extraction and separation of bioactive compounds from plants. *J Chromatogr B Analyt Technol Biomed Life Sci* 2012;904:1-21. doi: 10.1016/j.jchromb.2012.07.020

27. Herrero M, Mendiola JA, Cifuentes A, Ibanez E. Supercritical fluid extraction: Recent advances and applications. *J Chromatogr A* 2010;1217(16):2495-511. doi: 10.1016/j.chroma.2009.12.019

28. Fornari T, Vicente G, Vazquez E, Garcia-Risco MR, Reglero G. Isolation of essential oil from different plants and herbs by supercritical fluid extraction. *J Chromatogr A* 2012;1250:34-48. doi: 10.1016/j.chroma.2012.04.051

29. Richter BE, Jones BA, Ezzell JL, Porter NL, Avdalovic N, Pohl C. Accelerated solvent extraction: A technique for sample preparation. *Anal Chem* 1996;68(6):1033-9. doi: 10.1021/ac9508199

30. Motavalizadeh Ardakani A, Hashemi M, Safakish M, Alembagheri A, Shokohi SH, Mosadegh M. Cancer chemotherapy in Iranian traditional medicine. *J Islam IranTrad Med* 2012;3(1):3-18.

31. Ho WY, Yeap SK, Ho CL, Rahim RA, Alitheen NB. Development of multicellular tumor spheroid

(MCTS) culture from breast cancer cell and a high throughput screening method using the MTT assay. *PLoS One* 2012;7(9):e44640. doi: 10.1371/journal.pone.0044640

32. Al-Sheddi ES, Farshori NN, Al-Oqail MM, Musarrat J, Al-Khedhairy AA, Siddiqui MA. Portulaca Oleracea Seed Oil Exerts Cytotoxic Effects on Human Liver Cancer (HepG2) and Human Lung Cancer (A-549) Cell Lines. *Asian Pac J Cancer Prev* 2015;16(8):3383-7. doi: 10.7314/apjcp.2015.16.8.3383

33. Song JY, Kim BS. Rapid biological synthesis of silver nanoparticles using plant leaf extracts. *Bioprocess Biosyst Eng* 2009;32(1):79-84. doi: 10.1007/s00449-008-0224-6

34. Dimkpa CO, Calder A, Gajjar P, Merugu S, Huang W, Britt DW, et al. Interaction of silver nanoparticles with an environmentally beneficial bacterium, Pseudomonas Chlororaphis. *J Hazard Mater* 2011;188(1-3):428-35. doi: 10.1016/j.jhazmat.2011.01.118

35. Godipurge SS, Yallappa S, Biradar NJ, Biradar JS, Dhananjaya BL, Hegde G, et al. A facile and green strategy for the synthesis of Au, Ag and Au-Ag alloy nanoparticles using aerial parts of R. hypocrateriformis extract and their biological evaluation. *Enzyme Microb Technol* 2016;95:174-84. doi: 10.1016/j.enzmictec.2016.08.006

36. Yee MS, Khiew PS, Chiu WS, Tan YF, Kok YY, Leong CO. Green Synthesis of Graphene-Silver Nanocomposites and Its Application as a Potent Marine Antifouling Agent. *Colloids Surf B Biointerfaces* 2016;148:392-401. doi: 10.1016/j.colsurfb.2016.09.011

37. Dehghanizade S, Arasteh J, Mirzaie A. Green synthesis of silver nanoparticles using Anthemis atropatana extract: Characterization and *in vitro* biological activities. *Artif Cells Nanomed Biotechnol* 2018;46(1):160-8. doi: 10.1080/21691401.2017.1304402

38. Mandal D, Kumar Dash S, Das B, Chattopadhyay S, Ghosh T, Das D, et al. Bio-fabricated silver nanoparticles preferentially targets gram positive depending on cell surface charge. *Biomed Pharmacother* 2016;83:548-58. doi: 10.1016/j.biopha.2016.07.011

39. Priya RS, Geetha D, Ramesh PS. Antioxidant activity of chemically synthesized AgNPs and biosynthesized Pongamia pinnata leaf extract mediated AgNPs - A comparative study. *Ecotoxicol Environ Saf* 2016;134(Pt 2):308-18. doi: 10.1016/j.ecoenv.2015.07.037

40. Gopinath K, Kumaraguru S, Bhakyaraj K, Mohan S, Venkatesh KS, Esakkirajan M, et al. Green synthesis of silver, gold and silver/gold bimetallic nanoparticles using the Gloriosa superba leaf extract and their antibacterial and antibiofilm activities. *Microb Pathog* 2016;101:1-11. doi: 10.1016/j.micpath.2016.10.011

41. Vinopal S, Runal T, Kotrba P. Biosorption of Cd2+ and Zn2+ by cell surface-engineered Saccharomyces cerevisiae. *Int Biodeterior Biodegradation* 2007;60(2):96-102. doi: 10.1016/j.ibiod.2006.12.007

42. Kumar P, Malik HK, Ghosh A, Thangavel R, Asokan K. Bandgap tuning in highly c-axis oriented $Zn_{1-x}Mg_xO$ thin films. *J Appl Physics Let* 2013;102(22):221903-8. doi: 10.1063/1.4809575

43. Rodriguez-Gonzalez C, Velazquez-Villalba P, Salas P, Castano VM. Green synthesis of nanosilver-decorated graphene oxide sheets. *IET Nanobiotechnol* 2016;10(5):301-7. doi: 10.1049/iet-nbt.2015.0043

44. Syed B, Nagendra Prasad MN, Dhananjaya BL, Mohan Kumar K, Yallappa S, Satish S. Synthesis of silver nanoparticles by endosymbiont pseudomonas fluorescens CA 417 and their bactericidal activity. *Enzyme Microb Technol* 2016;95:128-36. doi: 10.1016/j.enzmictec.2016.10.004

45. Fouad H, Hongjie L, Yanmei D, Baoting Y, El-Shakh A, Abbas G, et al. Synthesis and characterization of silver nanoparticles using bacillus amyloliquefaciens and Bacillus subtilis to control filarial vector Culex pipiens pallens and its antimicrobial activity. *Artif Cells Nanomed Biotechnol* 2017;45(7):1369-78. doi: 10.1080/21691401.2016.1241793

46. Skladanowski M, Golinska P, Rudnicka K, Dahm H, Rai M. Evaluation of cytotoxicity, immune compatibility and antibacterial activity of biogenic silver nanoparticles. *Med Microbiol Immunol* 2016;205(6):603-13. doi: 10.1007/s00430-016-0477-7

19

Investigation of Effective Parameters on Size of Paclitaxel Loaded PLGA Nanoparticles

Fatemeh Madani[1,2], Seyedeh Sara Esnaashari[1], Basil Mujokoro[3], Farid Dorkoosh[4], Masood Khosravani[1]*, Mahdi Adabi[1]*

[1] Department of Medical Nanotechnology, School of Advanced Technologies in Medicine, Tehran University of Medical Sciences, Tehran, Iran.

[2] Student's Scientific Research Center, Tehran University of Medical Sciences, Tehran, Iran.

[3] Department of Medical Nanotechnology, School of Advanced Technologies in Medicine, International Campus, Tehran University of Medical Sciences, Tehran, Iran.

[4] Department of Pharmaceutics, Faculty of Pharmacy, Tehran University of Medical Sciences, Tehran, Iran.

Keywords:
- PLGA
- Paclitaxel
- Nanoparticle
- Size

Abstract

Purpose: The size of polymeric nanoparticles is considered as an effective factor in cancer therapy due to enterance into tumor tissue via the EPR effect. The purpose of this work was to investigate the effective parameters on poly(lactic-co-glycolic acid)-paclitaxel (PLGA – PTX) nanoparticles size.

Methods: We prepared PLGA-PTX nanoparticles via single emulsion and precipitation methods with variable paremeters including drug concentration, aqueous to organic phase volume ratio, polymer concentration, sonication time and PVA concentration.

Results: PLGA-PTX nanoparticles were characterized by dynamic light scattering (DLS) and scanning electron microscopy (SEM). The results exhibited that the diameter of nanoparticles enhanced with increasing drug, polymer and PVA concentrations whereas organic to aqueous phase volume ratio and sonication time required to the optimization for a given size.

Conclusion: The precipitation method provides smaller nanoparticles compared to emulsion one. Variable parameters including drug concentration, aqueous to organic phase volume ratio, polymer concentration, sonication time and PVA concentration affect diameter of nanoparticles.

Introduction

Cancer is a major global cause of morbidity and mortality which is estimated that the incidence of all new cancer cases will reach 22 million by 2030 in worldwide.[1] Chemotherapy is a versatile cancer treatment modality due to its application as first line,[2,3] adjuvant[4] and/or palliative therapy[5] in the fight against different cancers. In addition, chemotherapy is easier to administer and less invasive compared to other clinical cancer treatment modalities such as surgical removal and radiotherapy. Unfortunately, since the efficacy of most chemotherapeutic drugs is dose dependent, severe chemo-induced side events have been observed at higher doses.[6-8] Thus targeted delivery of drugs with minimum non-specific exposure is essential for successful chemotherapy. Tumor targeting chemotherapy can be accomplished by exploiting the diseases' pathophysiology such as unique or overexpressed molecules[9] and leaky tumor vasculature.[10]

Therapeutics can be passively targeted to the hyper-permeable tumor vasculature commonly observed on most cancers. Moreover, the absence of lymphatic drainage in tumors leads to retention of accumulated therapeutic agents within the tumor tissue.[11,12] This unusual extravasation, accumulation and retention of expediently sized therapeutic molecules within tumor tissue is called enhanced permeability and retention (EPR) effect.[13] In addition, nano-sized drug carriers can simultaneously deliver higher amounts of drugs with lower unspecific toxicity, without loss in therapeutic activity. Examples of these biocompatible nano-scale drug carriers include solid lipid nanoparticles (SLN),[14] liposomes,[15] micelles,[16] nanobubbles[17] and polymers.[18,19] Among these, an extensively studied family of materials in the fabrication of biocompatible nanostructures is polymers.[20,21] Polymeric nanostructures possesses several advantages such as simple synthesis techniques, ability to carry a wide payload of therapeutic agents and biodegradability.[22] A wide range of synthetic and natural polymers have been investigated for a variety of biomedical applications such as tissue engineering,[23,24]

*Corresponding authors: Masood Khosravani and Mahdi Adabi, Email: drkhosravani@tums.ac.ir, madabi@tums.ac.ir

bioimaging[25] biosensors[26-28] and drug delivery.[29,30] Synthetic polymers, notably, PLGA and its co-monomer PLA are widely used in the synthesis of nano-sized drug delivery systems. Flexible synthesis techniques enable the tailoring of nanoparticle properties such as size,[31] drug loading[32] and in-vivo drug release.[33]

Among a legion of anti-cancer drugs, paclitaxel is a potent chemo-agent used in the treatment of several solid tumors including ovarian cancer, breast cancer, AIDS related kaposi sarcoma and lung cancer. Further investigations on the efficacy of paclitaxel against gastrointestinal cancer,[34] glioblastoma[35] and pancreatic cancer[36] have yielded promising results. However, a major clinical limitation of paclitaxel is the drugs' poor solubility in water. Therefore biocompatible nano-sized colloidal structures offer safer alternative paclitaxel delivery vehicles.[37-40]

Since most synthesis nanoparticle and drug loading techniques are well established, current scientific focus is increasingly being directed towards optimization of various parameters to obtain effective formulations. Therefore, for EPR targeting, it is of great interest to determine the various input parameters which affect the diameter of nanoparticles. Meanwhile, it is also important to be cognizant of the rate limiting size-dependent physiological processes which may affect the intra-tumoral accumulation of nanoparticles. Nanoparticle sizes less than 30 nm are prone to renal filtration[41] whilst sizes larger than 250 nm are ideal candidates for phagocytosis.[42] Therefore, the effective therapeutic window for EPR targeting may be considered between 50 and 200 nm. Thus the aim of this work was investigate the various parameters which affect the diameter of PTX loaded PLGA nanoparticles for effective EPR targeting. PLGA nanoparticles were chosen for this study due the simplicity and flexibility of synthesis techniques such as nanoprecipitation and emulsion/solvent evaporation.[43,44]

Materials and Methods

Paclitaxel was purchased from sigma. PLGA (50:50, MW 30000 g mol^{-1}) was bought from Shenzhen Esun Industrial Co., China. Dichloromethane (DCM) and acetone (99%) supplied by Carol Erba. Polyvinyl alcohol (PVA), fully hydrolized (MW 60000 g mol^{-1}) was obtained from Merck (Germany). All solutions were prepared using deionized water.

Preparation of paclitaxel-loaded nanoparticles by single emulsion

Nanoparticles were prepared by single emulsion (O/W) method. The PVA polymer was dissolved in deionized water as aqueous phase under continuous magnetic stirring at 40 °C for 5 h to obtain a homogenous solution. Different amounts of paclitaxel and PLGA were dissolved in DCM and stirred for 1 h at room temperature. Then the organic phase poured in PVA solution (30 ml) and stirred for 30 min at room temperature. Then emulsion was sonicated using probe sonication (Top Sonics Ltd., Co., Iran) for 4 minute. After evaporation of the organic solvent overnight, the nanoparticles were collected by centrifugation (Eppendorf centrifuge) at 12000 rpm for 20 min at room temperature and washed twice with deionized water.

Preparation of paclitaxel-loaded nanoparticles by precipitation

The homogenous solutions of PVA were prepared. Specific amount of PLGA and paclitaxel was dissolved in acetone (5 ml) as the organic phase and stirred for 30 min at room temperature. Next, organic phase was added to the 20 ml of PVA solution while stirring. Afterward, organic phase was evaporated overnight and nanoparticles were collected by centrifugation at 12000 rpm for 20 min at room temperature and washed twice with deionized water.

Characterization of nanoparticles

Scanning Electron Microscopy (SEM)

The morphology and diameter of nanoparticles were carried out using SEM as an accelerating voltage of 20.0 kv (Philips XL-30) after sputtering with gold. The diameter of nanoparticles was measured by randomly choosing 30 nanoparticles by SemAfore (4.01 demo, JEOI., Finland) software as shown in Figure 1a.

Dynamic light scattering (DLS)

The hydrodynamic diameter and the median nanoparticles size were obtained using DLS (Scatter Scope) as shown in Figure 1b.

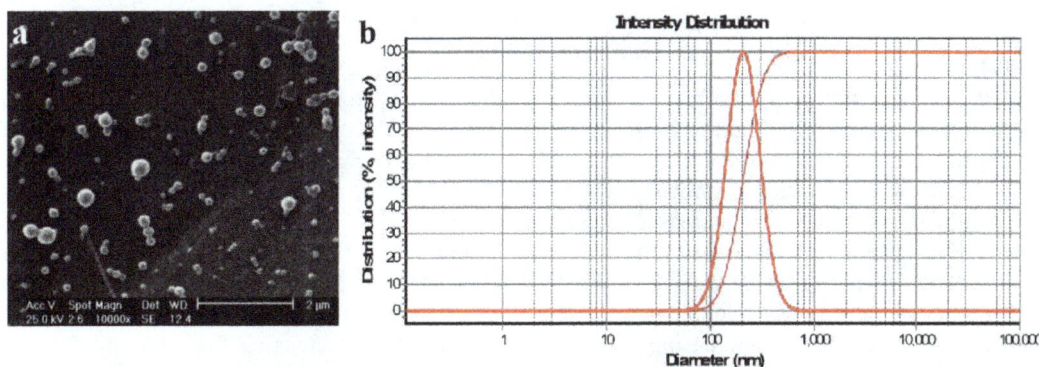

Figure 1. a) SEM image of PLGA-PTX nanoparticles **b)** DLS result of PLGA-PTX nanoparticles.

Results and Discussion
Comparison of two methods single emulsion and precipitation

Table 1 and 2 summarizes experiments conducted in this study to investigate drug and PLGA concentrations, the amounts of PVA and solvent and sonication time which affect PLGA nanoparticles size and morphology. Emulsion solvent evaporation and nanoprecipitation/interfacial deposition are the two most common methods for the preparation of polymeric nanoparticles. These two techniques were originally developed by Vanderhoff et al[45] and Fessi et al,[46] respectively. In an study PLGA incorporated with procaine nanoparticles was prepared via nanoprecipitaion technique with the size less than 210 nm.[32] In another study protein encapsulated in PLGA nanoparticles were prepared by phase separation method with the size

around 300 nm for biomedical application.[47] Commercial success of the various polymeric nanoformulation products developed by emulsion and nanoprecipitation were documented by Nava-Arzaluz et al[48] and Minost et al.[49] We investigated the effect of two methods of single emulsion and precipitation on nanoparticles size. The size of polymeric nanoparticles is particularly important in cancer therapy as drug delivery vehicles can enter into the tumor tissue via the EPR effect. Our results indicated that paclitaxel-loaded nanoparticles prepared with precipitation had smaller size (Table 2. No. 11) compare to single emulsion method (Table 1, No. 19). In addition, acetone is used in precipitation method which have less toxic effect than DCM applied in emulsion method.[50] Therefore, precipitation method is suggested for medical applications.

Table 1. Applied parameters for preparation of paclitaxel loaded PLGA nanoparticles using single emulsion

Number	PLGA (mg)	Solvent (ml)	Drug (mg)	PVA (W/V %)	Sonication time (min)	Mean Size (nm)
1	20	3	1	1%	4	250 ± 12
2	20	3	1.5	1%	4	270 ± 22
3	20	3	3	1%	4	353 ± 24
4	20	3	4.5	1%	4	371 ± 39
5	20	3	6	1%	4	402 ± 9
6	60	3	3	1%	2	548 ± 10
7	60	3	3	1%	4	303 ± 15
8	60	3	3	1%	5	546 ± 17
9	60	3	3	1%	6	598 ± 20
10	10	3	1.5	1%	4	250 ± 15
11	30	3	1.5	1%	4	327 ± 17
12	40	3	1.5	1%	4	354 ± 12
13	50	3	1.5	1%	4	381 ± 18
14	60	3	1.5	1%	4	414 ± 21
15	30	1	1	1%	4	478 ± 10
16	30	2	1	1%	4	381 ± 12
17	30	3	1	1%	4	300 ± 18
18	30	4	1	1%	4	412 ± 21
19	30	5	1	1%	4	469 ± 14
20	30	6	1	1%	4	491 ± 11

The effect of PVA
The function of PVA concentration as an effective factor on PLGA diameter is shown in Figure 2. In this experiment the applied concentrations of PVA were 0.25, 0.5, 1 and 2 W/V % whereas other parameters were constant. The nanoparticles diameter increased from about 130 nm to 378 nm (Table 2, Nos. 6-9) as the PVA concentration increased from 0.25 to 2 W/V%. It was observed that the size of the nanoparticles enhances in the precipitation method with increasing PVA concentration which can be associated with the deposition of PVA on the surface of paclitaxel-loaded

nanoparticles. An increase in nanoparticle size has also been reported as the concentration of PVA enhanced.[51]

The effect of drug concentration
The effect of the amount of drug was also examined on nanoparticles diameter. In this study the different amounts of drug were used whilst other parameters were constant by both emulsion (Table 1, Nos. 1-5) and precipitation (Table 2, Nos. 1-5) methods. As shown in Figure 3, by increasing the amount of drug from 1 to 6 mg, the nanoparticles diameter enhanced from 250 nm to 402 nm and from 210 nm to 342 nm using emulsion and

precipitation methods, respectively. This increase may be because of the more content of drug available in the emulsion droplets or adsorption of drug on surface of nanoparticles in single emulsion method. In addition, increase in the amount of paclitaxel leads to larger size of nanoparticles because more solid content form after evaporation in precipitation method. The literature also confirms that increase in content of drug results in larger size of nanoparticles.[52,53] Although some reports presented lack of relationship between size of nanoparticles and drug concentration.[50,54]

Table 2. Applied parameters for preparation of paclitaxel loaded PLGA nanoparticles using precipitation method

Number	PLGA (mg)	Solvent (ml)	Drug (mg)	PVA (W/V %)	Mean Size (nm)
1	20	5	1	1%	210 ± 17
2	20	5	1.5	1%	235 ± 10
3	20	5	3	1%	271 ± 16
4	20	5	4.5	1%	310 ± 32
5	20	5	6	1%	342 ± 9
6	20	5	1	0.25%	130 ± 70
7	20	5	1	0.5%	192 ± 21
8	20	5	1	1.5%	271 ± 16
9	20	5	1	2%	378 ± 29
10	10	5	1.5	1%	217 ± 14
11	30	5	1.5	1%	251 ± 12
12	40	5	1.5	1%	267 ± 21
13	50	5	1.5	1%	289 ± 18
14	60	5	1.5	1%	324 ± 17

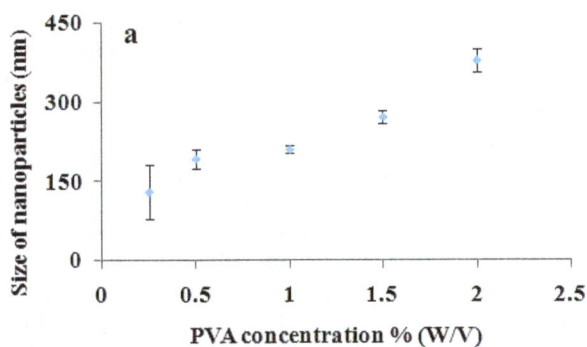

experiment, for nanoparticles prepared by emulsion method, probe sonicator was used for 2, 4, 5 and 6 min (Table 1, Nos. 6-9) and the trend of applied sonication time on mean nanoparticles size was investigated. As shown in Figure 4, the nanoparticles size decreased from 548 to 303 nm when applied sonication time increased from 2 to 4 min. It can be attributed to the high released energy in emulsification process, resulting in the formation of smaller droplets which affect the size of polymeric nanoparticles. In addition, by increasing sonication time from 4 to 6 min, the nanoparticles size increased from 303 to 598 nm. This increase may be because of de-emulsification process[56] or agglomeration.[57] In a study, size of drug loaded PLGA nanoparticles was optimized by varing sonication time.[58] Therefore, sonication time can be considered as a parameter for optimized size of nanoparticles.

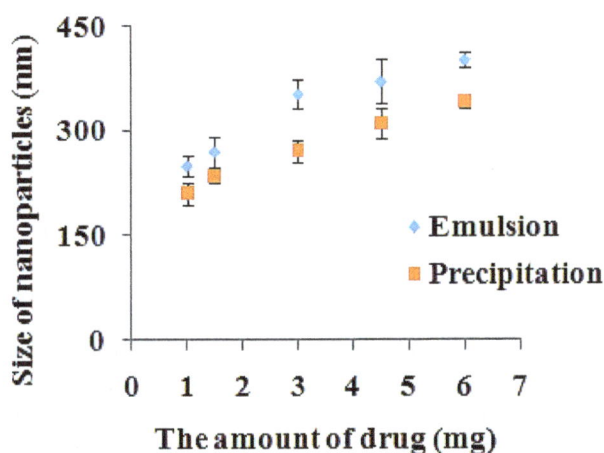

Figure 3. The effect of drug concentration on nanoparticles size by single emulsion and precipitation method.

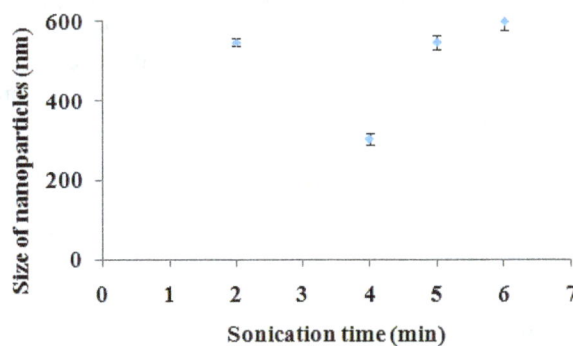

Figure 2. The effect of PVA concentration on nanoparticles size.

Figure 4. The effect of sonication time on nanoparticles size.

The effect of sonication time on nanoparticles size

Polymeric nanoparticles can be synthesized via two approaches; "bottom up" or "top down". In "bottom up", the nanoparticles are formed from continuous deposition of molecular growth species on a nanoparticle nuclei, that is, polymer aggregation. In "Top down" synthesis, external energy sources are used to break down colloidal polymer complex structures into nanoemulsions. A commonly applied technique in the "top down" synthesis is the use of ultra-sound homogenization.[55] In this

The effect of polymer concentration

In this experiment, by increasing the PLGA concentration from 10 to 60 mg, the mean size of nanoparticles enhanced from about 250 to 414 nm (Table 1, Nos. 2, 10-14) and from about 217 to 324 nm (Table 2, Nos. 2, 10-14) in emulsion and precipitation methods, respectively (Figure 5). In both techniques, it was observed that the size of the nanoparticles has a direct relationship with the PLGA concentration. In single emulsion method, this might be attributed to the increase in viscosity of dispersed phase, resulting in a reduction of the net shear stress and prompting bigger nanodroplets. Besides, PLGA solution cannot be rapidly dispersed into the aqueous phase as the viscosity increases and result in larger nanoparticles.[59,60] In precipitation method, frequency of collisions increase which leads to fusion of nanoparticles as concentration of polymer enhances.[61]

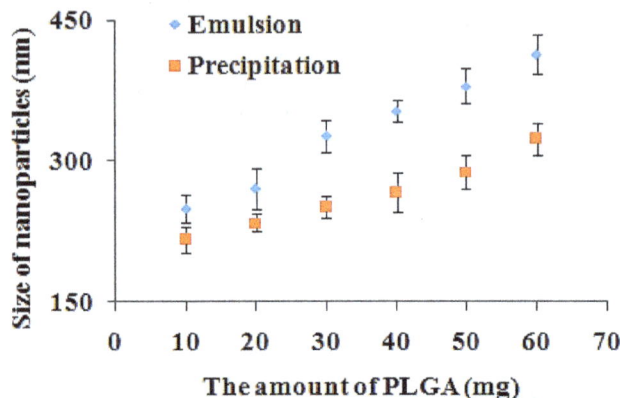

Figure 5. The effect of PLGA concentration on nanoparticles size prepared by single emulsion and precipitation method.

The effect of organic to aqueous phase volume ratio

In our experiments, the nanoparticles size demonstrated an initial decrease from 478 nm to 300 nm as the amount of the organic phase enhanced from 1 to 3 ml (as shown in Figure 6 and Table 1, Nos. 15-17). The reason why the nanoparticles size decreased from 478 nm to 300 may be attributed to viscosity of organic phase. Increasing organic phase results in decrease in concentration of polymer and consequently decreases in size. However, by further increasing the amount of the organic phase from 3 to 6 ml, the particle size enhanced from 300 nm to 491 nm (Table 1, Nos. 17-20). This may be because of an enhanced time for the evaporation of the organic phase. In other words, a higher amount of solvent may cause ostwald ripening of the nanoemulsions before solvent evaporation of organic phase.

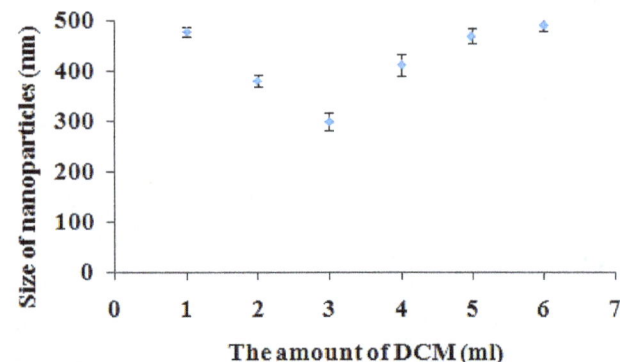

Figure 6. The effect of aqueous to organic phase volume ratio on nanoparticles size.

Conclusion

This study compared two methods for preparation of paclitaxel loaded PLGA nanoparticles including single emulsion and precipitation. The results indicated that precipitation method results in smaller nanoparticles compared to emulsion one. In addition, the effect of the various parameters on the size of the nanoparticles was investigated The results demonstrated that the concentration of the PLGA polymer, drug and PVA had a direct relationship with the size of nanoparticles whereas sonication time and organic phase to aqueous volume ratio needed to the optimization to obtain the nanoparticles with smaller sizes.

Acknowledgments
This work was supported by Tehran University of Medical Sciences, Grant No. 96-01-87-34138.

Ethical Issues
Not applicable.

Conflict of Interest
The authors declare no conflict of interests.

References
1. Bray F, Jemal A, Grey N, Ferlay J, Forman D. Global cancer transitions according to the human development index (2008-2030): A population-based study. *Lancet Oncol* 2012;13(8):790-801. doi: 10.1016/S1470-2045(12)70211-5
2. Goffin J, Lacchetti C, Ellis PM, Ung YC, Evans WK. First-line systemic chemotherapy in the treatment of advanced non-small cell lung cancer: A systematic review. *J Thorac Oncol* 2010;5(2):260-74. doi: 10.1097/JTO.0b013e3181c6f035
3. Mujokoro B, Adabi M, Sadroddiny E, Adabi M, Khosravani M. Nano-structures mediated co-delivery of therapeutic agents for glioblastoma treatment: A review. *Mater Sci Eng C Mater Biol Appl* 2016;69:1092-102. doi: 10.1016/j.msec.2016.07.080
4. Anampa J, Makower D, Sparano JA. Progress in adjuvant chemotherapy for breast cancer: An overview. *BMC Med* 2015;13:195. doi: 10.1186/s12916-015-0439-8
5. Tassinari D, Fochessati F, Arcangeli V, Sartori S, Agostini V, Fantini M, et al. Carboplatin and gemcitabine in the palliative treatment of stage iv non-small cell lung cancer: Definitive results of a phase ii trial. *Tumori* 2004;90(1):54-9.
6. Quasthoff S, Hartung HP. Chemotherapy-induced peripheral neuropathy. *J Neurol* 2002;249(1):9-17.
7. Monsuez JJ, Charniot JC, Vignat N, Artigou JY. Cardiac side-effects of cancer chemotherapy. *Int J Cardiol* 2010;144(1):3-15. doi: 10.1016/j.ijcard.2010.03.003
8. Partridge AH, Burstein HJ, Winer EP. Side effects of chemotherapy and combined chemohormonal therapy in women with early-stage breast cancer. *J Natl Cancer Inst Monogr* 2001;(30):135-42.
9. Kue CS, Kamkaew A, Burgess K, Kiew LV, Chung LY, Lee HB. Small molecules for active targeting in

cancer. *Med Res Rev* 2016;36(3):494-575. doi: 10.1002/med.21387

10. Matsumura Y, Kimura M, Yamamoto T, Maeda H. Involvement of the kinin-generating cascade in enhanced vascular permeability in tumor tissue. *Jpn J Cancer Res* 1988;79(12):1327-34.

11. Maeda H, Nakamura H, Fang J. The EPR effect for macromolecular drug delivery to solid tumors: Improvement of tumor uptake, lowering of systemic toxicity, and distinct tumor imaging in vivo. *Adv Drug Deliv Rev* 2013;65(1):71-9. doi: 10.1016/j.addr.2012.10.002

12. Greish K. Enhanced permeability and retention (EPR) effect for anticancer nanomedicine drug targeting. *Methods Mol Biol* 2010;624:25-37. doi: 10.1007/978-1-60761-609-2_3

13. Maeda H. Macromolecular therapeutics in cancer treatment: The EPR effect and beyond. *J Control Release* 2012;164(2):138-44. doi: 10.1016/j.jconrel.2012.04.038

14. Martins S, Tho I, Reimold I, Fricker G, Souto E, Ferreira D, et al. Brain delivery of camptothecin by means of solid lipid nanoparticles: Formulation design, in vitro and in vivo studies. *Int J pharm* 2012;439(1-2):49-62. doi: 10.1016/j.ijpharm.2012.09.054

15. Xiang Y, Liang L, Wang X, Wang J, Zhang X, Zhang Q. Chloride channel-mediated brain glioma targeting of chlorotoxin-modified doxorubicine-loaded liposomes. *J Control Release* 2011;152(3):402-10. doi: 10.1016/j.jconrel.2011.03.014

16. Kataoka K, Harada A, Nagasaki Y. Block copolymer micelles for drug delivery: Design, characterization and biological significance. *Adv Drug Deliv Rev* 2001;47(1):113-31.

17. Ayodele AT, Valizadeh A, Adabi M, Esnaashari SS, Madani F, Khosravani M, et al. Ultrasound nanobubbles and their applications as theranostic agents in cancer therapy: A review. *Biointerface Res Appl Chem* 2017;7(6):2253-62.

18. Shah M, Naseer MI, Choi MH, Kim MO, Yoon SC. Amphiphilic pha-mpeg copolymeric nanocontainers for drug delivery: Preparation, characterization and in vitro evaluation. *Int J Pharm* 2010;400(1-2):165-75. doi: 10.1016/j.ijpharm.2010.08.008

19. Maleki H, Dorkoosh F, Adabi M, Khosravani M, Arzani H, Kamali M. Methotrexate-loaded plga nanoparticles: Preparation, characterization and their cytotoxicity effect on human glioblastoma U87MG cells. *Int J Med Nano Res* 2017;4(1):020. doi:10.23937/2378-3664/1410020

20. Murthy SK. Nanoparticles in modern medicine: State of the art and future challenges. *Int J Nanomedicine* 2007;2(2):129-41.

21. Salata O. Applications of nanoparticles in biology and medicine. *J Nanobiotechnology* 2004;2(1):3. doi: 10.1186/1477-3155-2-3

22. Kumari A, Yadav SK, Yadav SC. Biodegradable polymeric nanoparticles based drug delivery systems. *Colloids Surf B Biointerfaces* 2010;75(1):1-18. doi: 10.1016/j.colsurfb.2009.09.001

23. Sell SA, Wolfe PS, Garg K, McCool JM, Rodriguez IA, Bowlin GL. The use of natural polymers in tissue engineering: A focus on electrospun extracellular matrix analogues. *Polymers* 2010;2(4):522-53. doi: 10.3390/polym2040522

24. Hosseinzadeh S, Mahmoudifard M, Mohamadyar-Toupkanlou F, Dodel M, Hajarizadeh A, Adabi M, et al. The nanofibrous pan-pani scaffold as an efficient substrate for skeletal muscle differentiation using satellite cells. *Bioprocess Biosyst Eng* 2016;39(7):1163-72. doi: 10.1007/s00449-016-1592-y

25. Kim JH, Park K, Nam HY, Lee S, Kim K, Kwon IC. Polymers for bioimaging. *Prog Polym Sci* 2007;32(8-9):1031-53. doi: 10.1016/j.progpolymsci.2007.05.016

26. Adabi M, Saber R, Faridi-Majidi R, Faridbod F. Performance of electrodes synthesized with polyacrylonitrile-based carbon nanofibers for application in electrochemical sensors and biosensors. *Mater Sci Eng C Mater Biol Appl* 2015;48:673-8. doi: 10.1016/j.msec.2014.12.051

27. Adabi M, Saber R, Naghibzadeh M, Faridbod F, Faridi-Majidi R. Parameters affecting carbon nanofiber electrodes for measurement of cathodic current in electrochemical sensors: An investigation using artificial neural network. *RSC Adv* 2015;5(99):81243-52. doi: 10.1039/C5RA15541J

28. Samadian H, Zakariaee SS, Adabi M, Mobasheri H, Azami M, Faridi-Majidi R. Effective parameters on conductivity of mineralized carbon nanofibers: An investigation using artificial neural networks. *RSC Adv* 2016;6(113):111908-18. doi: 10.1039/C6RA21596C

29. Pillai O, Panchagnula R. Polymers in drug delivery. *Curr Opin Chem Biol* 2001;5(4):447-51.

30. Kamali M, Dinarvand R, Maleki H, Arzani H, Mahdaviani P, Nekounam H, et al. Preparation of imatinib base loaded human serum albumin for application in the treatment of glioblastoma. *RSC Adv* 2015;5(76):62214-9. doi: 10.1039/C5RA08501B

31. Kulkarni SA, Feng SS. Effects of particle size and surface modification on cellular uptake and biodistribution of polymeric nanoparticles for drug delivery. *Pharm Res* 2013;30(10):2512-22. doi: 10.1007/s11095-012-0958-3

32. Govender T, Stolnik S, Garnett MC, Illum L, Davis SS. PLGA nanoparticles prepared by nanoprecipitation: Drug loading and release studies of a water soluble drug. *J Control Release* 1999;57(2):171-85. doi: 10.1016/S0168-3659(98)00116-3

33. Corrigan OI, Li X. Quantifying drug release from PLGA nanoparticulates. *Eur J Pharm Sci* 2009;37(3-4):477-85. doi: 10.1016/j.ejps.2009.04.004

34. Sakamoto J, Matsui T, Kodera Y. Paclitaxel chemotherapy for the treatment of gastric cancer. *Gastric Cancer* 2009;12(2):69-78. doi: 10.1007/s10120-009-0505-z

35. Terzis AJ, Thorsen F, Heese O, Visted T, Bjerkvig R, Dahl O, et al. Proliferation, migration and invasion of human glioma cells exposed to paclitaxel (taxol) in vitro. *Br J Cancer* 1997;75(12):1744-52. doi: 10.1038/bjc.1997.298

36. Safran H, Moore T, Iannitti D, Dipetrillo T, Akerman P, Cioffi W, et al. Paclitaxel and concurrent radiation for locally advanced pancreatic cancer. *Int J Radiat Oncol Biol Phys* 2001;49(5):1275-9. doi: 10.1016/S0360-3016(00)01527-3

37. Peltier S, Oger JM, Lagarce F, Couet W, Benoit JP. Enhanced oral paclitaxel bioavailability after administration of paclitaxel-loaded lipid nanocapsules. *Pharm Res* 2006;23(6):1243-50. doi: 10.1007/s11095-006-0022-2

38. Lee MK, Lim SJ, Kim CK. Preparation, characterization and in vitro cytotoxicity of paclitaxel-loaded sterically stabilized solid lipid nanoparticles. *Biomaterials* 2007;28(12):2137-46. doi: 10.1016/j.biomaterials.2007.01.014

39. Erdogar N, Esendagli G, Nielsen TT, Sen M, Oner L, Bilensoy E. Design and optimization of novel paclitaxel-loaded folate-conjugated amphiphilic cyclodextrin nanoparticles. *Int J Pharm* 2016;509(1-2):375-90. doi: 10.1016/j.ijpharm.2016.05.040

40. Gupta PN, Jain S, Nehate C, Alam N, Khare V, Dubey RD, et al. Development and evaluation of paclitaxel loaded PLGA:Poloxamer blend nanoparticles for cancer chemotherapy. *Int J Biol Macromol* 2014;69:393-9. doi: 10.1016/j.ijbiomac.2014.05.067

41. Balogh L, Nigavekar SS, Nair BM, Lesniak W, Zhang C, Sung LY, et al. Significant effect of size on the in vivo biodistribution of gold composite nanodevices in mouse tumor models. *Nanomedicine* 2007;3(4):281-96. doi: 10.1016/j.nano.2007.09.001

42. Nicolete R, dos Santos DF, Faccioli LH. The uptake of plga micro or nanoparticles by macrophages provokes distinct in vitro inflammatory response. *Int Immunopharmacol* 2011;11(10):1557-63. doi: 10.1016/j.intimp.2011.05.014

43. Yallapu MM, Gupta BK, Jaggi M, Chauhan SC. Fabrication of curcumin encapsulated plga nanoparticles for improved therapeutic effects in metastatic cancer cells. *J Colloid Interface Sci* 2010;351(1):19-29. doi: 10.1016/j.jcis.2010.05.022

44. Murakami H, Kobayashi M, Takeuchi H, Kawashima Y. Preparation of poly(DL-lactide-co-glycolide) nanoparticles by modified spontaneous emulsification solvent diffusion method. *Int J Pharm* 1999;187(2):143-52. doi: 10.1016/S0378-5173(99)00187-8

45. Vanderhoff JW, El-Aasser MS, Ugelstad J. Polymer emulsification process. Google Patents. 1979.

46. Fessi H, Puisieux F, Devissaguet JP, Ammoury N, Benita S. Nanocapsule formation by interfacial polymer deposition following solvent displacement. *Int J Pharm* 1989;55(1):R1-4. doi: 10.1016/0378-5173(89)90281-0

47. Swed A, Cordonnier T, Fleury F, Boury F. Protein encapsulation into plga nanoparticles by a novel phase separation method using non-toxic solvents. *J Nanomed Nanotechnol* 2014;5(6):241. doi: 10.4172/2157-7439.1000241

48. Nava-Arzaluz MG, Pinon-Segundo E, Ganem-Rondero A, Lechuga-Ballesteros D. Single emulsion-solvent evaporation technique and modifications for the preparation of pharmaceutical polymeric nanoparticles. *Recent Pat Drug Deliv Formul* 2012;6(3):209-23. doi: 10.2174/187221112802652633

49. Minost A, Delaveau J, Bolzinger MA, Fessi H, Elaissari A. Nanoparticles via nanoprecipitation process. *Recent Pat Drug Deliv Formul* 2012;6(3):250-8. doi: 10.2174/187221112802652615

50. Budhian A, Siegel SJ, Winey KI. Haloperidol-loaded plga nanoparticles: Systematic study of particle size and drug content. *Int J Pharm* 2007;336(2):367-75. doi: 10.1016/j.ijpharm.2006.11.061

51. Maaz A, Abdelwahed W, Tekko IA, Trefi S. Influence of nanoprecipitation method parameters on nanoparticles loaded with gatifloxacin for ocular drug delivery. *Int J Acad Sci Res* 2015;3(1):1-12

52. Krishnamachari Y, Madan P, Lin S. Development of pH- and time-dependent oral microparticles to optimize budesonide delivery to ileum and colon. *Int J Pharm* 2007;338(1-2):238-47. doi: 10.1016/j.ijpharm.2007.02.015

53. Snehalatha M, Venugopal K, Saha RN. Etoposide-loaded PLGA and PCL nanoparticles I: Preparation and effect of formulation variables. *Drug Deliv* 2008;15(5):267-75. doi: 10.1080/10717540802174662

54. Derman S. Caffeic acid phenethyl ester loaded PLGA nanoparticles: Effect of various process parameters on reaction yield, encapsulation efficiency, and particle size. *J Nanomater* 2015;2015:341848. doi: 10.1155/2015/341848

55. Sah E, Sah H. Recent trends in preparation of poly(lactide-co-glycolide) nanoparticles by mixing polymeric organic solution with antisolvent. *J Nanomater* 2015;2015:794601. doi: 10.1155/2015/794601

56. Español L, Larrea A, Andreu V, Mendoza G, Arruebo M, Sebastian V, et al. Dual encapsulation of hydrophobic and hydrophilic drugs in PLGA nanoparticles by a single-step method: Drug delivery and cytotoxicity assays. *RSC Adv* 2016;6(112):111060-9. doi: 10.1039/C6RA23620K

57. Tripathi A, Gupta R, Saraf SA. PLGA nanoparticles of anti tubercular drug: Drug loading and release studies of a water in-soluble drug. *Int J Pharm Tech Res* 2010;2(3):2116-23.

58. Dangi R, Shakya S. Preparation, optimization and characterization of PLGA nanoparticle. *Int J Pharm Life Sci* 2013;4(7):2810-8.

59. Song X, Zhao Y, Wu W, Bi Y, Cai Z, Chen Q, et al. PLGA nanoparticles simultaneously loaded with vincristine sulfate and verapamil hydrochloride: Systematic study of particle size and drug entrapment efficiency. *Int J Pharm* 2008;350(1-2):320-9. doi: 10.1016/j.ijpharm.2007.08.034

60. Mainardes RM, Evangelista RC. PLGA nanoparticles containing praziquantel: Effect of formulation variables on size distribution. *Int J Pharm* 2005;290(1-2):137-44. doi: 10.1016/j.ijpharm.2004.11.027

61. Mostafavi SH, Aghajani M, Amani A, Darvishi B, Noori Koopaei M, Pashazadeh AM, et al. Optimization of paclitaxel-loaded poly (d,l-lactide-co-glycolide-n-p-maleimido benzoic hydrazide) nanoparticles size using artificial neural networks. *Pharm Dev Technol* 2015;20(7):845-53. doi: 10.3109/10837450.2014.930487

20

Determination and Quantification of the Vinblastine Content in Purple, Red, and White *Catharanthus Roseus* Leaves Using RP-HPLC Method

Rohanizah Abdul Rahim*[1], Nor Hazwani Ahmad[1], Khaldun Mohammad Al Azzam*[2,3], Ishak Mat[4]

[1] *Advanced Medical & Dental Institute, Universiti Sains Malaysia, 13200 Kepala Batas, Pulau Pinang, Malaysia.*

[2] *Preparatory Year Department, Al-Ghad International Colleges for Applied Medical Sciences, Riyadh, Kingdom of Saudi Arabia.*

[3] *Department of Chemistry, Dalhousie University, Halifax, Nova Scotia, Canada.*

[4] *Unit Kanser MAKNA-USM, Advanced Medical & Dental Institute, Universiti Sains Malaysia, 13200 Kepala Batas, Pulau Pinang, Malaysia.*

Keywords:
· *Catharanthus roseus*
· HPLC
· Alkaloid
· Vinblastine
· Plant

Abstract

Purpose: To determine and quantify vinblastine in different varieties of *Catharanthus roseus* using reversed-phase HPLC method.

Methods: The liquid chromatographic separation was performed using a reversed phase C18, Microsorb - MV column (250 mm x 4.6 mm, 5 µm) at room temperature and eluted with a mobile phase containing methanol – phosphate buffer (5 mM, pH 6.0) – acetonitrile with different proportion gradient elution at a flow rate of 2.0 mL min^{-1} and detection at 254 nm.

Results: The HPLC method was utilized for the quantification of vinblastine in purple, red and white varieties of *Catharanthus roseus* leaves. The separation was achieved in less than 8 min. The peak confirmation was done based on the retention times and UV spectra of the reference substance. The method was validated with respect to linearity, precision, recovery, limit of detection and quantification. Results showed that the purple variety gives 1.2 and 1.5 times more vinblastine concentration compared to the white and pink varieties, respectively.

Conclusion: The obtained results from different varieties are thus useful for the purpose of vinblastine production from *Catharanthus roseus* plant.

Introduction

Catharanthus roseus, commonly known as Madagascar periwinkle which belongs to the Apocynaceae family. It grows naturally as a wild flower throughout Africa, America, Australia, Asia, Southern Europe and on some islands in the Pacific Ocean. The *Catharanthus roseus* is widely studied and used as plant due to its pharmaceutical value that comes from its diversity of useful terpenoid indole alkaloids. The most valuable bisindole alkaloids are vincristine and vinblastine due to their antineoplastic activity in the treatment of many types of cancers.[1]

The difference in color of its flowers indicates the varieties of the plants along with its different biological characteristics.[2] Aqueous extracts of *Catharanthus roseus* have also been used in traditional medicine for preventing some diseases such as bleeding problems, diabetes, fever, malaria, stomach problems, heart disease and cancer.[3]

The most two important alkaloids present in *Catharanthus roseus* as antitumor compounds are vinblastine (Figure 1) and vincristine which are a derivative of dimerization of vindoline and catharanthine in the vacuole of *Catharanthus roseus* leaves and stem cells.[4]

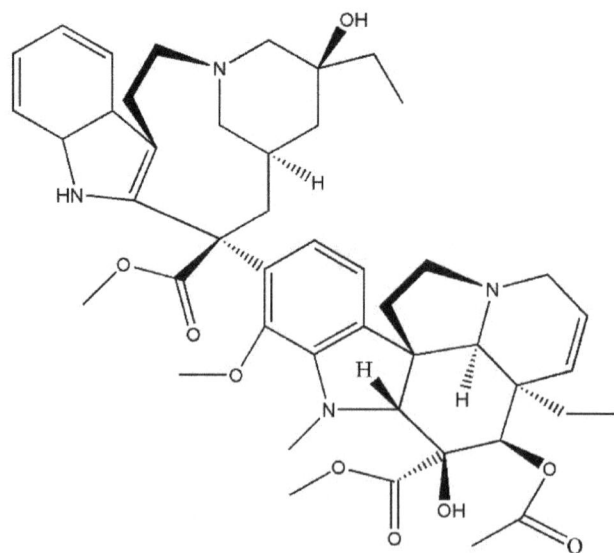

Figure 1. Chemical structure of vinblastine .

The conventional methods for extracting traditional herbal medicine products include soxhlet extraction,

Corresponding authors: Rohanizah Abdul Rahim, Email: rohanizah@usm.my; Khaldun Mohammad Al Azzam; Email: azzamkha@yahoo.com

ultrasonication and reflux. These extraction methods have some drawbacks such as the prolonged preparation time and low efficiency.[5]

Several studies have been conducted to identify these alkaloids using various methods such as high performance liquid chromatography (HPLC) either equipped with ultraviolet (UV)[6] or photodiode array (PDA) detector,[7,8] thin layer chromatography (TLC),[9] and capillary electrophoresis.[10]

To the best of our knowledge, there is no study reported on the vinblastine quantification in *Catharanthus roseus* with different varieties. In the present study, we investigated and compared the vinblastine content in the leaves from three wild local varieties of *Catharanthus roseus* which have purple, pink and white flowers. A simple and fast HPLC method was also developed and validated for the separation and determination of vinblastine in the aqueous extract.

Materials and Methods
Chemicals and reagents
All chemicals and solvents used were of analytical and chromatographic grade, respectively. Nanopure water (resistivity, 18.2 M Ω cm^{-1}) (Mili-Q18 Barnstead Sterling Ascent, USA) was used for the preparation of samples. Disodium hydrogen orthophosphate dihydrate, orthophosphoric acid (85%), HPLC grade of acetonitrile and methanol were purchased from Fisher Scientific (Darmstadt, Germany). Standard of vinblastine (99%) was purchased from Tocris (Northpoint Fourth Way, UK).

Preparation of standard solutions
Vinblastine stock solution was prepared at 100 µg mL^{-1} concentration by dissolving the vinblastine standard in the purified water in a universal bottle and stored at -20 °C. Standard of working solutions were prepared by diluting the stock solution in purified water at 56, 52, 48, 44, 40 and 32 µg mL^{-1} concentrations and filtered through 0.2 µm membrane cellulose filters (Advantec, Japan) for further analysis.

Samples
Green leaves of *Catharanthus roseus* of purple, pink and white flower were obtained from Melaka, Malaysia.

Extraction procedure
The leaves were dried using conventional oven (Sharp, Malaysia) at 40 °C for four days. 10 g of the dried leaves were placed in 200 mL water at 40 °C for 24 h in a covered container and placed in the shaker water bath (Memmert, Germany) to obtain the extracts. Once the dried leaves have been disintegrated, the extracts were then centrifuged at 3600 rpm for 30 min in order to yield the supernatants. The supernatants were then freeze dried in order to obtain the powder which was later kept in a refrigerator at -30°C (Sanyo, Japan) for further analysis. The procedure is summarized in Figure 2.

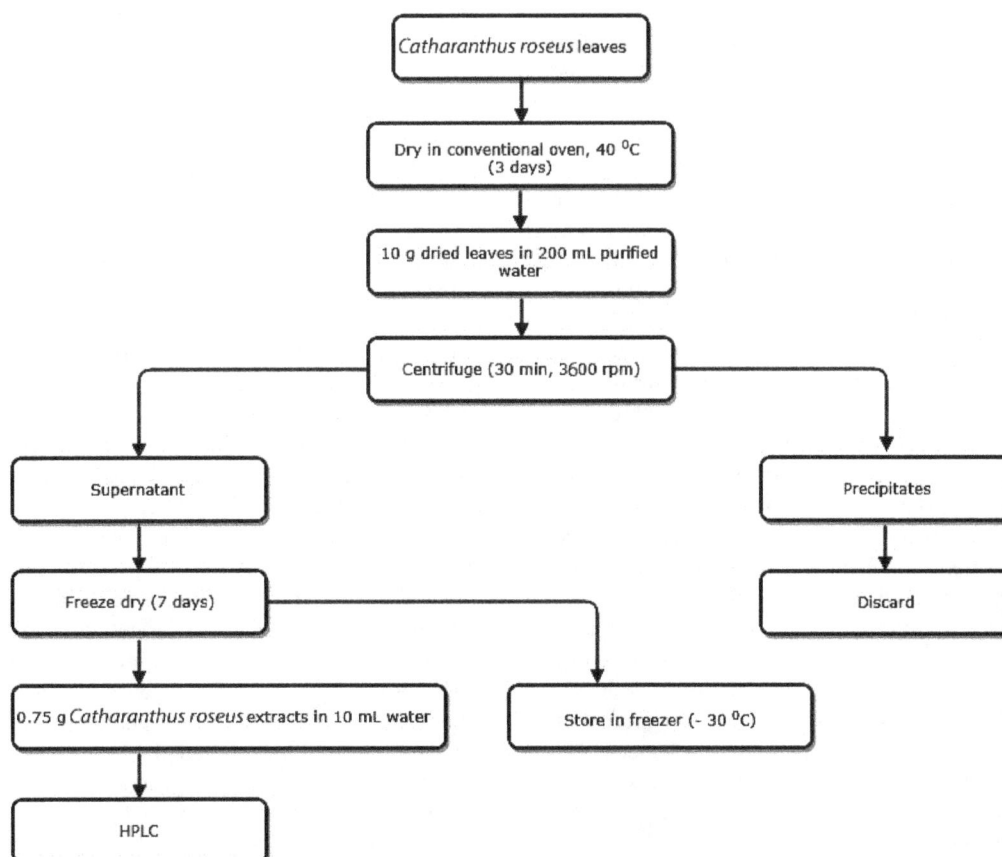

Figure 2. Schematic diagram for the extraction procedure of vinblastine from *Catharanthus roseus* plant.

HPLC analysis and chromatographic conditions
Preparation of samples
1 g of aqueous extract was dissolved in 10 mL purified water and filtered through 0.2 μm membrane filters to obtain the sample stock solution and then, diluted to the 75 mg mL^{-1} for HPLC analysis.

Identification and quantification of vinblastine in the leaf samples
HPLC System (Varians, USA) equipped with a Pro Star solvent delivery system (model 240), photodiode array detector (PDA) (model 335), rheodyne injector with a 20 μL sample loop (model 410) and the Galaxie LS WS software was used. The separation was achieved by using

Microsorb-MV C18 reversed phase column (150 mm x 4.6 mm lengths, 5 μm) at room temperature. A gradient mode with the following solvent systems that is A (methanol), B (5 mM phosphate buffer) and C (acetonitrile) was used. The buffer was filtered using nylon 0.2 μm membrane filter (Magna, China) and all solvents were degassed in a sonicator (Power Sonic 405, Korea) for 15 min prior to use. The flow rate was set at 2.0 mL min^{-1}. The elution profile starting from 25% A, 40% B, 35% C for 0 min; 35% A, 3% B, 30% C for 5 min; 30% A, 35% B, 35% C at 10 min and 30% A, 35% B, 35% at 15 min. Then the system was allowed to stabilize for 5 min under the initial conditions. The UV detection was conducted at 254 nm instead of 220 nm because it provides a better baseline (Figure 3(A & B)).

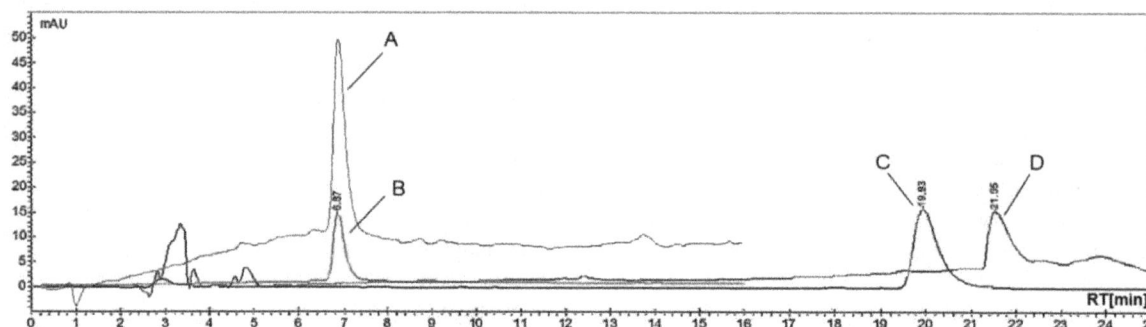

Figure 3. Typical HPLC chromatograms of vinblastine standard at (40 μg mL^{-1}). A) 220 nm B) 254 nm using isocratic elution (acetonitrile and phosphate buffer); C) Gradient elution (methanol, acetonitrile and ammonium acetate buffer); D) Gradient elution (acetonitrile and phosphate buffer).

Results and Discussion
Experimental data were analyzed using *t*-test (SPSS Version 13.0, USA). Throughout the analysis, F-values ($P < 0.05$) were considered significant.

Sample preparation
The leaves were dried before the extraction procedure to ensure the total removal of water from the leaves. The percentage of water in purple, pink and white were 75.8, 85.5 and 85.6%, respectively. The dried leaves were ground until homogenous to ensure that it can improve the kinetic of the analytes in the extraction process.[5] The extraction method as described by Ferreres *et al.*[3] and Tickhomiroff and Jolicoeur[11] was chosen as it involved the same matrix plant. Slight modification was done to the previous method where in the present study, we used temperature at 40°C and non-toxic solvent (water) instead of boiling water and toxic alcoholic solvent (methanol).[3] In this study, aqueous extracts is preferable and more importantly, it is safe to be used as a cure or disease prevention in the field of medicine.
The extraction yield of vinblastine was 88% when they used single methanol extraction.[11] However, aqueous extraction method, allows us to retain higher extracts from the leaves as reported in this study, and this procedure has succeeded to yield about 95 – 103% of vinblastine extracts. The samples were frozen, dried after the extraction procedure in order to reduce the volume of aqueous used without denaturing the alkaloids.[6]

Method optimization and development of HPLC conditions
The HPLC method was optimized using different proportions of mobile phase such as acetonirile, methanol, sodium phosphate and ammonium acetate buffer. A previous study conducted by Singh *et al.*[12] showed that the separation of alkaloid can be achieved using isocratic elution. Therefore, initially the most straight forward isocratic elution conditions have been investigated using acetonitrile - phosphate buffer (pH 6.0; 5 mM) (1:1, v/v) at a flow rate of 2.0 mL min^{-1}. However, the isocratic conditions showed that there was a peak tailing to vinblastine peak.
Other studies done by Tickhomiroff and Jolicoeur[11] used phosphate buffer and Choi *et al.*[13] used ammonium acetate showed that the separation of alkaloids also can be improved by using gradient elution. Therefore, the gradient elution mode was further investigated. The elution process involved the use of A (acetonitrile) and B (5 mM sodium phosphate buffer) at a flow rate of 2.0 mL min^{-1}. The mobile phase started with 20% A at 0 min, 80% A at 20 min, 20% A at 25 min and 80% A at 40 min. It was found that the detection of vinblastine standard takes a longer time, which is around 21.55 min (Figure 3(D)) than in the previous study.[11,13] Therefore, ammonium acetate buffer with acetonitrile has also been tried, but it gave late elution of vinblastine which was around 19.93 min (Figure 3(C)).
The determination and separation of vinblastine were done using gradient elution in three mobile phases consisted of 5 mM sodium phosphate buffer with pH 6.6 and organic solvents of acetonitrile and methanol. Phosphate buffer was used in this analysis to minimize the peak tailing. Results

showed that vinblastine elutes faster, which is around 6.87 min (Figure 3 (B)) compared to the previous methods which are around 15.2 min[11] and 21 min.[13]

Linearity, limit of detection and limit of quantification

Good linear regression ($r^2 > 0.999$) was achieved by injecting triplicate of six concentrations of vinblastine standard (32 - 56 µg mL^{-1}) into the HPLC system.

The limit of detection (LOD) and limit of quantification (LOQ) were calculated based on the formula of Shabir:[14] LOD = 3.3 (SD/S), while LOQ = 10 (SD/S), whereby SD is the standard deviation of response and *S* is the slope in the calibration curve. The value of LOD was 0.0230 µg mL^{-1}, while LOQ 0.0698 µg mL^{-1}.

Precision

Repeatability and reproducibility of the method were determined by injecting six times each of the standard solutions (36, 44 and 52 µg mL^{-1}) on the same day (intra-day) and over six days (inter-day), respectively. The results showed good repeatability of both the peak area (% RSD, 1.11 - 2.37%) and retention times (% RSD, 0.41 - 3.02%) as shown in Table 1. Student *t*-test was done and the results are statistically significant (Table 1).

Table 1. Intra and inter-day precision for the determination of vinblastine.

Amount (µg mL^{-1})	RSD (%) (Area)	RSD (%) (Retention time)
Intra-day precision (n=9)	-	-
36	1.11	0.74
44	2.21	0.41
52	1.19	1.12
Inter-day precision (n = 27)	-	-
36	1.14	1.59
44	1.33	2.22
52	2.37	3.02

Key to abbreviation; RSD: Relative Standard Deviation

Recovery

Recovery studies were carried out by spiking three concentrations (36, 44 and 52 µg mL^{-1}) of vinblastine standard to the samples. The mixtures were extracted and the supernatants were freeze-dried. The obtained aqueous extracts were dissolved in water and injected into the HPLC column. Recovery for each sample was varied from 95 to 103% (CV, 0.5234 - 2.4498%), 95 to 99% (CV, 3.0316 to 4.0754%) and 96 to 101% (RSD, 0.05774 - 0.7069%) for purple, pink and white variety, respectively. The results for recovery are statistically significant as shown in Table 2.

Table 2. Accuracy results for the determination of varieties of *Catharanthus roseus* which have purple, pink and white flowers.

Concentration Level (µg mL^{-1})	% Recovery*		
	(Purple Flower) (Mean ± SD)	(White Flower) (Mean ± SD)	(Pink Flower) (Mean ± SD)
36	103.0 ± 2.71	98.0 ± 2.71	101.0 ± 3.14
44	95.0 ± 1.28	95.0 ± 2.22	98.0 ± 1.28
52	100.0 ± 2.87	99.0 ± 1.08	96.0 ± 1.28

*Indicates mean of six determinations (n=6); SD: Standard deviation.

Analysis of sample

The peak identification of vinblastine was based on the comparison between retention times and UV spectra of vinblastine standard. We further confirmed the identification by spiking standards to the samples. Vinblastine standard was detected at the retention time around 6.80 min at wavelength 254 nm (Figure 3(B)). The method was applied for the determination of vinblastine in the leaves of three local varieties of *Catharanthus roseus*. The highest concentration of vinblastine was found in purple variety with (0.7320 mg in 1 g) (Figure 4(A)) compared to the white variety (0.5890 mg in 1 g) (Figure 4(B)) and pink variety (0.4920 mg in 1 g) (Figure 4(C)).

Our work provides a simple extraction method with a simple and rapid HPLC analytical method using a PDA detector. Moreover, the HPLC method also was proposed because it can be scaled-up to the preparative HPLC in the next study and used to isolate pure compounds for biological assays.

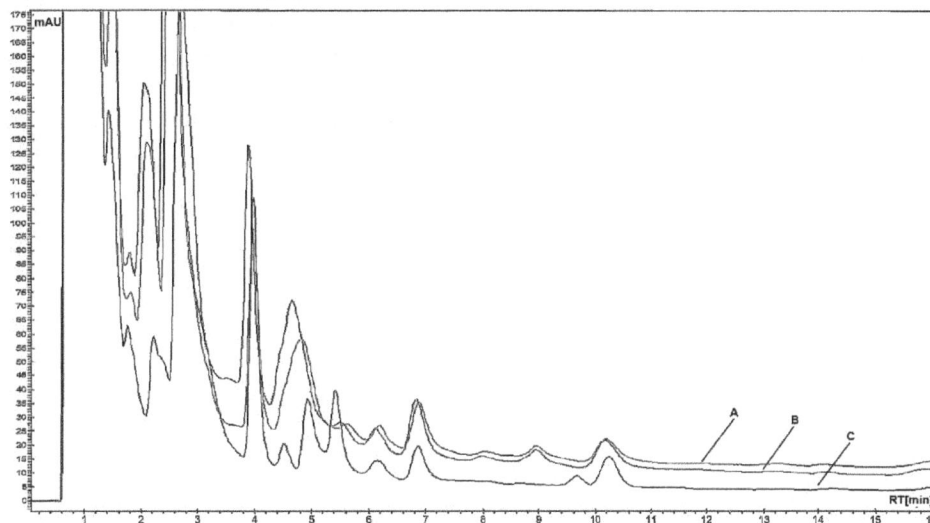

Figure 4. Typical HPLC chromatograms of (A) Purple variety (B) White variety (C) Pink variety.

Conclusion

This study proved the existence of vinblastine in *Catharanthus roseus* leaves using reversed-phase HPLC method. Purple variety has 1.2 times and 1.5 times more vinblastine concentrations as compared to the white variety and pink variety, respectively. A simple extraction procedure had effectively yielded vinblastine after separation in crude *Catharanthus roseus* aqueous extracts.

Acknowledgments

This work has been supported by the Majlis Kanser Nasional (MAKNA).

Ethical Issues

Not applicable

Conflict of Interest

All authors declare that she has no conflict of interest.

References

1. Aslam J, Mujib A, Seikh AN, Maheshwar PS. Screening of vincristine in ex vitro and in vitro somatic embryos derived plantlets of *Catharanthus roseus* L. (G) Don. *Sci Horic* 2009;119(3):325-9. doi: 10.1016/j.scienta.2008.08.018

2. Jaleel CA, Gopi R, Gomathinayagam M, Panneerselvam R. Traditional and non-traditional plant growth regulators alters phytochemical constituents in *Catharanthus roseus*. *Process Biochem* 2009;44(2): 205-9. doi: 10.1016/j.procbio.2008.10.012

3. Ferreres F, Pereira DM, Valentao P, Oliveira JM, Faria J, Gaspar L, et al. Simple and reproducible hplc-dad-esi-ms/ms analysis of alkaloids in catharanthus roseus roots. *J Pharm Biomed Anal* 2010;51(1):65-9. doi: 10.1016/j.jpba.2009.08.005

4. Pan Q, Chen Y, Wang Q, Yuan F, Xing S, Tian Y, et al. Effect of plant growth regulators on the biosynthesis of vinblastine, vindoline and catharanthine in *Catharanthus roseus*. *Plant Growth Regul* 2010; 60(2): 133 - 41. doi: 10.1007/s10725-009-9429-1

5. Ong ES. Extraction methods and chemical standardization of botanicals and herbal preparations. *J Chromatogr B Analyt Technol Biomed Life Sci* 2004;812(1-2):23-33. doi: 10.1016/j.jchromb.2004.07.041

6. Hisiger S, Jolicoeur M. Analysis of *Catharanthus roseus* alkaloids by HPLC. *Phytochem Rev* 2007;6(2-3): 207 - 34. doi: 10.1007/s11101-006-9036-y

7. Aslam J, Mujib A, Fatima Z, Sharma MP. Variations in vinblastine production at different stages of somatic embryogenesis, embryo, and field-grown plantlets of *Catharanthus roseus* L. (G) Don, as revealed by HPLC. *In Vitro Cell Dev Biol Plant* 2010; 46(4):348 - 53. doi: 10.1007/s11627-010-9290-y

8. Uniyal GC, Bala S, Mathur AK, Kulkarni RN. Symmetry c18 column: A better choice for the analysis of indole alkaloids of catharanthus roseus. *Phytochem Anal* 2001;12(3):206-10. doi: 10.1002/pca.575

9. Lourdes Miranda-Ham M, Islas-Flores I, Vazquez-Flota AF. Accumulation of monoterpenoid indole alkaloids in periwinkle seedlings (catharanthus roseus) as a model for the study of plant-environment interactions. *Biochem Mol Biol Educ* 2007;35(3):206-10. doi: 10.1002/bmb.60

10. Stockigt J, Sheludk Y, Unger M, Gerasimenko I, Warzecha H, Stockigt D. High-performance liquid chromatographic, capillary electrophoretic and capillary electrophoretic-electrospray ionisation mass spectrometric analysis of selected alkaloid groups. *J Chromatogr A* 2002;967(1):85-113.

11. Tikhomiroff C, Jolicoeur M. Screening of catharanthus roseus secondary metabolites by high-performance liquid chromatography. *J Chromatogr A* 2002;955(1):87-9

12. Singh DV, Maithy A, Verma RK., Gupta MM, Kumar S. Simultaneous determination of *Catharanthus alkaloids* using reversed phase high performance liquid chromatography. J Liq Chromatogr Relat Technol 2000; 23(4), 601-7. doi:10.1081/JLC-100101476

13. Choi YH, Yoo KP, Kim J. Supercritical fluid extraction and liquid chromatography-electrospray mass analysis of vinblastine from catharanthus roseus. *Chem Pharm Bull (Tokyo)* 2002;50(9):1294-6.

14. Shabir GA. Validation of high-performance liquid chromatography methods for pharmaceutical analysis. Understanding the differences and similarities between validation requirements of the us food and drug administration, the us pharmacopeia and the international conference on harmonization. *J Chromatogr A* 2003;987(1-2):57-66.

21

Porous Microparticles Containing Raloxifene Hydrochloride Tailored by Spray Freeze Drying for Solubility Enhancement

Seyyed Pouya Hadipour Moghaddam[1,2], Sajjad Farhat[3], Alireza Vatanara[3]*

[1] Department of Pharmaceutics and Pharmaceutical Chemistry, School of Pharmacy, University of Utah, Salt Lake City, UT 84112, USA.
[2] Utah Center for Nanomedicine, Nano Institute of Utah, University of Utah, Salt Lake City, UT 84112, USA.
[3] Department of Pharmaceutics, School of Pharmacy, Tehran University of Medical Sciences, Tehran, Iran.

Keywords:
· Dissolution profile
· Porous microparticles
· Raloxifene
· Solubility
· Spray freeze drying

Abstract

Purpose: The goal of this study was to improve the solubility and dissolution behavior of Raloxifene Hydrochloride (RH) using Spray Freeze Drying (SFD) technique.

Methods: For achieving this goal, series of samples containing RH with polyvinylpyrrolidone (PVP) or hydroxypropyl beta cyclodextrin (HPβCD) used as solubility enhancers were prepared and microparticles were formed *via* SFD. The resultant microparticles were physicochemically characterized. Morphology of the microparticles were observed using Scanning Electron Microscopy (SEM). High Performance Liquid Chromatography (HPLC) was used for analyzing the solubility and dissolution profile of the samples.

Results: Fourier Transmission Infrared (FTIR) spectra showed that SFD processed compositions did not affect chemical structure of RH. SEM and Thermal Gravimetric Analysis (TGA) revealed that the fabricated spherical and highly porous microparticles were in amorphous state. SFD processed powders showed superior solubility and dissolution behavior; where, 80% of the drug was dissolved within 5 minutes.

Conclusion: SFD method can be a promising alternative for enhancing the solubility of poorly water soluble compounds.

Introduction

Raloxifene Hydrochloride (RH) is a Selective Estrogen Receptor Modulator (SERM) acts as an agonist on bone and liver. However, Raloxifene shows antagonistic effects on breast and uterus. Hence, Raloxifene has been approved for the prevention of osteoporosis as well as reducing the risk of invasive breast cancer in post-menopausal women.[1] RH shows very low oral bioavailability (*c.a.* 2% of the given dose) which is mostly due to its extensive first pass hepatic metabolism *via* glucuronide conjugation as well as incomplete dissolution as the drug is poorly water-soluble.[2,3] This drug is categorized as class II of Biopharmaceutical Classification System (BCS).[4] Accordingly, its low bioavailability seems to be enhanced by increasing its solubility.[5,6]

Several techniques can be used to improve solubility of drugs such as co-grinding, salt formation, spray drying, and supercritical fluid processing.[7-10] In order to increase the solubility of RH, different methods have been investigated to date. Co-grinding of RH with different superdisintegrants such as polyvinylpyrrolidone (PVP), hydroxypropylmethyl cellulose, crospovidone, croscarmellose sodium, and sodium starch glycolate have been reported and resulted in considerable improvement of drug solubility in most cases.[7,11] Spray freeze drying (SFD) is relatively a novel technique for pharmaceutical

particle engineering and drying of foods as well as bioproducts.[12,13] In this process, a feed solution is atomized by a nozzle over/in a cryogenic medium and frozen droplets are lyophilized in low pressure and temperature. In comparison to other particle engineering processes, SFD grants better control on different aspects of particle properties. This method can produce highly porous and low density particles. It has been reported that SFD could create particles forty times higher in specific surface area and one ninth lower in density versus spray drying technique.[14] Consequently, SFD is now an authentic approach for enhancement of particle properties like surface area and increasing dissolution of different drugs.

Many factors can influence particle characteristics produced by this method such as composition, total solid content of liquid feed solution, spraying rate of liquid feed, distance between nozzle, and cryogenic liquid surface.[15,16]

In the present study, the effect of SFD method on dissolution rate of RH was studied in the presence of PVP and HPβCD as solubility enhancers. PVP has been widely used for solubility improvement of water-insoluble drugs such as piroxicam, furosemide, praziquantel, and celecoxib.[17-20] Cyclodextrin (CD) derivatives are cyclic oligosaccharides comprise hydrophilic outer part and hydrophobic internal cavity which can form a complex with various drugs. CDs have been used to increase water solubility and dissolution rate of low water soluble drugs such as miconazole, doxorubicin, and naproxen.[21-23] Complexation of RH with Hydoxybutenyl beta Cyclodextrin (HBenβCD) has been shown to be effective in increasing solubility and dissolution rate of the drug.[24,25]

Materials and Methods
RH was received from Glochem (India). PVP K30 and HPβCD were purchased from Sigma Aldrich (Germany). Ethanol and acetonitrile of HPLC grade were obtained from Merck (Germany) and the liquid nitrogen were received from Sabalan (Iran).

Formation of RH Microparticles via SFD Method
Hydroethanolic (4:1) solvent was selected to dissolve the drug and excipients. Samples were prepared in compositions according to the Table 1. To produce spray freeze dried powders, the feed solution was loaded into the solution cell and sprayed 10 cm above the surface of 300 mL liquid nitrogen through a two-fluid nozzle with a flow rate of 6 and 12 mL/min at the pressure of 6 bars provided by an air pump. Figure 1 indicates a schematic diagram of the spraying set up used in this study. The resultant suspension (frozen droplets of the solution in liquid nitrogen) was transferred into the freeze dryer (Christ, The Netherlands). Vacuum was applied as soon as all nitrogen was evaporated. During the first 24 h, the pressure was set at 0.005 mbar and the shelf temperature was fixed at -70 °C. During the second 24 h, the shelf temperature was gradually raised to 20 °C. After removing the samples from the freeze drier, they were stored over silica gel in a desiccator at room temperature.

Table 1. Composition of spray freeze dried formulations

Run No.	RH (mg)	HPβCD (mg)	PVP (mg)	Flow Rate (mL/min)
F₁	112.50			6
F₂	75			6
F₃	56.25	225	-	6
F₄	112.50			12
F₅	75			12
F₆	56.25			12
F₇	112.50			6
F₈	75			6
F₉	56.25	-	225	6
F₁₀	112.50			12
F₁₁	75			12
F₁₂	56.25			12

RH: Raloxifene Hydrochloride
HPβCD: Hydroxypropyl Beta Cyclodextrin
PVP: Polyvinylpyrrolidone

Thermal Analysis
Thermal analysis of RH, HPβCD, PVP, and selected SFD processed samples were performed using a PL-DSC apparatus (polymer laboratories, UK). Approximately, 5 mg of the samples were sealed firmly and scanned under dry nitrogen atmosphere at the heat rate of 10 °C per minute from 10 to 350 °C.

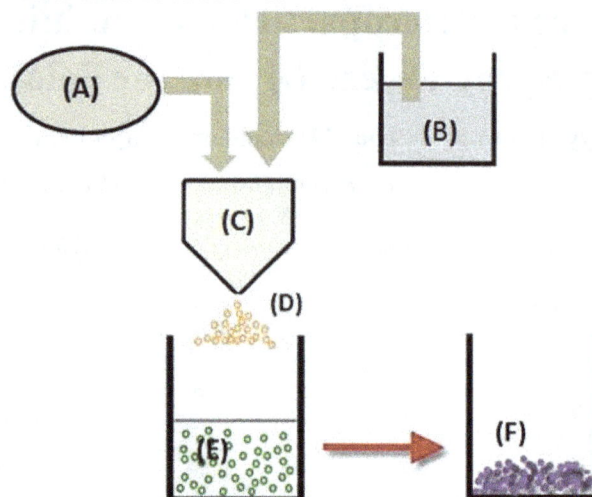

Figure 1. Schematic diagram of spray freeze drying apparatus. (A) Compressed air inlet, (B) Solution cell, (C) Two fluid nozzle, (D) Drug containing droplets, (E) Frozen particles in liquid nitrogen, and (E) Powder collected after freeze drying.

Scanning Electron Microscopy (SEM)
A Philips Model XL30 scanning electron microscope (Philips, The Netherlands) was used to obtain the SEM images. The samples were glued onto aluminum stages using double adhesive carbon conducting tape and coated with gold–palladium at room temperature before the examination. The accelerator voltage for scanning was 25.0 kV.

Fourier Transform Infrared Spectroscopy (FTIR)
FTIR spectra were recorded with a spectrophotometer (Mega-IR, 550, Nicolet, USA) in the range of 400-4000 cm⁻¹, using a resolution of 4.000 cm⁻¹ and 4 scans. Samples were diluted with KBr at concentration of 1% and pressed to obtain self-supporting disks.

Solubility and Dissolution Studies
An excess amount of RH formulations was added to 20 mL of freshly prepared deionized water and rotated at 100 rpm in a water bath (Dorsa, Iran) for 150 min. Then, the samples were filtered and analyzed by reversed-phase High Performance Liquid Chromatography (HPLC) system (Waters, USA) on a Nucleosil C18 column (Macherey Nagel, Germany). The mobile phase was a mixture of acetonitrile and 0.05 M phosphate buffer (pH= 3; 35:65 v/v) with the flow rate of 0.7 mL/min. Detection was carried out at 287 nm with 20-50 μL injection volume.

The in-vitro dissolution studies of selected formulations and two physical mixtures (PMs) were performed by dissolving the same amount of samples (700 mg) in pure water previously heated to 37 °C. 100 μL of samples were collected in 0, 5, 10, 25, 35, 60, and 90 min. Afterwards, samples were analyzed by mentioned HPLC method.

Results and Discussion

Series of microparticles containing solid dispersions of RH, HPβCD or PVP were produced by SFD process according to Table 1. Micrographs of the resultant particles (Figure 2) showed numerous pores in the structure of spherical microparticles that could be attributed to the voids remained after sublimation of ice crystals. This process showed that *via* SFD technique, the atomized droplets were completely frozen in contact with liquid nitrogen and their shapes as well as sizes were preserved during freeze drying. Morphology and particle size of the microparticles were in a similar range in samples containing PVP and HPβCD. In terms of particle size, comparisons between F_2 and F_5 revealed that increasing the solution flow rate may result in formation of asymmetrical particles. The same results were obtained when F_8 and F_{11} were compared. Higher flow rate may affect degree of atomization and level of freezing in droplets.

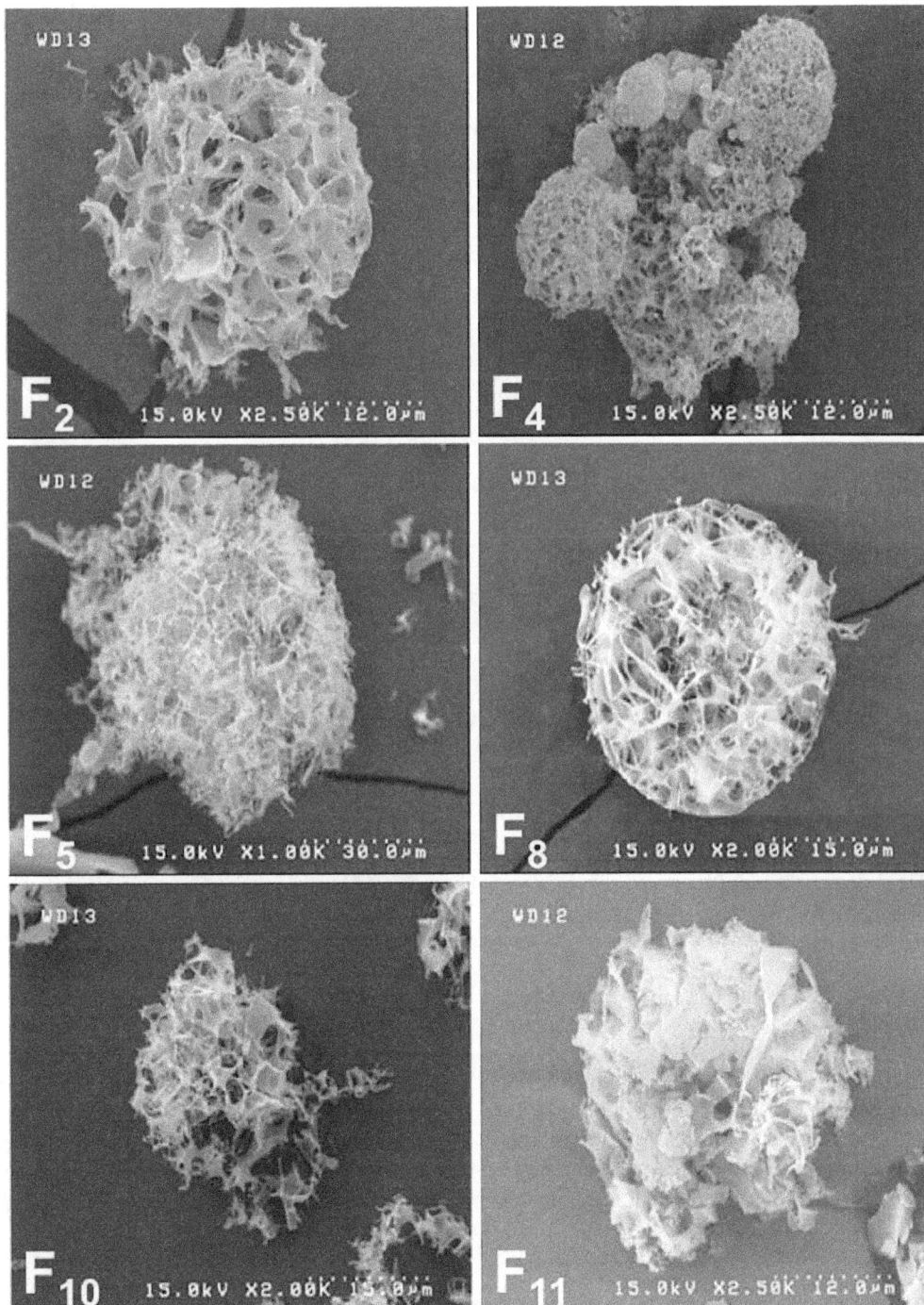

Figure 2. SEM images of Raloxifene Hydrochloride-loaded samples after spray freeze drying. The porous structure of the microparticles is shown in these SEM images.

FTIR studies indicated that there was no important interaction between RH and solubility enhancers. As shown in Figure 3, the amide bond of PVP at 1690 cm^{-1} overlapped with carbonyl bond of RH; however, the stretch of C-O-C bond of RH was observed in 1600 cm^{-1} of F_{11} spectra. The broad 3400 cm^{-1} stretch and 1034

vibrating wave in F_6 spectra confirmed the presence of hydroxyl group in HPβCD. Similarly, the 1462 cm^{-1} stretch in S-benzothiofuran of RH was observable in F_5 sample. No wave shift was seen with pure HPβCD spectrum.

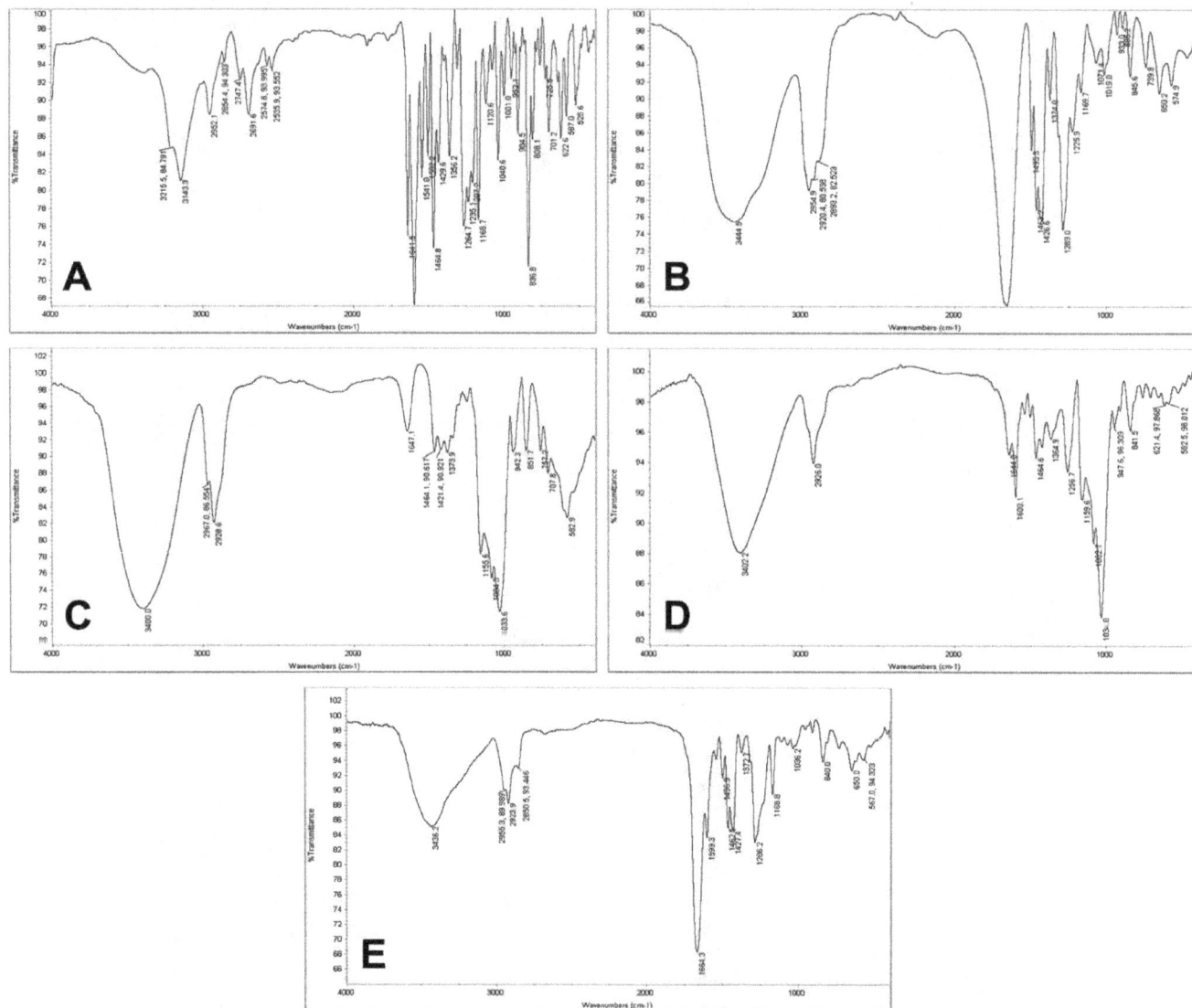

Figure 3. FTIR spectra for different formulations. (A) Raloxifene Hydrochloride, (B) PVP, (C) HPβCD, (D) F_4, and (E) F_{11}.

Thermograms of F_2 and F_8 formulations were compared with unprocessed RH, PVP, and HPβCD to investigate the thermal behavior of SFD processed microparticles (Figure 4). Pure RH exhibited a single sharp endotherm at 267 °C that was completely disappeared in both SFD processed samples and revealed amorphous state of the drug in SFD processed particles. Rapid freezing and high sublimation rate in drying step caused formation of amorphous solid dispersion in SFD method.[26]

The solubility saturation of the processed samples was compared with raw RH and physical mixtures in Figure 5. In all SFD processed samples, the solubility of drug was extremely higher than pure RH and their physical mixtures. Amorphous and porous nature of the particles can improve wettability and solubility of insoluble drugs.[15] Higher ratios

of solubility enhancers caused higher solubility levels; however, samples containing PVP showed considerably higher solubility versus HPβCD containing microparticles. The highest solubility of the samples was observed in F_9 formulation with RH concentration of 36.65 mg/mL in comparison to 24.15 mg/mL in F_3. This difference could be attributed to the formation of intermolecular bonding between RH and PVP.[27]

Dissolution rate of F_2, F_5, F_8, F_{11}, and two physical mixtures are illustrated in Figure 6. Each sample contained RH to solubility enhancer in 1:3 weight ratios. After adding the sample to the dissolution medium for 10 minutes, only 2% of RH-PVP and about 1% of RH-HPβCD physical mixtures were dissolved. On the other hand, at least 40% of the drug in SFD processed samples was dissolved within 10 minutes. Among all the samples, F_8 and F_{11} demonstrated considerably higher dissolution rate than all the other samples and more than 83% and 77% of the drug was dissolved, respectively. These findings emphasized that dissolution rate of samples containing PVP was much faster than HPβCD processed ones due to superior wettability of PVP.

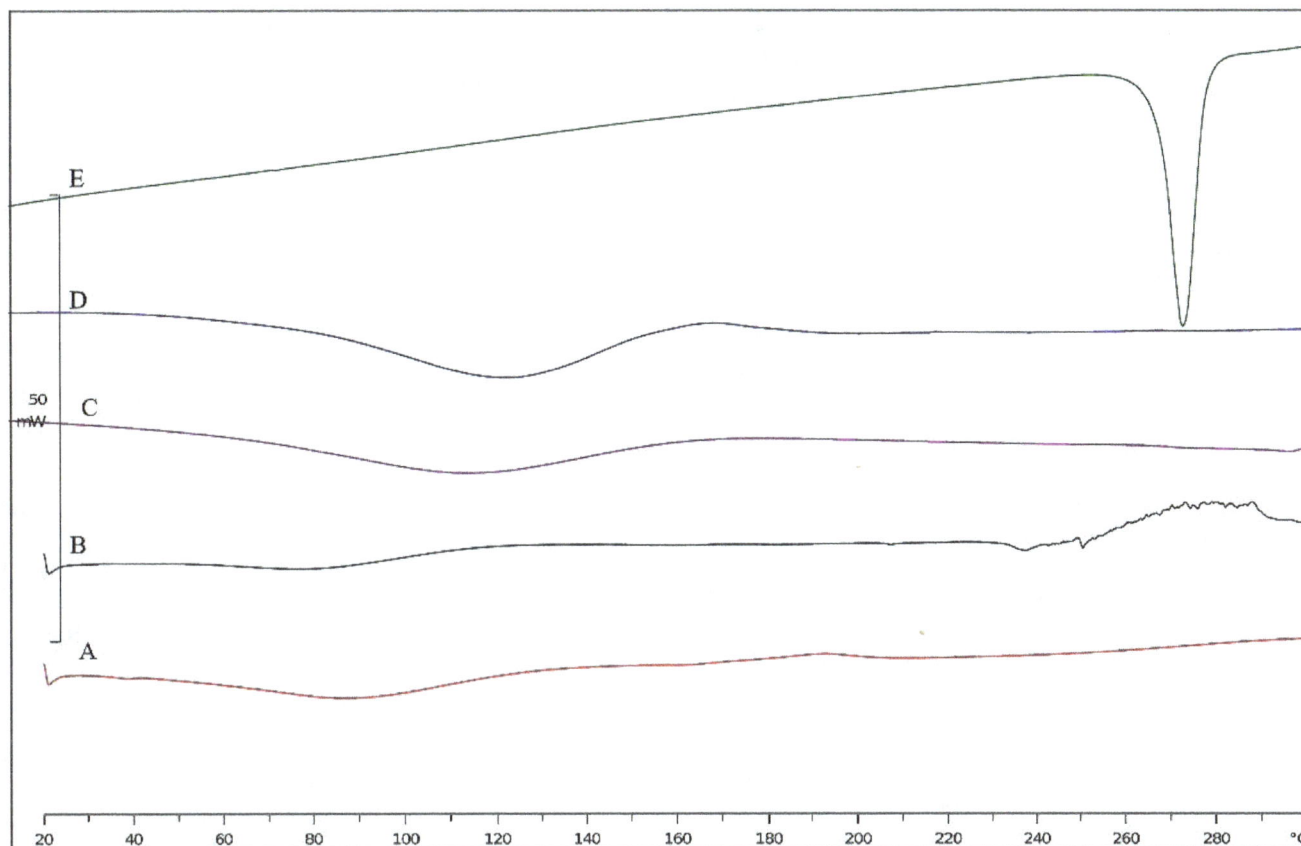

Figure 4. DSC thermograms for different formulations. (A) F_2, (B) F_8, (C) HPBCD, (D) PVP, and (E) Raw Raloxifene Hydrochloride.

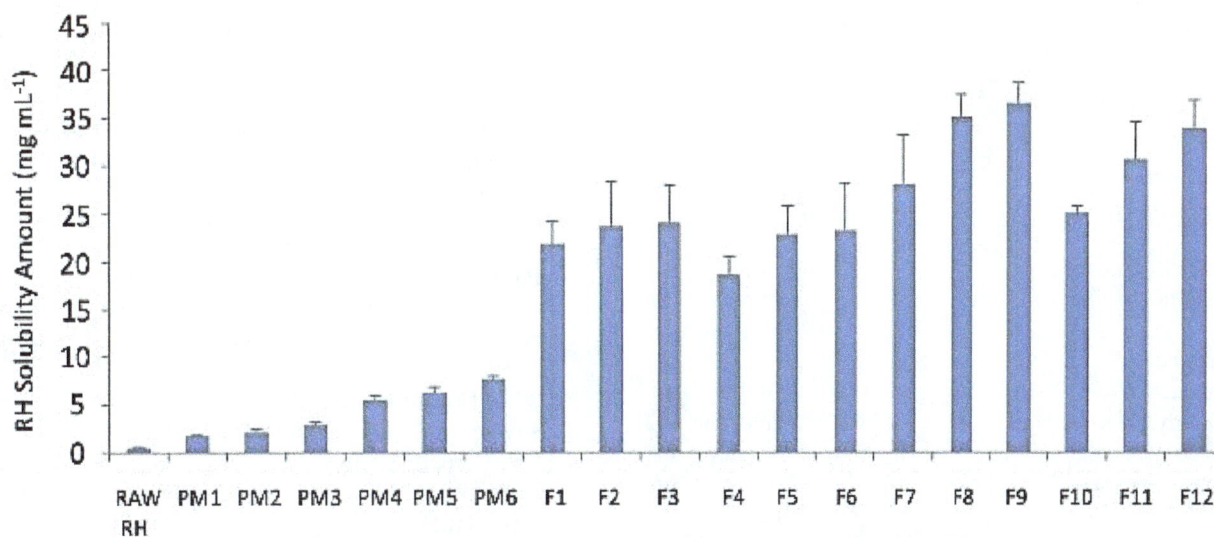

Figure 5. Water solubility of spray freeze dried formulations compared with Raw Raloxifene Hydrochloride and physical mixtures (PMs). PM_1 (Raloxifene Hydrochloride:HPβCD 1:2), PM_2 (Raloxifene Hydrochloride: HPβCD 1:3), PM_3 (Raloxifene Hydrochloride: HPβCD 1:4), PM_4 (Raloxifene Hydrochloride:PVP 1:2), PM_5 (Raloxifene Hydrochloride:PVP 1:3), and PM_6 (Raloxifene Hydrochloride:PVP 1:4). The highest water solubility of the samples was observed in F_9 formulation.

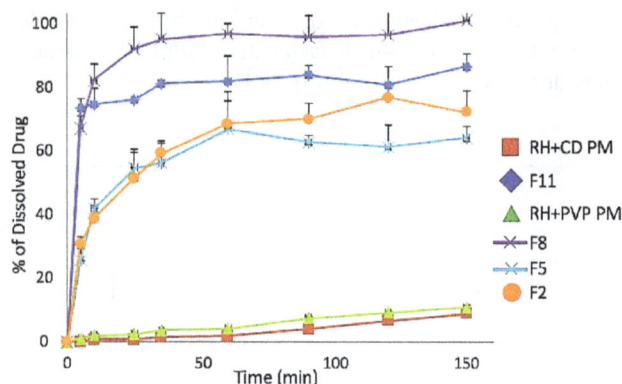

Figure 6. Dissolution profile of various Raloxifene Hydrochloride complexes. F_8 and F_{11} demonstrated significantly higher dissolution rate than all the other samples and more than 83% and 77% of the drug was dissolved, respectively.

Spray freeze drying of RH with PVP and HPβCD as solubility enhancers produced amorphous and highly porous microparticles. They exhibited superior solubility and dissolution rate compared to raw RH and physical mixtures. The highest solubility was achieved by F_9 sample with more than 70 folds increase in drug solubility. Samples containing PVP showed higher solubility versus HPβCD containing microparticles. Samples produced with lower flow rate conditions, showed higher solubility and dissolution rate.

Conclusion
The results indicated that SFD could be an effective particle engineering approach for improving dissolution rate of poorly water soluble drugs used in oral drug delivery such as Raloxifene.

Acknowledgments
This research was part of a PharmD student thesis (Thesis Number: 5212) and has been financially supported by Tehran University of Medical Sciences (TUMS).

Ethical Issues
Not applicable.

Conflict of Interest
There is no conflict of interest.

References
1. Barrett-Connor E, Mosca L, Collins P, Geiger MJ, Grady D, Kornitzer M, et al. Effects of raloxifene on cardiovascular events and breast cancer in postmenopausal women. *N Engl J Med* 2006;355(2):125-37. doi: 10.1056/NEJMoa062462

2. Patel BD, Modi RV, Thakkar NA, Patel AA, Thakkar PH. Development and characterization of solid lipid nanoparticles for enhancement of oral bioavailability of raloxifene. *J Pharm Bioallied Sci* 2012;4(Suppl 1):S14-6. doi: 10.4103/0975-7406.94121

3. Thakkar H, Nangesh J, Parmar M, Patel D. Formulation and characterization of lipid-based drug delivery system of raloxifene-microemulsion and self-microemulsifying drug delivery system. *J Pharm Bioallied Sci* 2011;3(3):442-8. doi: 10.4103/0975-7406.84463

4. Patil PH, Belgamwar VS, Patil PR, Surana SJ. Solubility enhancement of raloxifene using inclusion complexes and cogrinding method. *J Pharm (Cairo)* 2013;2013:527380. doi: 10.1155/2013/527380

5. Nabi-Meibodi M, Vatanara A, Najafabadi AR, Rouini MR, Ramezani V, Gilani K, et al. The effective encapsulation of a hydrophobic lipid-insoluble drug in solid lipid nanoparticles using a modified double emulsion solvent evaporation method. *Colloids Surf B Biointerfaces* 2013;112:408-14. doi: 10.1016/j.colsurfb.2013.06.013

6. Wu CY, Benet LZ. Predicting drug disposition via application of bcs: Transport/absorption/ elimination interplay and development of a biopharmaceutics drug disposition classification system. *Pharm Res* 2005;22(1):11-23.

7. Jagadish B, Yelchuri R, K B, Tangi H, Maroju S, Rao VU. Enhanced dissolution and bioavailability of raloxifene hydrochloride by co-grinding with different superdisintegrants. *Chem Pharm Bull (Tokyo)* 2010;58(3):293-300.

8. Pandit NK M, Strykowski J, Shtohryn L. The effect of salts on the distribution and solubility of an acidic drug. *Int J Pharm* 1989;50(1):7-13. doi: 10.1016/0378-5173(89)90174-9

9. Vogt M, Kunath K, Dressman JB. Dissolution enhancement of fenofibrate by micronization, cogrinding and spray-drying: Comparison with commercial preparations. *Eur J Pharm Biopharm* 2008;68(2):283-8. doi: 10.1016/j.ejpb.2007.05.010

10. Kerc J, Srcic S, Knez Z, Sencar-Bozic P. Micronization of drugs using supercritical carbon dioxide. *Int J Pharm* 1999;182(1):33-9.

11. Garg A, Singh S, Rao VU, Bindu K, Balasubramaniam J. Solid state interaction of raloxifene hcl with different hydrophilic carriers during co-grinding and its effect on dissolution rate. *Drug Dev Ind Pharm* 2009;35(4):455-70. doi: 10.1080/03639040802438365

12. Padma Ishwarya S, Anandharamakrishnan C. Spray-freeze-drying approach for soluble coffee processing and its effect on quality characteristics. *J Food Eng* 2015;149:171-80. doi: 10.1016/j.jfoodeng.2014.10.011

13. Ishwarya SP, Anandharamakrishnan C, Stapley AGF. Spray-freeze-drying: A novel process for the drying of foods and bioproducts. *Trends Food Sci Technol* 2015;41(2):161-81. doi: 10.1016/j.tifs.2014.10.008

14. Maa YF, Nguyen PA, Sweeney T, Shire SJ, Hsu CC. Protein inhalation powders: Spray drying vs spray freeze drying. *Pharm Res* 1999;16(2):249-54.

15. Hu J, Rogers TL, Brown J, Young T, Johnston KP, Williams RO, 3rd. Improvement of dissolution rates of poorly water soluble apis using novel spray

freezing into liquid technology. *Pharm Res* 2002;19(9):1278-84.

16. Elversson J, Millqvist-Fureby A, Alderborn G, Elofsson U. Droplet and particle size relationship and shell thickness of inhalable lactose particles during spray drying. *J Pharm Sci* 2003;92(4):900-10. doi: 10.1002/jps.10352

17. Tantishaiyakul V, Kaewnopparat N, Ingkatawornwong S. Properties of solid dispersions of piroxicam in polyvinylpyrrolidone k-30. *Int J Pharm* 1996;143(1):59-66. doi: 10.1016/S0378-5173(96)04687-X

18. Doherty C, York P. Mechanisms of dissolution of frusemide/pvp solid dispersions. *Int J Pharm* 1987;34(3):197-205. doi: 10.1016/0378-5173(87)90180-3

19. El-Arini SK, Leuenberger H. Dissolution properties of praziquantel–PVP systems. *Pharm Acta Helv 1998*;73(2):89-94. doi: 10.1016/S0031-6865(97)00051-4

20. Gupta P, Kakumanu VK, Bansal AK. Stability and solubility of celecoxib-pvp amorphous dispersions: A molecular perspective. *Pharm Res* 2004;21(10):1762-9.

21. Pedersen M, Edelsten M, Nielsen VF, Scarpellini A, Skytte S, Slot C. Formation and antimycotic effect of cyclodextrin inclusion complexes of econazole and miconazole. *Int J Pharm* 1993;90(3):247-54. doi: 10.1016/0378-5173(93)90197-N

22. Brewster ME, Loftsson T, Estes KS, Lin J-L, Fridriksdóttir H, Bodor N. Effect of various cyclodextrins on solution stability and dissolution rate of doxorubicin hydrochloride. *Int J Pharm* 1992;79(1-3):289-99. doi: 10.1016/0378-5173(92)90121-H

23. Mura P, Faucci MT, Bettinetti GP. The influence of polyvinylpyrrolidone on naproxen complexation with hydroxypropyl-beta-cyclodextrin. *Eur J Pharm Sci* 2001;13(2):187-94.

24. Buchanan CM, Buchanan NL, Edgar KJ, Lambert JL, Posey-Dowty JD, Ramsey MG, et al. Solubilization and dissolution of tamoxifen-hydroxybutenyl cyclodextrin complexes. *J Pharm Sci* 2006;95(10):2246-55. doi: 10.1002/jps.20710

25. Wempe MF, Wacher VJ, Ruble KM, Ramsey MG, Edgar KJ, Buchanan NL, et al. Pharmacokinetics of raloxifene in male wistar-hannover rats: Influence of complexation with hydroxybutenyl-beta-cyclodextrin. *Int J Pharm* 2008;346(1-2):25-37. doi: 10.1016/j.ijpharm.2007.06.002

26. Rogers TL, Johnston KP, Williams RO, 3rd. Solution-based particle formation of pharmaceutical powders by supercritical or compressed fluid co2 and cryogenic spray-freezing technologies. *Drug Dev Ind Pharm* 2001;27(10):1003-15. doi: 10.1081/ddc-100108363

27. Tran TH, Poudel BK, Marasini N, Chi SC, Choi HG, Yong CS, et al. Preparation and evaluation of raloxifene-loaded solid dispersion nanoparticle by spray-drying technique without an organic solvent. *Int J Pharm* 2013;443(1-2):50-7. doi: 10.1016/j.ijpharm.2013.01.013

22

Assessing the Effect of High Performance Inulin Supplementation via KLF5 mRNA Expression in Adults with Type 2 Diabetes: A Randomized Placebo Controlled Clinical Trail

Abed Ghavami[1], Neda Roshanravan[2], Shahriar Alipour[3], Meisam Barati[4], Behzad Mansoori[5], Faezeh Ghalichi[1], Elyas Nattagh- Eshtivan[1], Alireza Ostadrahimi[6]*

[1] Department of Nutrition, School of Nutrition, Tabriz University of Medical Sciences, Tabriz, Iran.
[2] Cardiovascular Research Center, Tabriz University of Medical Sciences, Tabriz, Iran.
[3] Department of Molecular Medicine, Nutrition Research Center, Tabriz University of Medical Sciences, Tabriz, Iran.
[4] Department of Nutrition, School of Nutrition, Shahid beheshti University of Medical Sciences, Tehran, Iran.
[5] Immunology Research Center, Tabriz University of Medical Sciences, Tabriz, Iran.
[6] Nutrition Research Center, Tabriz University of Medical Sciences, Tabriz, Iran.

Keywords:
· Diabetes
· Inulin
· KLF5
· miR-375
· Fasting plasma glucose

Abstract

Purpose: The worldwide prevalence of metabolic disorders such as diabetes is increasing rapidly. Currently, the complications of diabetes are the major health concern. The aim of this study was to investigate the effect of high performance (HP) inulin supplementation on glucose homeostasis via KLF5 mRNA expression in adults with type 2 diabetes.

Methods: In the present clinical trial conducted for a duration of 6 weeks, 46 volunteers diabetic patients referring to diabetes clinic in Tabriz, Iran, were randomly assigned into intervention (n= 23, consuming 10 gr/ d HP inulin) and control groups (n= 23, consuming 10 gr/ d starch). We assessed glycemic and anthropometric indices, blood lipids and plasmatic level of miR-375 as well as KLF5 mRNA expression before and after the intervention.

Results: Findings indicated that inulin supplementation significantly decreased fasting plasma glucose (FPG) in comparison to the placebo group (P<0.001). Also Intra-group and between group results showed that inulin supplementation resulted in significant decrease in KLF5 mRNA expression in peripheral blood mononuclear cells (PBMCs) (Fold change: 0.61± 0.11; P-value= 0.001) and significant increase in plasmatic level of miR-375 (Fold change: 3.75± 0.70; P-value=0.004).

Conclusion: Considering the improvements of FPG level in diabetic patients, it seems that HP inulin supplementation may be beneficial in controlling diabetes via the expression of some genes. However, further studies are needed to achieve concise conclusions.

Introduction

Diabetes mellitus (DM) as a complex metabolic disorder influenced by various environmental and genetic factors has become a common health problem in the entire world.[1] According to recent reports it is estimated that by the year 2030, at least 366 million people will suffer from diabetes.[2] Recent scientific advances point to manipulation of gut microbiota as contributing factors for preventing or controlling diabetes.[2,3]

The intestinal microbiota is a vital organ with trillions of commensally microorganisms which is involved in host metabolism. Nowadays, dietary components, particularly prebiotics are considered as functional foods that provide beneficial health effects on the intestinal tract. Prebiotics are defined as " non-viable food components that confer health benefits on the host in association with modulation of the microbiota".[4]

Inulin- type fructans are a kind of prebiotic fibers that have received much attention in the last decade. Inulin (a mixture of fructo oligo- and polysaccharides) is a very interesting functional ingredient, present as storage carbohydrate in more than 30,000 vegetables and fruits such as garlic, chicory root, wheat and banana.[5,6] High performance (HP) inulin, the highly refined kind of inulin, is the average rate of polymerization which consists of 25 monosaccharide units. This form of inulin has many advantages with minimum gastrointestinal side effects such as abdominal tension.[7,8] The beneficial health effects of inulin-type fructans have been previously studied. It has been showed that inulin may modulate glucose homeostasis by direct and indirect mechanisms. Alteration in gene expression and its effect

*Corresponding author: Alireza Ostadrahimi, Email: ostadrahimi@tbzmed.ac.ir

on the gut microbiota at different taxonomic levels are few of the beneficial effects of inulin.[9,10]

Recent evidences showed an elaborate network of certain transcription factors coordinate with the expression of hundreds of genes which are responsible for the beneficial effects of inulin.[11,12] The Kruppel Like Factor (KLF) is a kind of zinc finger transcriptional factor which encodes proteins that bind directly to a specific recognition motif in the promoters of target genes. KLF5, a member of the KLF family known as Gut-Enriched Kruppel-Like Factor (GKLF) has been characterized as a transcription factor which is expressed in high amounts in the cells of the intestinal epithelium.[13] Previous studies reported an intense association between KLF5 overexpression and some metabolic disorders such as cardiovascular disease and diabetes.[14] It has been proved that the translation of KLF5 is controlled by microRNAs (miRNAs).[15]

MiRNAs are small (~ 22 nucleotides), single strand, noncoding RNAs which are important regulators of gene expression via base pairing with 3′- untranslated regions of messenger RNA (mRNA).[16] In fact, MiRNAs could possibly lead to degradation of mRNA or protein translation inhibition.[17] Pioneering studies showed that the expression of miR-375 is able to prohibit the translation of KLF5.[18] As the miRNA expression is very high in the human intestine,[19] we supposed that mediation of the gut microbiota with inulin supplementation may promote glucose homeostasis via overexpression of miR-375 in adult diabetic patients. Thus, the objective of this study was to evaluate the effect of HP inulin supplementation on glucose homeostasis via KLF5 mRNA expression in type II diabetic patients in the form of a randomized, double-blind, placebo-controlled clinical trial.

Materials and Methods
Participants
In the current randomized, double-blind, placebo-controlled trial, 46 volunteer diabetic adult patients referring to diabetes clinics in East Azerbaijan, Iran, during September 2016 and November 2016, were recruited. With Confidence Interval: 95% & Power: 90%, calculation of the sample size was accomplished based on the fasting insulin parameter.[20] The formula: n = [(Z1 − α/2 + Z1 − β) 2 (SD12 +S D22)]/Δ2 was used to estimate the 23 samples allocated for each group while considering 6 patients for withdrawal. The inclusion criteria were having diabetes mellitus for more than 6 months; aged 30 to 50 years; body mass index) BMI) greater than 25 and less than 35 kg/m². Exclusion criteria were having kidney disease; liver failure; heart failure; rheumatic diseases inflammatory diseases of the gastrointestinal tract; lactose intolerance; insulin injection and consuming drugs such as: estrogen, progesterone, corticosteroids; smoking; breast feeding and pregnancy; vitamin, mineral, omega-3 and antibiotic supplementation for three weeks before the beginning of the study. These

subjects (46 patients) were randomly allocated using randomized block procedure, to one of the 2 treatment groups (A, or B) by computer-generated allocation schedule (Random Allocation Software) in which A was inulin group, B was placebo. Participants were also matched by type of consumed drugs (glucose lowering and anti- hyperlipidemia drugs) and disease duration in this trial.

Study design
After stratifying patients based on gender and age, subjects were randomly allocated into HP inulin (n=23) and placebo groups (n=23). The randomization process was not disclosed to the researchers and diabetic patients until the main analyses were completed. Also, during the study, none of the researchers and patients was aware of the drug randomization procedure. A study technician accomplished the randomization allocation procedure and allocated the participants into two groups. The HP inulin group received 10 g per day HP inulin powder (Sensus, Borchwef 3, 4704 RG Roosendaal the Netherlands) and the placebo group obtained 10g starch powder as placebo for 6 consecutive weeks. The components used for supplementation were sequenced into equal doses (5 grams) which were prescribed to consume before breakfast and dinner for 6 weeks. HP inulin powder and placebo (starch powder) were manufactured by Sensus Company, Netherlands. The HP inulin powder and placebo were in the same appearance such as colour, shape and packaging, which were coded by the producer to guarantee blinding. The participants were encouraged to avoid changing the dose and drugs consuming in order to prevent potential effects on the results of the study. Compliance to the HP inulin was assessed via asking participants to return the medication packages. Subjects were controlled weekly for possible side effects.

Physical activity and dietary intake assessments
For evaluating physical activity level before and after the intervention The International Physical Activity Questionnaire (IPAQ) was used for assessing physical activity level at baseline and end of intervention. According to the categorical scoring guidelines of the concluded form of IPAQ, participants were classified as highly, moderate and/or low physical activity level. we grouped our participants into high, moderate or low physical activity levels.[21] Dietary intake was determined using a 24-hour food recall method for 2 average working days and 1 weekend day a week before and at the end of intervention. The dietary recalls were analyzed using the Nutritionist IV software (First Databank, San Bruno, CA, USA) adjusted for Iranian foods. Subjects were informed to continue their usual intake and physical activity until the end of the trial.

RNA extraction and quantitative real-time PCR for gene and miRNA

Peripheral blood mononuclear cells (PBMCs) separation was accomplished by Ficoll-Histopaque solution gradient (ficoll- paque, GmbH) centrifugation. Total RNA was extracted from PBMCs using ambion Trizol LS reagent. Thermo Fisher scientific revertaid first strand cDNA synthesis kit was used for the synthesis of cDNA. The level of KLF5 mRNA were evaluated by SYBR Green Master mix (Thermo Fisher Scientific, USA). The primer sequences were designed using PrimerBank. The amount of the mRNA normalized against the β-actin mRNA and $-2^{\Delta\Delta C_T}$ method[22] was used for relative mRNA abundance. For miR-375 expression evaluation, complementary DNA was synthesized from isolated total RNA obtained from 200-μL plasma using the Universal cDNA synthesis kit (EXIQON, Denmark). Quantitative reverse transcription PCR (qRT-PCR) was prepared using ExiLENT SYBER Green Master mix (Exiqon) against LNA based primer sets (Exiqon) and comparative $-2^{\Delta\Delta C_T}$ method was used to prove the relative quantitative level of miRNAs using Endogenous Control Primer miR-191 (Exiqon) for miRNA normalization.[23,24] All samples were run in duplicate. Fold change of the parameters was computed as relative expression post intervention/control. The primers sequences of KLF5, β-actin, miR- 375 and miR-191 are illustrated as following: KLF5: Forward TCATCTTTCTGTCCCTACCC, Reverse TCCATTGCTGCTGTCTGA, Forward GGTGAAGGTGACAGCAGT, Reverse TGGGGTGGCTTTTAGGAT Hsa-miR-375 (5'-3') UUUGUUCGUUCGGCUCGCGUGA, Hsa-miR-191-5p (5'-3') CAACGGAAUCCCAAAAGCAGCUG.

Anthropometric measurements

At the onset and end of the trial, anthropometric indices such as body weight (BW), height, waist and hip circumferences (WC and HC respectively), waist to hip ratio (WHR) and body mass index (BMI) were recorded. Weight was measured via a calibrated scale (Itin Scale Co., Inc. Germany) with least clothing and 0.1 kg accuracy. Also, height was measured in a standing position next to ruler attached to the wall. For calculating BMI, the following equation was used: weight (kg) / height^2 (m). Waist circumference (WC) was obtained by measuring the smallest area below the rib cage and above the umbilicus. Standing HC was measured at the inter trochantric level.[25] Waist to hip ratio (WHR) was measured by dividing mean WC to mean HC.

Biochemical Assessment

For biochemical assessment, 7 ml blood sample was collected at baseline and at the end of the trial after 12h overnight fasting for measuring fasting plasma glucose (FPG), fasting insulin, glycated hemoglobin (HbA1c), total Cholestrol (TC), Triglycerides (TG), High density lipoprotein cholesterol (HDL-C) and Low density lipoprotein cholesterol (LDL-C). Auto-analyzer (Mindray Auto Hematology Analyzer, China) was used

for biochemical analysis as well as platinum enzyme-linked immunosorbent assay (ELISA) kit (Monobind, Iran) for measuring fasting insulin. Also, NycoCard kit (NycoCard, Norway) was used for measuring HbA1c. Based on the Homeostatic model assessment of insulin resistance (HOMA-IR method, insulin resistance was measured: Fasting Glucose (mg/dL) × fasting insulin (mU/L)/450.

Statistical analysis

The Kolmogorov-Smirnov test was used for testing the normal distribution all of variables. Numerical variables were compared by Student t test and reported as mean ± standard deviation (SD). The Pearson chi-square test was used for comparing categorical variables and reported as number (%). Within group comparisons were determined by paired-sample t test. After adjusting for baseline values, Analysis of Covariance (ANCOVA) was applied to identify any differences between two groups at the end of the study. Statistically significant variables had p-value less than, 0.05 and were analyzed using the SPSS software version 23 (SPSS Inc., Chicago, Illinois, USA).

Results

The study flowchart is shown in Figure 1. A total of 46 diabetic patients completed the study and were interred in the final analyses. No adverse side-effects were reported by diabetic patients following the HP inulin or placebo supplementation. General characteristics (demographic variables and baseline values of anthropometric indices) of the participants are presented in Table 1. None of the demographic and anthropometric variables were different between the study groups, at baseline (P>0.05). As specified in Table 2, no differences were seen in the percent changes of few of the variables such as HbA1c, Weight, BMI, anthropometric indices (WC, HC and WHR) and blood lipids (TC, TG, HDL-C, LDL-C) after Inulin supplementation compared to the placebo group (P>0.05). However, Inulin supplementation significantly decreased FPG in comparison to the placebo group (P<0.001). Also, a statistically insignificant increase was observed in fasting insulin level after inulin supplementation. Intra-group statistical analysis indicated that Inulin supplementation significantly reduced FPG, WC and HC (P<0.05). Inulin supplementation significantly decreased WC from 97.47± 8.41 to 96.28±8.03 (p=0.009).

Dietary intake of study participants is shown in Table 3 demonstrates subject's dietary intake. Within group ad between group differences for dietary intake of energy and macro-nutrients such as carbohydrates, proteins, fats and dietary fiber was not statistically significant. There were no within-or between-group differences observed for dietary intake of total energy, carbohydrates, proteins, fats and dietary fiber.

Intra-group and between-group statistical analysis revealed that Inulin supplementation resulted in significant decrease in KLF5 mRNA expression of KLF5 (Fold change: 0.61± 0.11; P-value= 0.001) (Figure 2). Additionally, Inulin supplementation significantly increased miR-375 level (Fold change: 3.75± 0.70; P-value=0.004) (Figure 3).

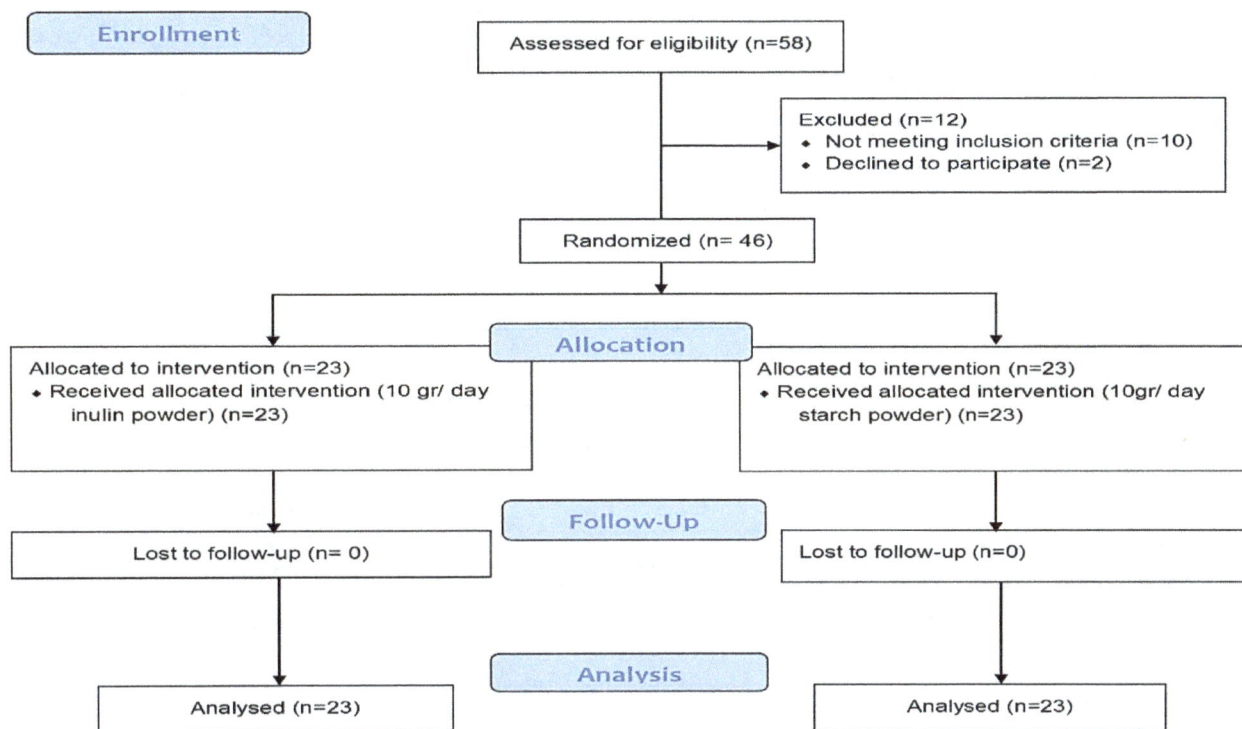

Figure 1. Trial flow diagram

Table 1. Baseline characteristics of the study subjects

Variable	HP inulin group (n=23)	Placebo group (n=23)	P-value[b]
Male/Female	10/13	10/13	1.00
Age(year)	41.50±6.27	42.73±5.95	0.509
Weight(kg)	81.87± 11.46	79.91± 14.60	0.624
Height(cm)	168.68± 8.83	164.09± 10.10	0.116
BMI(kg/m^2)	27.71± 4.60	28.79±4.77	0.444
WC(cm)	97.47± 8.41	93.84± 11.16	0.467
HC(cm)	108.04± 7.39	104.50± 10.70	0.455
WHR	0.90±0.08	0.88±0.07	0.455
Diabetes duration(year)	8.78± 4.67	9.86± 4.95	0.546
Physical activity level n(%)			0.459
Low	14(60.87)	15(65.23)	
Moderate	7(30.44)	7(30.43)	
High	2(8.69)	1(4.34)	

Abbreviations: BMI, body mass index; WC, waist circumference; HC, hip circumference; WHR, waist To hip ratio. [a] Variables are expressed as mean ± SD. And number (percentage). [b] p-values resulted from independent t tests for quantitative and Chi-square for qualitative variables between the two groups.

Table 2. The effect of HP inulin supplementation on anthropometric indices and biochemical in patient with diabetes.

Variable	HP inulin group(n=23)		placebo group(n=23)		P-value[a]
	mean±sd	Change	mean±sd	Change	
Weight (kg)					
Baseline	81.87± 11.46	-0.61	79.91± 14.60	-0.47	0.317
End of trial	81.46± 11.39		79.40± 13.91		
P-value[b]	0.362		0.259		
BMI(kg/m²)					
Baseline	30.37±2.47	-0.710	30.86±2.41	-0.62	0.792
End of trial	30.15±2.73		30.64±2.24		
P-value[b]	0.104		0.084		
WC(cm)					
Baseline	97.47±8.41	-1.17	93.84±11.16	-0.003	0.952
End of trial	96.28±8.03		93.68±9.98		
P-value[b]	0.009		0.846		
HC(cm)					
Baseline	108.04±7.39	-1.93	104.50±10.70	-1.17	0.687
End of trial	106.01±8.23		103.22±10.47		
P-value[b]	0.004		0.061		
WHR(cm)					
Baseline	0.90±0.08	-0.21	0.88±0.07	-1.28	0.192
End of trial	0.90±0.08		0.87±0.05		
P-value[b]	0.744		0.135		
Insulin(μU/ml)					
Baseline	4.99±1.41	7.54	5.42±1.56	-0.57	0.817
End of trial	5.20±1.75		5.38±1.56		
P-value[b]	0.546		0.598		
FPG(mg/dl)					
Baseline	130±36.25	-7.46	127.64±24.19	1.93	<0.001
End of trial	119.28±30.75		130.36±27.85		
P-value[b]	0.001		0.216		
HOMA-IR					
Baseline	1.53±0.53	1.05	1.71± 0.60	1.47	0.815
End of trial	1.55±0.69		1.72± 0.61		
P-value[b]	0.974		0.568		
HbA1c (%)					
Baseline	8.04±2.45	-0.69	7.02±1.60	-2.52	0.128
End of trial	7.62±1.85		7.79± 1.29		
P-value[b]	0.389		0.156		
TG(mg/dl)					
Baseline	177.16±72.02	-0.80	186.73± 74.64	-0.40	0.136
End of trial	168.58±53.50		185.45± 7.74		
P-value[b]	0.299		0.402		
TC(mg/dl)					
Baseline	201.38±73.43	-7.77	174.27± 42.35	2.97	0.819
End of trial	178.24±55.01		176.18±31.02		
P-value[b]	0.122		0.742		
HDL-C(mg/dl)					
Baseline	41.18±9.23	4.79	41.64±8.75	1.49	0.388
End of trial	42.95±9.19		42.09± 9.42		
P-value[b]	0.091		0.681		
LDL-C(mg/dl)					
Baseline	111.81±48.54	-8.32	107.20±30.96	6.52	0.070
End of trial	97.57±44.05		112.32±32.60		
P-value[b]	0.183		0.169		

Abbreviations: ANCOVA, analysis of co-variance; BMI, body mass index; HDL-C, High density lipoprotein cholesterol; LDL, low density lipoprotein cholesterol; TG, triglycerides; TC, total cholesterol; WC, waist circumference; HC, hip circumference; WHR, waist to hip ratio; FPG, fasting plasma glucose; HbA1c, glycosylated hemoglobin; HOMA-IR, homeostasis model assessment of insulin resistance;[a] obtained from ANCOVA adjusted for baseline value. [b]obtained from paired T test.

Table 3. Dietary intake of study participants at Baseline and End of trial[a]

Variable	HP inulin group (n=23)	Placebo group(n=23)	P-value[b]
Energy(Kcal/day)			
Baseline	1680.24±387.81	1739.57±421.05	0.603
End of trial	1786.84±495.04	1666.15±458.37	0.370
P-value[c]	0.213	0.505	
Carbohydrate(g/day)			
Baseline	242.92±62.84	255.25±77.19	0.536
End of trial	259.25±80.20	242.38±60.06	0.398
P-value[c]	0.18	0.58	
Protein(g/day)			
Baseline	66.95±19.01	70.73±19.83	0.491
End of trial	74.35±24.41	67.69±19.14	0.283
P-value[c]	0.13	0.45	
Fat(g/day)			
Baseline	50.73±15.90	51.05±16.50	0.944
End of trial	50.55±13.38	47.56± 18.79	0.518
P-value[c]	0.96	0.37	
Dietary fiber(g/day)			
Baseline	18.35± 6.62	17.60± 4.60	0.519
End of trial	17.92± 3.95	16.95±4.30	0.109
P-value[c]	0.231	0.401	

[a] Variables are expressed as mean ± SD,). [b] p-values resulted from independent T tests. [c] obtained from paired T test.

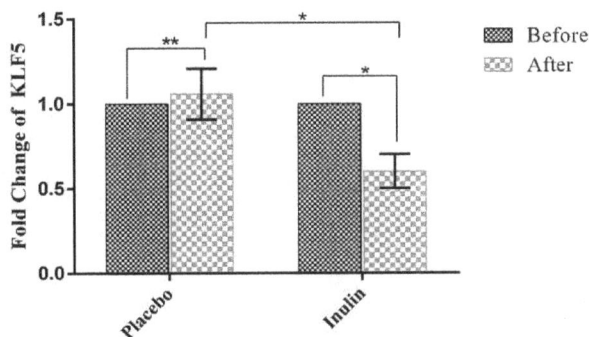

Figure 2. The PBMC levels of KLF5. X-axis represents the study groups and Y-axis shows fold changes of KLF5. Statistical analysis was done by One Sample T test and Independent Sample T test. Each point representsmean±SD. * P-value< 0.05; ** P-value> 0.05.

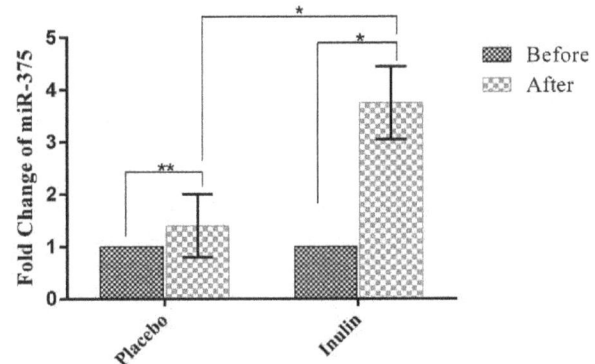

Figure 3. The plasma levels of miR-375. X-axis represents the study groups and Y-axis shows fold changes of miR-375. Statistical analysis was done by One Sample T test and Independent Sample T test. Each point represents mean±SD. * P-value< 0.05; ** P-value> 0.05.

Discussion

Our findings provide strong evidence for modulation of glycemic indices via miR-375 as an important regulator for KLF5 mRNA expression in type 2 diabetic patients after HP inulin supplementation. The findings of the present study indicated that HP inulin supplementation decreased FPG and KLF5 mRNA expression significantly. Interestingly, miR-375 expression increased remarkably in the intervention group compared with the placebo group. Additionally, our study revealed that the levels of FPG, WC and HC decreased in inulin group compared to the placebo one.

Based on our understanding, the present study is the first study that investigated the effects of HP inulin supplementation on KLF5 mRNA expression via miR-375 up-regulation. The decrease of FPG level in our study is in agreement with earlier results.[26,27] In contrast, in some previous studies no beneficial effects were reported for FPG level after inulin- type fructans supplementation in diabetic patients.[28,29] These conflicting effects could be due to different ethnic background, various doses and time intervals of inulin supplementation. Regarding the effect of inulin supplementation on fasting insulin, HbA1c and HOMA-IR indices we did not observe any significant changes in line with pioneering studies.[30,31] According to a new systematic review and meta- analysis, there were no significant improvement in fasting insulin after inulin-type fructans' supplementation.[32]

Similar to few previous studies[8,33,34] we observed no statistical significant changes in lipid profile following HP inulin supplementation. Nevertheless, in few studies positive effects of prebiotics on lipid profile were reported.[35,36] The contradictory results obtained from several studies may be due to the diversity in type and dose of supplements and differences in baseline values of lipid profile.

Other studies have shown that fructooligosaccharides' consumption was associated with anthropometric indices improvement and the promotion of weight loss.[20,37-40] However, conflicting results have also been reported.[30] In this study inulin supplementation resulting in WC, HC decreases in intra-group analysis but in between-group assessments no significant differences were observed.

An interesting finding was the effect of inulin supplementation on KLF5 mRNA expression. It has been previously indicated that plasmatic level of miR-375 is considered as a biomarker for β-cell function. This miRNA is a key regulator for securing intestinal epithelium safety and multiple metabolic processes via controlling various gene expression.[41] Indeed, KLF5 is a target gene for miR-375 and has been implicated in glucose homeostasis.[42] In the present study, we focused on conserved intestinal evolutionary miRNA (miR-375) in order to evaluate glucose homeostasis. In fact, we found a relation between modulation of gut microbiota and overexpression of miR-375 following inulin consumption by suppressing the KLF5 expression in PBMCs. Interestingly, KLF5 is one of the essential transcriptional factors communicating with inflammatory conditions and may contribute to the improvement of glucose homeostasis and diminution of inflammatory cytokines like Tumor necrosis factor alpha (TNF-α) through chemoattractant protein-1 (MCP-1) and transcription factor Nuclear factor-kappa B (NF- κB) pathways.[43]

Although the exact mechanisms by which inulin- type fructans act on glucose metabolism remain unclear, however several proposed mechanisms have been reported, including:

I. Changes in gut microbiota composition particularly increased the number of bifidobacteria and butyrate-producing colon bacteria after feeding inulin.[44]

II. Fermentation of inulin- type fructans in the large bowel into short chain fatty acids(SCFAs) such as acetate, butyrate and propionate modulate inflammation by preventing the production of TNF-α and NF- κB.[45]

III. Butyrate and propionate induce intestinal gluconeogenesis which thereby improves glucose homeostasis.[32]

IV. Increased production of short chain fatty acids in colon may control the expression of some genes and miRNAs which are involved in glucose homeostasis.[46]

No study is without limitations and the limitations of this study include the small sample size and lack of measurement of some related factors such as inflammatory markers, serum levels of short-chain fatty acids and other genes expression related to glucose homeostasis. The strength of this study is that it was the first study investigating the beneficial effects of inulin supplementation on KLF5 and miR-375 expression in diabetic patients. In order to obtain further conclusive results and determine the exact related mechanisms, more studies with larger sample sizes are needed.

Conclusion

According to the effectiveness of inulin supplementation on glucose homeostasis through effective mechanisms like genes expression, this survey can be considered as a novel therapeutic approach in controlling diabetes. Our results revealed new insights into how KLF5 functions play a role in controlling diabetes. The newly identified KLF5- miR-375 pathway may contribute to diabetes progression. Inhibiting KLF5 may be a potential pharmacological intervention in controlling diabetes. With descriptions above, inulin supplementation maybe considered an adjunctive therapy for diabetic patients.

Acknowledgments

The authors would like to thank all the study participants, as well as nurses and doctors in the diabetes clinics in East Azerbaijan, Iran for their collaboration. The present study did not achieve any grants.

Ethical Issues

The Ethics committee of Tabriz University of Medical Science (Ethic code: IR.TBZMED.REC.1395.671) approved the research protocol of the study and a written informed consent document was obtained from all patients. The study was registered in the Iranian Registry of Clinical Trials website (IRCT ID: IRCT201610212017N31).

Conflict of Interest

The authors would like to gratitude the individuals who participated in this study.

Abbreviations

HP: high performance; KLF5: kruppel like factor 5; FPG: fasting plasma glucose; PBMCs: Peripheral blood mononuclear cells.

References

1. Qin J, Li Y, Cai Z, Li S, Zhu J, Zhang F, et al. A metagenome-wide association study of gut microbiota in type 2 diabetes. *Nature* 2012;490(7418):55-60. doi: 10.1038/nature11450

2. Pourghassem Gargari B, Dehghan P, Aliasgharzadeh A, Asghari Jafar-abadi M. Effects of high performance inulin supplementation on glycemic control and antioxidant status in women with type 2

diabetes. *Diabetes Metab J* 2013;37(2):140-8. doi: 10.4093/dmj.2013.37.2.140

3. Qin HL, Zheng JJ, Tong DN, Chen WX, Fan XB, Hang XM, et al. Effect of lactobacillus plantarum enteral feeding on the gut permeability and septic complications in the patients with acute pancreatitis. *Eur J Clin Nutr* 2008;62(7):923-30. doi: 10.1038/sj.ejcn.1602792

4. FAO Technical Meeting on Prebiotics. Food Quality and Standards Service (AGNS), Food and Agriculture Organization of the United Nations (FAO). Rome: FAO Technical Meeting Report; 2007.

5. Apolinario AC, de Lima Damasceno BP, de Macêdo Beltrão NE, Pessoa A, Converti A, da Silva JA. Inulin-type fructans: A review on different aspects of biochemical and pharmaceutical technology. *Carbohydr Polym* 2014;101:368-78. doi: 10.1016/j.carbpol.2013.09.081

6. Vogt L, Meyer D, Pullens G, Faas M, Smelt M, Venema K, et al. Immunological properties of inulin-type fructans. *Crit Rev Food Sci Nutr* 2015;55(3):414-36. doi: 10.1080/10408398.2012.656772

7. Franck A. Technological functionality of inulin and oligofructose. *Br J Nutr* 2002;87(S2):S287-91. doi: 10.1079/BJNBJN/2002550

8. Roshanravan N, Mahdavi R, Alizadeh E, Jafarabadi MA, Hedayati M, Ghavami A, et al. Effect of butyrate and inulin supplementation on glycemic status, lipid profile and glucagon-like peptide 1 level in patients with type 2 diabetes: A randomized double-blind, placebo-controlled trial. *Horm Metab Res* 2017;49(11):886-91. doi: 10.1055/s-0043-119089

9. Tsurumaki M, Kotake M, Iwasaki M, Saito M, Tanaka K, Aw W, et al. The application of omics technologies in the functional evaluation of inulin and inulin-containing prebiotics dietary supplementation. *Nutr Diabetes* 2015;5:e185. doi: 10.1038/nutd.2015.35

10. Kumar M, Verma V, Nagpal R, Kumar A, Gautam SK, Behare PV, et al. Effect of probiotic fermented milk and chlorophyllin on gene expressions and genotoxicity during AFB(1)-induced hepatocellular carcinoma. *Gene* 2011;490(1-2):54-9. doi: 10.1016/j.gene.2011.09.003

11. Wu Z, Wang S. Role of kruppel-like transcription factors in adipogenesis. *Dev Biol* 2013;373(2):235-43. doi: 10.1016/j.ydbio.2012.10.031

12. Forchielli ML, Walker WA. The role of gut-associated lymphoid tissues and mucosal defence. *Br J Nutr* 2005;93(S1):S41-8.

13. McConnell BB, Kim SS, Yu K, Ghaleb AM, Takeda N, Manabe I, et al. Kruppel-like factor 5 is important for maintenance of crypt architecture and barrier function in mouse intestine. *Gastroenterology* 2011;141(4):1302-13, 1313 e1-6. doi: 10.1053/j.gastro.2011.06.086

14. Shindo T, Manabe I, Fukushima Y, Tobe K, Aizawa K, Miyamoto S, et al. Kruppel-like zinc-finger transcription factor KLF5/BTEB2 is a target for angiotensin II signaling and an essential regulator of cardiovascular remodeling. *Nat Med* 2002;8(8):856-63. doi: 10.1038/nm738

15. Runtsch MC, Round JL, O'Connell RM. MicroRNAs and the regulation of intestinal homeostasis. *Front Genet* 2014;5:347. doi: 10.3389/fgene.2014.00347

16. Ventriglia G, Nigi L, Sebastiani G, Dotta F. MicroRNAs: Novel players in the dialogue between pancreatic islets and immune system in autoimmune diabetes. *BioMed Res Int* 2015;2015:749734. doi: 10.1155/2015/749734

17. Lorenzen J, Kumarswamy R, Dangwal S, Thum T. MicroRNAs in diabetes and diabetes-associated complications. *RNA Biol* 2012;9(6):820-7. doi: 10.4161/rna.20162

18. Masotti A. Interplays between gut microbiota and gene expression regulation by miRNAs. *Front Cell Infect Microbiol* 2012;2:137. doi: 10.3389/fcimb.2012.00137

19. Wu F, Zhang S, Dassopoulos T, Harris ML, Bayless TM, Meltzer SJ, et al. Identification of microRNAs associated with ileal and colonic crohn's disease. *Inflamm Bowel Dis* 2010;16(10):1729-38. doi: 10.1002/ibd.21267

20. Guess ND, Dornhorst A, Oliver N, Bell JD, Thomas EL, Frost GS. A randomized controlled trial: The effect of inulin on weight management and ectopic fat in subjects with prediabetes. *Nutr Metab (Lond)* 2015;12:36. doi: 10.1186/s12986-015-0033-2

21. IPAQ Group. Guidelines for Data Processing and Analysis of the International Physical Activity Questionnaire (IPAQ) – Short and Long Forms. IPAQ Group, 2005.

22. Livak KJ, Schmittgen TD. Analysis of relative gene expression data using real-time quantitative PCR and the 2− δδCT method. *Methods* 2001;25(4):402-8. doi: 10.1006/meth.2001.1262

23. Peltier HJ, Latham GJ. Normalization of microRNA expression levels in quantitative RT-PCR assays: Identification of suitable reference RNA targets in normal and cancerous human solid tissues. *RNA* 2008;14(5):844-52. doi: 10.1261/rna.939908

24. Pescador N, Pérez-Barba M, Ibarra JM, Corbatón A, Martínez-Larrad MT, Serrano-Ríos M. Serum circulating microRNA profiling for identification of potential type 2 diabetes and obesity biomarkers. *PLoS One* 2013;8(10):e77251. doi: 10.1371/journal.pone.0077251

25. Nagila A, Bhatt M, Poudel B, Mahato P, Gurung D, Prajapati S, et al. Thyroid stimulating hormone and its correlation with lipid profile in the obese nepalese population. *J Clin Diagn Res* 2008;2(4):932-7.

26. Yamashita K, Kawai K, Itakura M. Effects of fructo-oligosaccharides on blood glucose and serum lipids in diabetic subjects. *Nut Res* 1984;4(6):961-6. doi: 10.1016/S0271-5317(84)80075-5

27. Dehghan P, Gargari BP, Jafar-Abadi MA, Aliasgharzadeh A. Inulin controls inflammation and

metabolic endotoxemia in women with type 2 diabetes mellitus: A randomized-controlled clinical trial. *Int J Food Sci Nutr* 2014;65(1):117-23. doi: 10.3109/09637486.2013.836738

28. Alles MS, de Roos NM, Bakx JC, van de Lisdonk E, Zock PL, Hautvast JG. Consumption of fructooligosaccharides does not favorably affect blood glucose and serum lipid concentrations in patients with type 2 diabetes. *Am J Clin Nutr* 1999;69(1):64-9. doi: 10.1093/ajcn/69.1.64

29. Luo J, Rizkalla SW, Alamowitch C, Boussairi A, Blayo A, Barry JL, et al. Chronic consumption of short-chain fructooligosaccharides by healthy subjects decreased basal hepatic glucose production but had no effect on insulin-stimulated glucose metabolism. *Am J Clin Nutr* 1996;63(6):939-45. doi: 10.1093/ajcn/63.6.939

30. Dewulf EM, Cani PD, Claus SP, Fuentes S, Puylaert PG, Neyrinck AM, et al. Insight into the prebiotic concept: Lessons from an exploratory, double blind intervention study with inulin-type fructans in obese women. *Gut* 2013;62(8):1112-21. doi: 10.1136/gutjnl-2012-303304

31. Luo J, Van Yperselle M, Rizkalla SW, Rossi F, Bornet FR, Slama G. Chronic consumption of short-chain fructooligosaccharides does not affect basal hepatic glucose production or insulin resistance in type 2 diabetics. *J Nutr* 2000;130(6):1572-7. doi: 10.1093/jn/130.6.1572

32. Liu F, Prabhakar M, Ju J, Long H, Zhou HW. Effect of inulin-type fructans on blood lipid profile and glucose level: A systematic review and meta-analysis of randomized controlled trials. *Eur J Clin Nutr* 2017;71(1):9-20. doi: 10.1038/ejcn.2016.156

33. Pedersen A, Sandström B, Van Amelsvoort JM. The effect of ingestion of inulin on blood lipids and gastrointestinal symptoms in healthy females. *Br J Nutr* 1997;78(2):215-22.

34. Letexier D, Diraison F, Beylot M. Addition of inulin to a moderately high-carbohydrate diet reduces hepatic lipogenesis and plasma triacylglycerol concentrations in humans. *Am J Clin Nutr* 2003;77(3):559-64. doi: 10.1093/ajcn/77.3.559

35. Dehghan P, Pourghassem Gargari B, Asgharijafarabadi M. Effects of high performance inulin supplementation on glycemic status and lipid profile in women with type 2 diabetes: A randomized, placebo-controlled clinical trial. *Health Promot Perspect* 2013;3(1):55-63. doi: 10.5681/hpp.2013.007

36. Russo F, Chimienti G, Riezzo G, Pepe G, Petrosillo G, Chiloiro M, et al. Inulin-enriched pasta affects lipid profile and Lp(a) concentrations in italian young healthy male volunteers. *Eur J Nutr* 2008;47(8):453-9. doi: 10.1007/s00394-008-0748-1

37. Genta S, Cabrera W, Habib N, Pons J, Carillo IM, Grau A, et al. Yacon syrup: Beneficial effects on obesity and insulin resistance in humans. *Clin Nutr* 2009;28(2):182-7. doi: 10.1016/j.clnu.2009.01.013

38. Pedersen C, Lefevre S, Peters V, Patterson M, Ghatei MA, Morgan LM, et al. Gut hormone release and appetite regulation in healthy non-obese participants following oligofructose intake. A dose-escalation study. *Appetite* 2013;66:44-53. doi: 10.1016/j.appet.2013.02.017

39. Cicek B, Arslan P, Kelestimur F. The effects of oligofructose and polydextrose on metabolic control parameters in type-2 diabetes. *Pak J Med Sci* 2009;25(4):573-8.

40. Kaminskas A, Abaravičius JA, Liutkevičius A, Jablonskienė V, Valiūnienė J, Bagdonaitė L, et al. Quality of yoghurt enriched by inulin and its influence on human metabolic syndrome. *Vet Med Zoot* 2013;64(86):23-8.

41. Biton M, Levin A, Slyper M, Alkalay I, Horwitz E, Mor H, et al. Epithelial microRNAs regulate gut mucosal immunity via epithelium-t cell crosstalk. *Nat Immunol* 2011;12(3):239-46. doi: 10.1038/ni.1994

42. Gutiérrez-Aguilar R, Benmezroua Y, Vaillant E, Balkau B, Marre M, Charpentier G, et al. Analysis of klf transcription factor family gene variants in type 2 diabetes. *BMC Med Genet* 2007;8:53. doi: 10.1186/1471-2350-8-53

43. Kumekawa M, Fukuda G, Shimizu S, Konno K, Odawara M. Inhibition of monocyte chemoattractant protein-1 by kruppel-like factor 5 small interfering RNA in the tumor necrosis factor- α-activated human umbilical vein endothelial cells. *Biol Pharm Bull* 2008;31(8):1609-13. doi: 10.1248/bpb.31.1609

44. Delzenne NM, Daubioul C, Neyrinck A, Lasa M, Taper HS. Inulin and oligofructose modulate lipid metabolism in animals: Review of biochemical events and future prospects. *Br J Nutr* 2002;87(S2):S255-9. doi: 10.1079/BJNBJN/2002545

45. Place RF, Noonan EJ, Giardina C. HDAC inhibition prevents NF-κB activation by suppressing proteasome activity: Down-regulation of proteasome subunit expression stabilizes IκBα. *Biochem Pharmacol* 2005;70(3):394-406. doi: 10.1016/j.bcp.2005.04.030

46. Roshanravan N, Mahdavi R, Jafarabadi MA, Alizadeh E, Ghavami A, Saadat YR, et al. The effects of sodium butyrate and high-performance inulin supplementation on the promotion of gut bacterium Akkermansia muciniphila growth and alterations in miR-375 and KLF5 expression in type 2 diabetic patients: A randomized, double-blind, placebo-controlled trial. *Eur J Integr Med* 2018;18:1-7. doi: 10.1016/j.eujim.2017.12.011

23

Enhanced Lymphatic Uptake of Leflunomide Loaded Nanolipid Carrier via Chylomicron Formation for the Treatment of Rheumatoid Arthritis

Yadhu Krishnan, Shilpa Mukundan, Suresh Akhil, Swati Gupta, Vidya Viswanad*

Amrita School of Pharmacy, Amrita Institute of Medical Sciences and Research Centre, Amrita Vishwa Vidyapeetham, Kochi – 682041, India.

Keywords:
· Rheumatoid arthritis
· Lymphatic uptake
· Nano lipid carriers
· Leflunomide
· Chylomicron

Abstract

Purpose: The current study aims the lymphatic delivery of leflunomide loaded nanostructured lipid carriers (LNLC) for the treatment of rheumatoid arthritis, mainly focussed to enhance the lymphatic delivery via chylomicron formation, improved bioavailability and reduced systemic toxicity.

Methods: Melt emulsification ultra-sonication method was used to formulate the nanostructured lipid carrier (NLC) containing leflunomide. Four batches were prepared by using various concentration of surfactants (tween 80 and poloxmer 188) and lipid mixtures (stearic acid and oleic acid). All the formulations were studied for various physiochemical properties

Results: The formulation with increased concentration of lipid and surfactants showed highest entrapment efficiency ($93.96 \pm 0.47\%$) and better drug release (90.35%) at the end of 48 hrs. In vivo tests were carried out to determine the antiarthritic potential of the formulation in Sprague-dawley rats for a duration of 30d. The effect was evaluated by measuring the reduction in knee thickness. LNLC showed a marked reduction in inflammation compared to standard drug. Intestinal lymphatic uptake studies of LNLC were performed by intraduodenal administration and compared with leflunomide drug solution. The mesenteric lymph node was analysed by HPLC method and the concentration of drug was estimated. It showed that LNLC having highest uptake (40.34µg/ml) when compared with leflunomide drug solution (10.04µg/ml). Radiographic analysis and histopathological studies showed the formation of healthy cartilage after treatment period.

Conclusion: The results suggested that LNLC has the potential to reduce the systemic toxicities associated with conventional therapy along with improved efficacy in the treatment of rheumatoid arthritis.

Introduction

Rheumatoid arthritis (RA) is an autoimmune disease, which results in disabilities due to progressive inflammation & destruction of joints.[1] It is characterized by inflammation of synovial joint, production of auto antibodies, bone & cartilage deformities. The cause of RA is unknown, but it is believed that both genetic & environmental factors contribute RA.[2] Advances in understanding the pathogenesis involved in RA & developing drugs which target them brought a revolution in the treatment of RA. Different classes of drugs are used for the treatment, in which some are used to ease the symptoms & others are used to slow or stop the disease activity. Non-steroidal anti-inflammatory drugs (NSAIDs), disease modifying anti-rheumatic drugs (DMARDs), corticosteroids & biologic agents are the drug classes used for the treatment of RA. DMARDs are a class of anti-rheumatic drugs which not just treats the symptoms associated with the disease but acts on the immune system & modify the disease itself.[3,4] The treatment of RA with currently available DMARDs is based only on empirical observations.[5] Methotrexate, leflunomide, sulfasalazine & hydroxychloroquine are the most commonly prescribed DMARDs.[6] Leflunomide, a pyrimidine synthesis inhibitor, is a leading drug among DMARDs.[7] Leflunomide acts by modifying the inflammatory processes, particularly in RA.[8] The primary challenge in the treatment of RA with leflunomide is its systemic side effects including hepatotoxicity, allergic reactions etc. A site specific delivery of the drug can reduce these systemic side effects. Lymphatic system, which plays a great role in the pathogenesis of RA, is considered to be one of the effective delivery sites for the treatment of RA. A site specific delivery into the lymphatic system can be achieved by nano based drug delivery systems unlike conventional delivery systems. Thus the systemic and unwanted side effects can be avoided.[9]

For patient compliance, oral route of drug administration is mostly preferred.[10] But the oral route is having some limitations due to the physicochemical properties of the drugs including low permeability & solubility, instability & rapid metabolism which results in decreased

*Corresponding author: Vidya Viswanad, Email: vidyaviswanad@aims.amrita.edu

bioavailability. Most of the newly discovered drugs are having low solubility & high permeability belonging to BCS class-II. The bioavailability of orally administered lipophilic drugs is limited due to these characteristics.[11] The oral delivery of drug can be improved by drug transport through intestinal lymphatic system. NLCs, SLNs, liposomes & emulsomes are novel drug delivery systems designed to deliver drugs through the lymphatic systems & lipid based drug delivery systems are considered to be the best.[12]

Materials and Methods
Leflunomide was obtained as a gift sample from aarti pharmaceuticals, mumbai. Stearic acid as solid lipid purchased from nice chemicals, kerala, oleic acid as liquid lipid & tween 80 as surfactant was purchased from loba chemie pvt. Ltd. mumbai. Poloxamer 188 used as surfactant was purchased from research lab fine chem industries, mumbai. Methanol from nice chemicals, kerala. Adult female Sprague dawley rats weighing 200-250 g was obtained from central lab animal facility, AIMS, kochi.

Formulation of leflunomide loaded NLC
LNLC was prepared by melt emulsification ultrasonication method.[13] In this method the aqueous & oil phases were prepared separately & then mixed together. Aqueous phase was prepared by dissolving desired amount of surfactants in water under heating at 80°C with continuous stirring. Simultaneously lipid phase was prepared by melting a blend of solid lipid and liquid lipid at 80°C & the drug was dissolved in the melted lipid. Then the aqueous phase was added drop wise into the lipid phase at the same temperature by the aid of agitation at 600 rpm for 10 m & the pre emulsion obtained is further sonicated using a probe sonicator to form NLC. The optimization of the formulation was carried out using different ratios of lipids and surfactants which is mentioned in Table 1. To compare the particle size and zeta potential a formulation of leflunomide loaded SLN was also prepared by the same method without the incorporation of liquid lipid.

Table 1. Composition, particle size, zeta potential, polydispersivity index and percentage entrapment efficiency of drug loaded LNLC

Batch code	Drug (mg)	Stearic acid (%)	Oleic acid (%)	Tween 80 (%)	Poloxamer188 (%)	Particle size (nm)	PDI	Zeta potential	Entrapment efficiency (%)
F1	10	3.5	1.5	0.75	0.75	91.93±0.02	0.381±0.02	-25.3±2.7	93.96 ± 0.47
F2	10	3.5	1.5	0.25	0.75	92.54±17.00	0.607±0.12	-17.4±1.4	89.40 ± 0.50
F3	10	3	1.5	0.75	0.75	177.33±13.05	0.378±0.01	-21.8±4.0	91.86 ± 0.26
F4	10	3	1.5	0.25	0.25	45.66±3.34	0.0.452±0.06	-10.2±1.7	85.98 ± 0.52

Characterization of leflunomide loaded NLC
Particle size and Zeta potential
Particle size and zeta potential of LNLC was determined by differential light scattering (DLS) using a computerized inspection system by zeta sizer.[14] A particle size ranging 10-100 nm is found to be optimal for lymphatic uptake and retention in lymph node.[15]

Scanning electron microscopy and X-Ray diffraction
The morphological evaluation of LNLC was done by using scanning electron microscope (SEM). Information about the surface composition and topography of the samples will be obtained from the images produced by SEM. The sample was diluted & a drop of it was mounted on an aluminium stub with double sided adhesive carbon tape, it was dried & evaluated with SEM. The crystallinity and melting behaviour of the lipid nanoparticles were analyzed by DSC. Leflunomide API and LNLC were subjected to DSC analysis. The analysis was performed at a heating rate of 10°C/min between 30.0-300.0°C. XRD (X-ray diffraction) provide information on unit cell dimension used for phase identification of crystalline material. XRD analysis leflunomide API and lyophilized LNLC powder was performed in the range 2 θ. XRD data confirms the results of DSC analysis.

Determination of Entrapment efficiency
The entrapment efficiency was calculated by the indirect method in which the concentration of free drug in the aqueous phase of the dispersion was determined.

$$\text{Entrapment efficiency (\%)} = \frac{C_t - C_f}{C_t} \times 100$$

C_t – concentration of total amount of the drug added
C_f – concentration of free drug
In this technique, the LNLC was centrifuged at 10000 rpm at 5°C for 1 hr. After centrifugation, the supernatant obtained was diluted with 5ml methanol & the concentration of free drug (leflunomide) in the solution was quantified by UV spectroscopy analysis at 260nm. The study was performed in triplicate & the value was expressed as mean standard deviation.[11]

In vitro release study
In vitro drug release of entrapped drug (leflunomide) in NLCs was studied in phosphate buffer saline (PBS) of pH 7.4 using dialysis membrane. The dialysis membrane was activated by washing with running water for 3-4 h and treated with 0.3% sodium sulphide for 1m at 80°C followed by washing with hot water at 60°C for 2 m and acidified with 0.2% w/v sulphuric acid for a period of 1 m and finally rinse with hot water and stored in distilled water at refrigerated condition. PBS 7.4 was used as the dissolution medium. In order to determine the cumulative drug release, formulation containing 1mg of drug (2.5ml) was placed in an open end dialysis tube suspended in 30ml of phosphate buffer solution pH 7.4 at 37±1°C which was stirred at 50rpm. At predetermined time intervals, the samples were withdrawn and replaced with same amount of fresh medium. The withdrawn

samples were analysed spectrophotometrically at 260 nm.[14] Triplicate measurements were taken and results are expressed as mean standard deviation. The values that are obtained from the *in vitro* drug release study can be quantitatively analysed by using different mathematical formulae. The data obtained from *in vitro* drug release studies were plotted in various kinetic models: - Zero order drug release kinetics, first order release kinetics, Higuchi model and Korsmeyer peppas model.

Stability study

The optimized LNLC formulation was stored at room temperature (at 25°C) and refrigerator temperature (4-8°C) for a period of one month. Then the formulation was analysed for particle size (PS), polydispersity index (PDI) and entrapment efficiency (EE).

Haemocompatibility Analysis

The blood samples (5ml) was collected from healthy donor & immediately mixed with acid citrate dextrose (750µl) to prevent clotting. Then the blood sample was diluted with phosphate buffer saline (pH 7.4) in the ratio of 1:9. To the diluted blood samples different concentrations of nanoparticle formulation was added & incubated for 24 h. After 24 h, the sample was centrifuged at 3500 rpm for 10 min at 4°C. The supernatant was collected & transferred to a micro titre plate & taken absorbance at 540 nm using an Elisa plate reader. 0.1% triton X-100 treated blood sample was used as positive control.[15]

In vivo anti-inflammatory studies

In vivo anti-inflammatory studies were conducted on adult female Sprague dawley rats weighing 200-250 g. Four groups of animals having six each were housed in polypropylene cages, temperature maintained at 23±2°C. Lighting has to be controlled to supply 12 hrs light & 12 hrs dark for each 24 hr period. Chronic Arthritis will be induced by an intra-articular injection of 0.1 ml, of concentration 1 mg/ml complete freund's adjuant (CFA). Procedures were performed under isoflurane anaesthesia. After the development of arthritis-carrier, drug and formulation (0.1% w/v each) will be administered orally twice a week with an interval of 3 d between the doses for a period of 30 d to group II, III & IV respectively. The knee circumference (mm) of each group was measured from Day 1 - Day 30 using a digital micro meter. Data obtained was used to calculate percentage inflammation at different time points.[16]

Lymphatic uptake study by HPLC method

Sprague-dawley rats were selected for the *in vivo* intestinal lymphatic uptake study. The animals were divided into two groups, group-1 administered with standard leflunomide solution and group-2 with optimized leflunomide NLC formulation (LNLC) (F1). The tail vein of each rat was cannulated with a polyethylene tube under isoflurane anaesthesia. A small incision was made in the abdomen, the duodenum is located, and the LNLC formulation and drug solution was injected directly using a 1 mL syringe with a 31-gauge needle. The whole gastrointestinal tract will be then carefully replaced in the abdominal cavity, and the incision closed using clamps and kept moist by covering with gauze pads pre-soaked in normal saline. The rat was warmed using a lamp, and normal saline was infused at a rate of 1.5 mL per h during the experiment to rehydrate the rats. 1 h after administration of the LNLC and leflunomide drug solution, the rats were sacrificed, and isolate mesenteric lymph node. The mesenteric lymph nodes obtained was weighed and homogenized with four volumes of phosphate buffered saline using a homogenizer. After centrifugation, 200 µL aliquots of homogenate transferred to a new 2 mL tube, and add 1.5 mL of methanol.[17]

Estimation of liver enzymes (ALT, AST and ALP)

Liver injury can be diagnosed by certain biochemical markers like alanine aminotransferase [ALT], aspartate aminotransferase [AST] and alkaline phosphatase [ALP]. The blood samples for liver function test were given at merit labs, palarivatton, kochi, kerala. Elevations in serum enzyme levels are taken as the relevant indicators of liver toxicity. In this study, the liver toxicity was estimated based on the level of liver enzymes by using liver function test. Macroscopic and in particular histopathological observations and investigation of additional clinical biochemistry parameters allows confirmation of hepatotoxicity.

Histopathological studies

Histopathological analysis of liver samples of control, standard and test animals were carried out to confirm the ability of leflunomide NLC in reducing the liver toxicity, the systemic toxicity problem associated with pure drug. At the end of the study (after 30 d) the knee joints of standard and test group was subjected to histopathological analysis and compared with that of a normal animal's knee joint in order to confirm the better effectiveness of LNLC as anti-arthritic drug than leflunomide API.

Results and Discussion
Particle size and Zeta potential

Leflunomide loaded NLC was prepared by melt emulsification ultra-sonication method. A particle size of 10-100 nm was observed to be optimal for lymphatic uptake & due to the net negative charge of interstitial matrix, negatively charged lipid based drug delivery systems are reported to be showing higher lymphatic uptake compared to neutral & positively charged surfaces. The retention time of particles in lymph node increases with increase in negative charge.[18] In this study, F1 NLC formulation is found to be having a better PDI with an average particle size of 91.93 ± 4.70 nm and zeta potential -30 mV. As mentioned in Table 1 particle size is increased with high lipid content and increased surfactant concentration leading to higher viscosity of continuous phase resulting broadness of size distribution.[19] The prepared SLN were found to have a particle size of 257.14 ± 5.14nm and zeta potential of -26mV.

Scanning electron microscopy
The morphological characters of the optimized formulation F1 was evaluated using scanning electron

microscopy (SEM) analysis. Figure 1A shows the SEM photograph of LNLC which indicates that the particles were spherical and no drug crystals were visible. NLC aggregation has led to a particle size of 250nm while observed under SEM. Figure 1B shows the SEM photograph of LSLN with a particle size of more than 500nm due to aggregation.

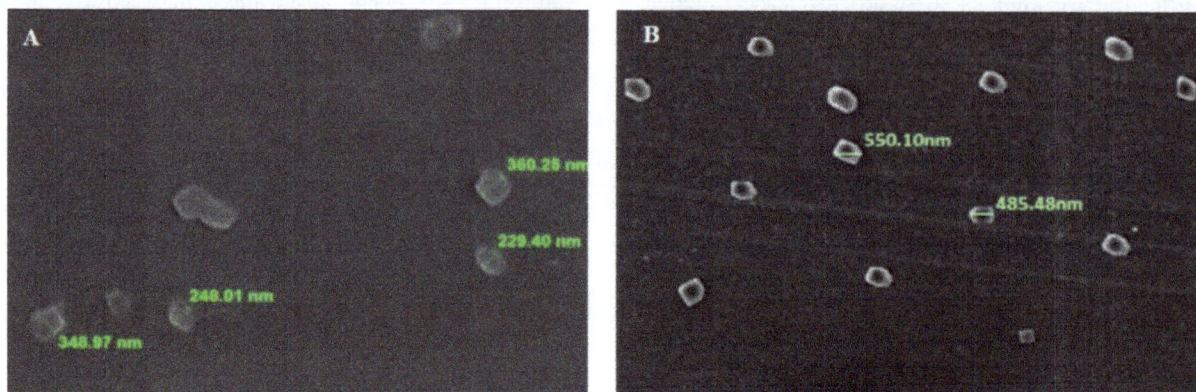

Figure 1. A: SEM image of leflunomide NLC and B: SEM image of leflunomide SLN

Differential scanning calorimetry and X-ray diffraction
The sharp peak at 167.03°C corresponds the melting peak of leflunomide was shown in Figure 2. The absence of endothermic peak within the melting range of leflunomide in the thermogram of LNLC formulation. Figure shows a complete solubilization of leflunomide in lipid matrix or transformation of leflunomide crystal to amorphous form that has been dispersed in the lipid matrix.[20]

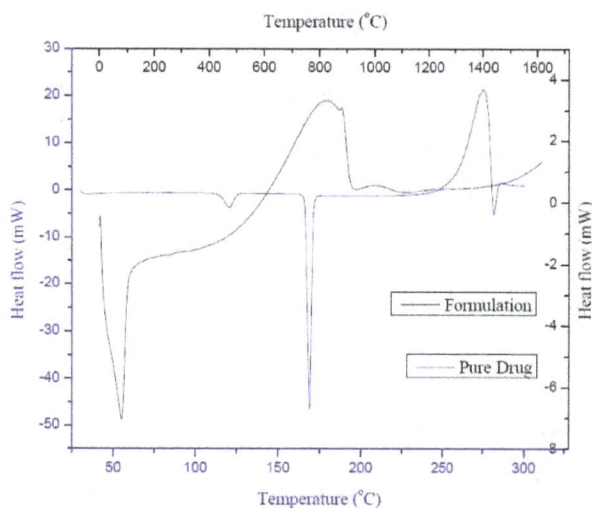

Figure 2. Differential scanning calorimetry of pure drug and drug loaded NLC formulation

The XRD of leflunomide in Figure 3 exhibits intense lines and characteristic peaks which indicates its crystallinity whereas XRD of lyophilized LNLC of F1 formulation in figure shows declined peaks indicating the possibility of converting crystalline to amorphous form.[21]

Entrapment efficiency
The percentage entrapment efficiency of the four different formulations (F1, F2, F3 and F4) was

determined and mention in Table 1. Formulation F1 is having the highest entrapment efficiency of 93.96 ± 0.47%. Entrapment efficiency of the formulations was found to be increased with increase in concentration of lipids and surfactants, because an increase in lipid content provide more space for incorporation of drugs and also reduces the tendency of drugs to escape into the external phase.[17] Surfactants increases the solubility of drugs in lipids, therefore entrapment efficiency will be increased with an increased concentration of surfactants.[18]

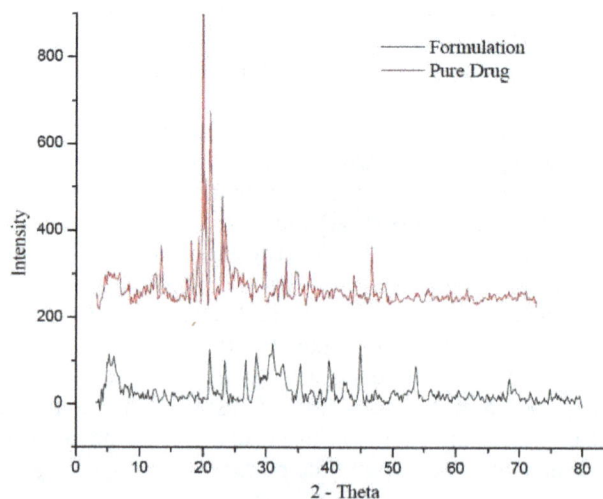

Figure 3. X-ray diffraction analysis of pure drug and drug loaded NLC formulation (F1)

In vitro release study
The in vitro release study of LNLC in phosphate buffer (pH 7.4) was studied for 48 h. The cumulative drug release was calculated and plotted against time. In the present study, the drug was entrapped or solubilized in the lipid matrix and thus lipid enhances absorption and bioavailability of the drug.[22] Here the highest amount of

drug release was observed with formulations having higher lipid concentration. Concentration of surfactants also plays an important role in drug release, since the drug release is found to be increased with an increase in surfactant concentration. The release rate of formulation F2 was found to be decreased with a reduction in concentration of tween-80 showing the significance of surfactants in drug release. Formulation F1 shows a better drug release with 90.35% release rate at 48 hrs. Based on the *in vitro* release studies, formulation F1 was found to be the best formulation for delivering leflunomide into the lymphatic system. Figure 4 shows the *in vitro* drug release of formulations F1, F2, F3 and F4. The data obtained from *in-vitro* drug release study was evaluated by fitting the data into zero order, first order, higuchi model and koresmeyer peppas model based on the R^2 value the release of the optimised formulation F1 was best fitted in higuchi model and the possible mechanism of drug release might be diffusion of drug from the matrix erosion resulting from degradation of lipids. The n value derived from koresmeyer peppas equation suggest that the mechanism of release follows a diffusion controlled model.

Stability Study

The purpose of stability study was to provide evidence that the product remains stable for a specified period of time. The particle size (PS), polydispersivity index (PDI)

and entrapment efficiency (EE) was measured to ensure that the product characteristics and drug content of the product remain unchanged. At room temperature after seven d, the product shows significant variation in the particle size, PDI and entrapment efficiency whereas at refrigerated temperature after 1 month, product did not show any significant variation. Therefore, from the results, which are mentioned in Table 2, we can say that LNLC formulation is more stable at refrigerated conditions whereas at room temperature it was not found to be stable.[23,24]

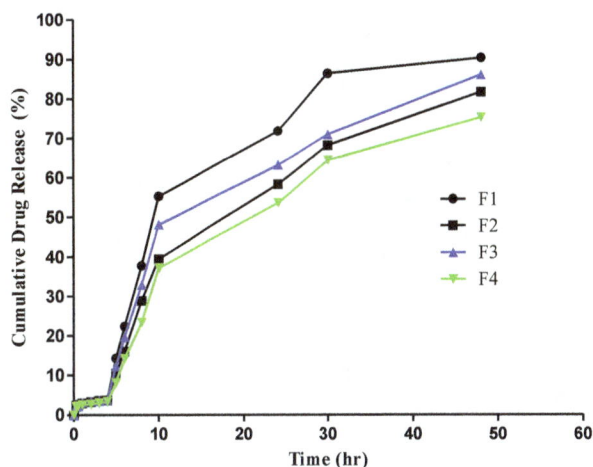

Figure 4. *In vitro* drug release of formulations F1, F2, F3 and F4

Table 2. Particle size, PDI and % entrapment of optimized formulation F1 on storage

Storage condition	Particle size (PS)	Polydispersity index (PDI)	Entrapment efficiency (EE)
At the time of preparation	86.90 ± 0.327	0.359 ± 0.034	90.62 ± 0.640
Room temperature (RT)	125.80 ± 0.543	0.475 ± 0.294	84.56 ± 0.587
Refrigerated temperature	97.21 ± 0.247	0.379 ± 0.095	87.28 ± 0.810

Haemocompatibility test

Haemocompatibility test is carried out to check the compatibility of the drug and formulation with blood, since it came in contact with the blood on *in vivo* administration. The test looks for bursting red blood cells. The degree of haemolysis is a sensitive indicator of the extent of damage to RBC. In the present study, different concentrations of optimized formulation F1 were tested and showed no evidence of haemolysis (<0.5%) after incubation for specified time period.[25,26] All the concentrations of F1 meet the standard, the data confirmed the optimized formulation F1 provides an acceptable level of haemolysis as shown in Figure 5.

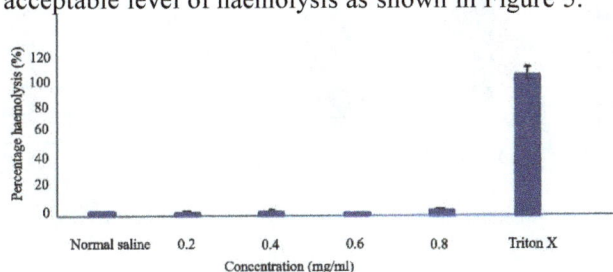

Figure 5. Percentage haemolysis of different concentration of optimized leflunomide loaded nlc in human blood

In vivo anti- inflammatory study

In vivo anti-inflammatory study was carried out in Sprague-dawley rats by complete freund's adjuant (CFA)[27] induced arthritis for a period of 30 d. The anti-arthritic potential of leflunomide NLC was evaluated by analysing its ability in inhibiting CFA induced knee edema. After the intra-articular injection of 1mg/ml of CFA, inflammation was developed in the left leg, it was then treated by using 0.1 % w/v of leflunomide NLC formulation twice weekly. The effect of the treatment was then evaluated by measuring the reduction in knee thickness which indicates anti-inflammatory action. Knee thickness was measured using digital micrometre was showed in Figure 6. The results of percentage knee edema after 30 d treatment was calculated and results shown in Figure 7. The standard and test group showed a marked reduction in inflammation over 30 d. Whereas the control and carrier group didn't show a significant reduction in inflammation. Test group showed more reduction in swelling compared to standard group which indicates leflunomide NLC is more effective in anti-arthritic activity than leflunomide drug solution.

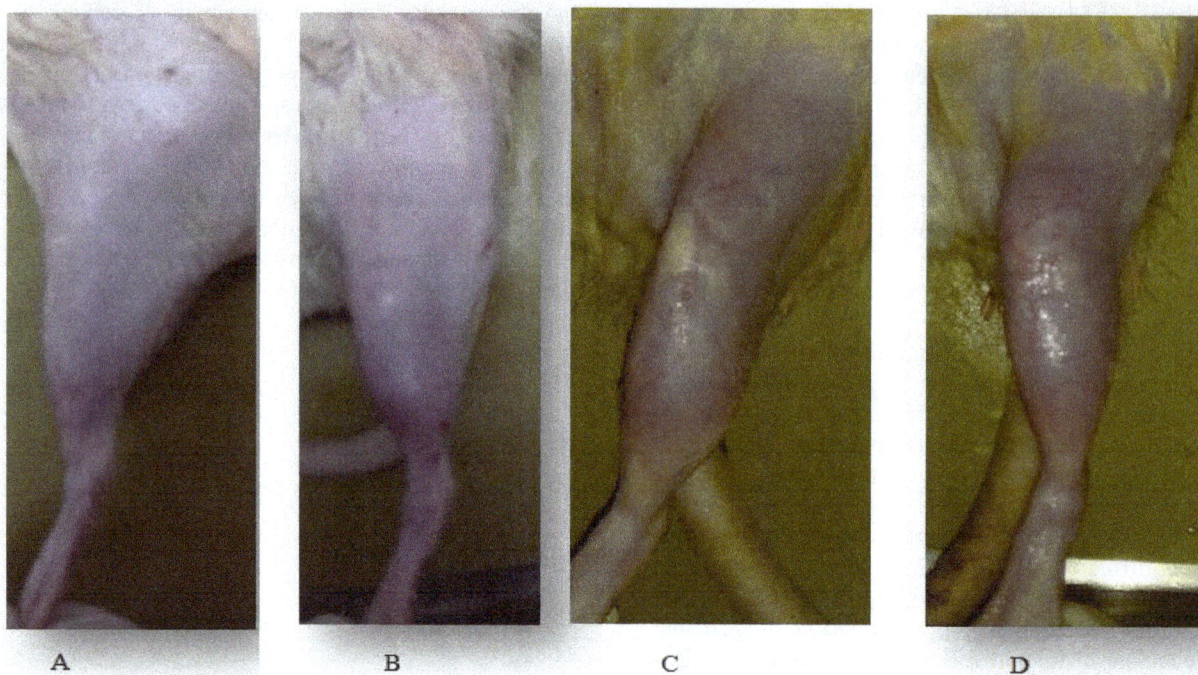

Figure 6. *In vivo* anti inflammatory studies for A) Control (no treatment), B) Carrier (NLC without drug), C) Standard (leflunomide drug solution), D) Test (optimized NLC formulation F1)

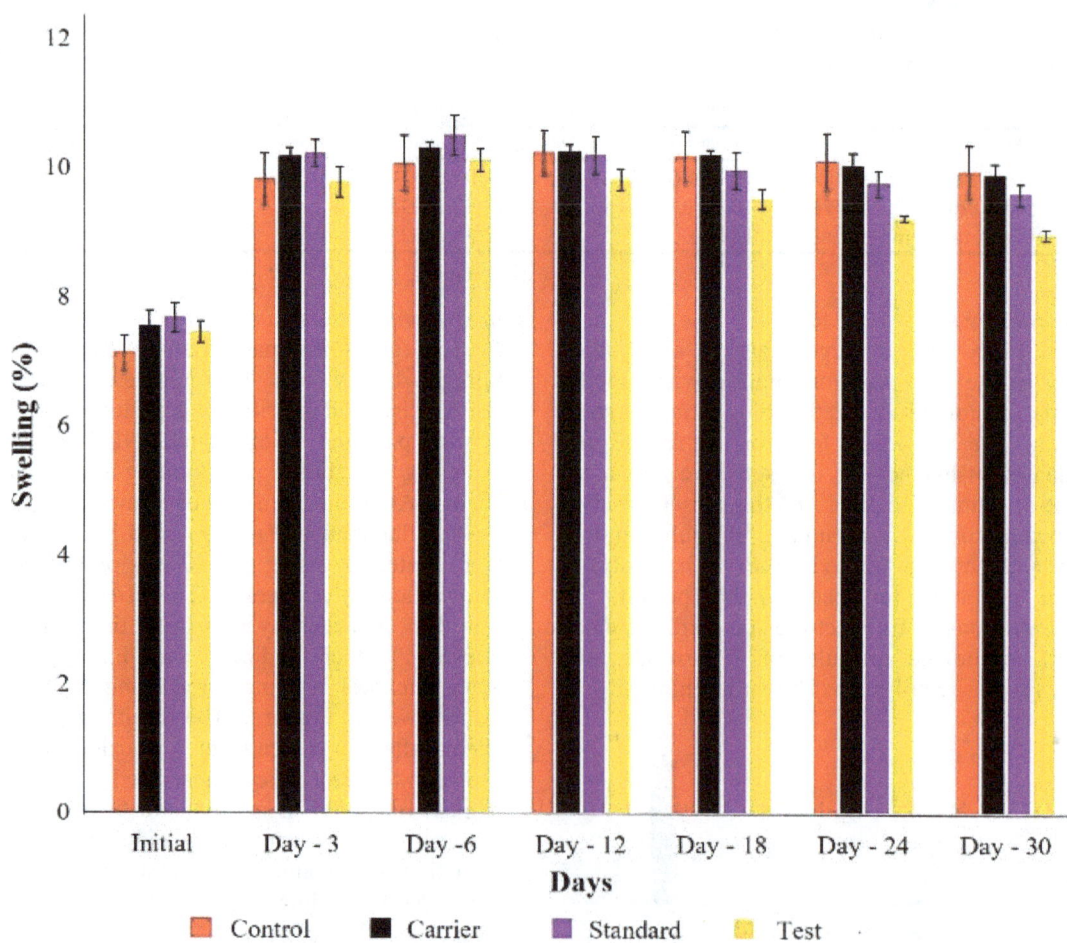

Figure 7. Percentage swelling in CFA induced inflammation

Determination of Lymphatic uptake by HPLC method

To evaluate the intestinal lymphatic uptake of leflunomide from NLC, the leflunomide content recovered from the mesenteric lymph node at specified time periods after intraduodenal administration of optimized leflunomide NLC formulations to Sprague-dawley rats was measured. The mesenteric lymph node is then analysed by HPLC method and the concentration of drug in the mesenteric lymph node at 1 hr after intraduodenal injection of leflunomide drug solution and leflunomide loaded NLC formulation was found to be 10.04μg/ml and 40.34μg/ml respectively. These results suggest that nano lipid carriers enhance the lymphatic uptake of leflunomide. It is well established that oral NLC facilitate the lymphatic uptake of drugs mainly via chylomicron formation. The results obtained from Figure 8A and 8B showed the significance of NLCs for site specific delivery of drugs into the lymphatic system.

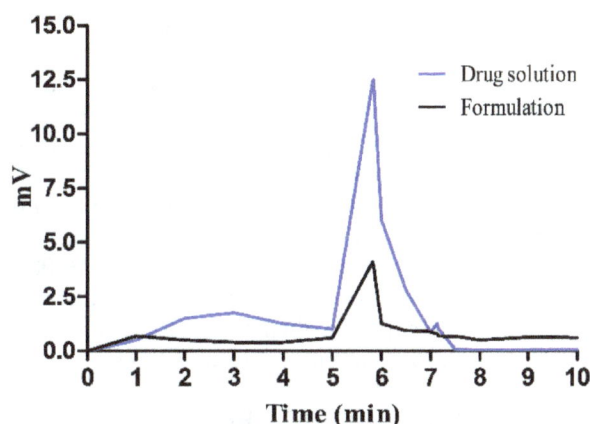

Figure 8. HPLC peak of pure drug solution and drug loaded NLC after lymphatic uptake study

Estimation of liver enzymes (ALT, AST and ALP)

Liver function test (LFT) was carried out in control animals and those administered with leflunomide loaded formulation (F1). Since the variation in the normal range of liver enzymes- alkaline phosphatase (ALP), serum glutamic oxalo transaminase (SGOT) or AST and serum glutamic pyruvic transaminase (SGPT) or ALT is an indication of liver toxicity, animals are subjected to LFT. The results as mentioned in Table 3, showed that the ALP and SGPT level found to be elevated in the standard group (leflunomide solution) compared to the test group (leflunomide NLC formulation F1) which indicates that leflunomide drug solution cause damage to the liver whereas in the optimized formulation (F1), the extent of inflammation was reduced and also the effect of leflunomide on liver was found to be in the normal level.

Table 3. ALT, AST and ALP level of standard and test group

Animal group	SGOT or AST (IU/L)	SGPT or ALT (IU/L)	ALP (IU/L)
Normal range in rats	85 - 123	25 - 36	136 - 188
Standard	128.9±9.02	40.1±5.8	209.3±10.4
LNLC	110.6±12	31.5±5.3	181.1±10.5

Histopathological studies

The histopathogical analysis of liver samples shows no evidence of liver toxicity in test group and the section of standard group shows liver damage since about 30% of hepatocytes show vacuolated cytoplasm, remaining hepatocytes are normal. Small necrotic areas are seen; these areas are replaced by inflammatory cells. Sinusoidal spaces appear congested whereas the section of test group shows normal structure. Portal traids and hepatic veins are normal. Some of the hepatocytes are vacuolated. Sinusoidal spaces and kupffer cells appear normal (Figure 9).

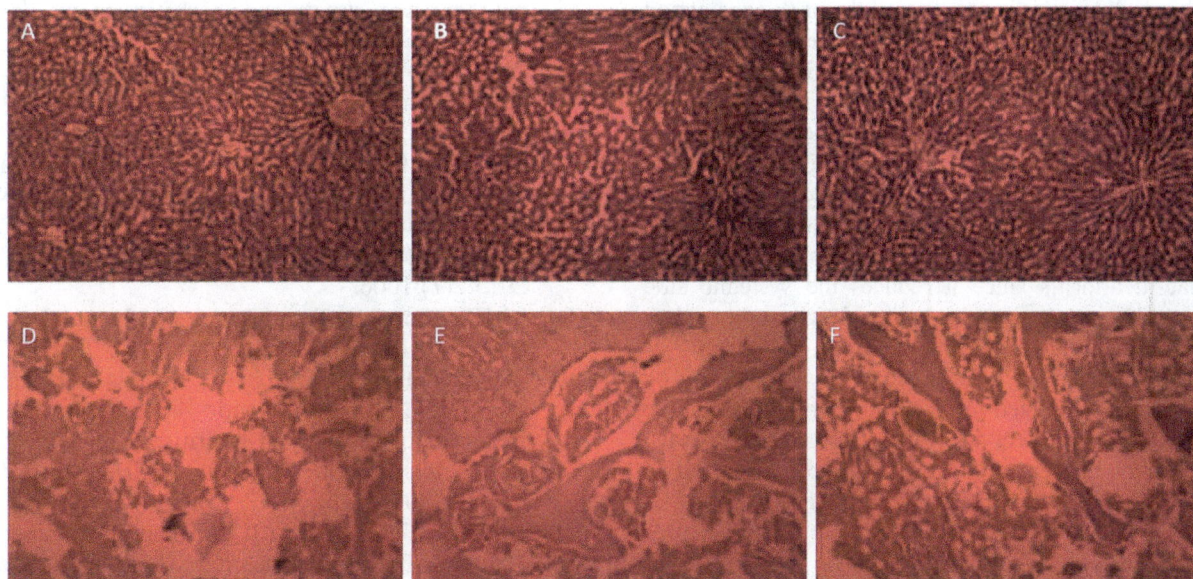

Figure 9. Histopathological analysis of liver samples of Control group (A), Standard group (B) showing liver damage, Test group (C) showing no liver damage. Histopathological analysis of knee joints of Normal group (D), Standard group (E) and Test group (F) seems to be more close to normal when compared with standard.

The histopathological study of a normal knee joint of Sprague dawley rat and that of standard and test group was carried out and the results shows the better efficacy of leflunomide NLC in the test group compared to the standard group. In the histopathological section of normal knee joint shows bony tissue with thin bony trabeculae. Osteocytes are normal. Cartilage also appears normal. Marrow is normocellular. Perosteum and surrounding tissue appear normal. Section of standard group shows thin bony trabeculae. Osteocytes are normal. Covering cartilage tissue also appear normal. Peristeum shows fibrosis and there are many collections of lymphocytes, plasma cells and polymorphs and in the test group, section shows bony trabeculae with normal osteocytes. Covering of cartilaginous tissue appear normal. Periosteal tissue shows fatty tissue with dense infiltrate of lymphocytes, plasma cells and polymorphs. The histopathology results of knee joints in Figure 9 shows that the test group section gives similar observations as that of the normal knee joint section compared to standard group.

Conclusion
Leflunomide is a disease modifying anti-rheumatic drug, which is reported to be equally effective as methotrexate in the treatment of rheumatoid arthritis. Conventional dosage forms of leflunomide are associated with systemic adverse effects and undergo first pass metabolism on oral delivery. In this study, leflunomide loaded nano lipid carrier (LNLC) for site specific delivery into lymphatic system through oral route was prepared, characterized and studied for various *in vitro* and *in vivo* evaluations. The study showed that, the lipids and surfactants used in the preparation has significant impact on particle size and surface charge which further influence the lymphatic uptake of the formulation. *In vitro* drug release studies confirmed the prolonged action and *in vivo* anti-inflammatory study proved the ability of drug loaded formulation to reduce systemic toxicities and improved anti-arthritic activity compared to conventional dosage form. The drug uptake study in mesenteric lymph node provides evidence for the capability of NLC for delivering drugs into intestinal lymphatics through oral route. It can be concluded that leflunomide loaded nano lipid carriers (LNLC) are better candidates for treating rheumatoid arthritis since it reduces the systemic side effects and improve the treatment efficacy compared to conventional dosage form of leflunomide.

In future, the synovial cell line study on SW982 can be done with the optimized formulation F1 to determine the anti-inflammatory effect of the drug. Through the *in vivo* animal study fluorescent imaging can be carried out to confirm the lymphatic uptake of drug loaded nano lipid carrier.

Ethical Issues
Animal approval was obtained from Central lab animal facility, AIMS, kochi. CPCSEA\Reg No 527\02\A\CPCSEA Dt 21\01\2002, renewal number – 527\PO\ReBi-S\Re-L\02\CPCSEA Dt 30\03\2017 (Ref No: IAEC\2016\1\7).

Conflict of Interest
The authors declare no conflict of interest. Authors are thankful to Amrita institute of medical sciences and research centre for proving the facilities for doing the work.

References
1. Lee EB, Fleischmann R, Hall S, Wilkinson B, Bradley JD, Gruben D, et al. Tofacitinib versus methotrexate in rheumatoid arthritis. *N Engl J Med* 2014;370(25):2377-86. doi: 10.1056/NEJMoa1310476
2. Choy E. Understanding the dynamics: Pathways involved in the pathogenesis of rheumatoid arthritis. *Rheumatology (Oxford)* 2012;51 Suppl 5:v3-11. doi: 10.1093/rheumatology/kes113
3. Cunninghame Graham DS, Morris DL, Bhangale TR, Criswell LA, Syvanen AC, Ronnblom L, et al. Association of ncf2, ikzf1, irf8, ifih1, and tyk2 with systemic lupus erythematosus. *PLoS Genet* 2011;7(10):e1002341. doi: 10.1371/journal.pgen.1002341
4. Kahlenberg JM, Fox DA. Advances in the medical treatment of rheumatoid arthritis. *Hand Clin* 2011;27(1):11-20. doi: 10.1016/j.hcl.2010.09.002
5. Emery P, Panayi G, Sturrock R, Williams B. Targeted therapies in rheumatoid arthritis: The need for action. *Rheumatology (Oxford)* 1999;38(10):911-2.
6. Singh JA, Furst DE, Bharat A, Curtis JR, Kavanaugh AF, Kremer JM, et al. 2012 update of the 2008 american college of rheumatology recommendations for the use of disease-modifying antirheumatic drugs and biologic agents in the treatment of rheumatoid arthritis. *Arthritis Care Res (Hoboken)* 2012;64(5):625-39. doi: 10.1002/acr.21641
7. Sultana N, Arayne MS, Khan MM, Afzal M. Synthesis Characterization and Anti-inflammatory Activity of Metal Complexes of 5-MethylN-[4-(Trifluoromethyl) Phenyl] Isoxazole-4-Carboxamide on Carrageenan Induced Arthritic Rats. *JSM Chem* 2013;2(1):1006.
8. LI EK, Tam LS, Tomlinson B. Leflunomide in the treatment of rheumatoid arthritis. *Clin Ther* 2004;26(4):447-59.
9. Pham CT. Nanotherapeutic approaches for the treatment of rheumatoid arthritis. *Wiley Interdiscip Rev Nanomed Nanobiotechnol* 2011;3(6):607-19. doi: 10.1002/wnan.157
10. Khan S, Baboota S, Ali J, Khan S, Narang RS, Narang JK. Nanostructured lipid carriers: An emerging platform for improving oral bioavailability of lipophilic drugs. *Int J Pharm Investig* 2015;5(4):182-91. doi: 10.4103/2230-973x.167661

11. Chaudhary S, Garg T, Murthy RS, Rath G, Goyal AK. Development, optimization and evaluation of long chain nanolipid carrier for hepatic delivery of silymarin through lymphatic transport pathway. *Int J Pharm* 2015;485(1-2):108-21. doi: 10.1016/j.ijpharm.2015.02.070

12. Chaudhary S, Garg T, Murthy RS, Rath G, Goyal AK. Recent approaches of lipid-based delivery system for lymphatic targeting via oral route. *J Drug Target* 2014;22(10):871-82. doi: 10.3109/1061186x.2014.950664

13. Zheng M, Falkeborg M, Zheng Y, Yang T, Xu X. Formulation and characterization of nanostructured lipid carriers containing a mixed lipids core. *Colloid Surf A Physicochem Eng Asp* 2013;403:76-84. doi: 0.1016/j.colsurfa.2013.03.070

14. Rajendran S, Ramesh S, Kumar S, Rao SR. In vitro release kinetics of simvastatin from methyl cellulose gel. *Int J Pharm Pharm Sci* 2015;7(10):106-10.

15. Dhanalakshmi V, Nimal TR, Sabitha M, Biswas R, Jayakumar R. Skin and muscle permeating antibacterial nanoparticles for treating staphylococcus aureus infected wounds. *J Biomed Mater Res B Appl Biomater* 2016;104(4):797-807. doi: 10.1002/jbm.b.33635

16. Levy AS, Simon O, Shelly J, Gardener M. 6-shogaol reduced chronic inflammatory response in the knees of rats treated with complete freund's adjuvant. *BMC Pharmacol* 2006;6:12. doi: 10.1186/1471-2210-6-12

17. Cho HJ, Park JW, Yoon IS, Kim DD. Surface-modified solid lipid nanoparticles for oral delivery of docetaxel: Enhanced intestinal absorption and lymphatic uptake. *Int J Nanomedicine* 2014;9:495-504. doi: 10.2147/ijn.s56648

18. Ali Khan A, Mudassir J, Mohtar N, Darwis Y. Advanced drug delivery to the lymphatic system: Lipid-based nanoformulations. *Int J Nanomedicine* 2013;8:2733-44. doi: 10.2147/ijn.s41521

19. Velmurugan R, Selvamuthukumar S. Unsatisfied processing conditions in making ifosfamide nanostructured lipid carriers: Effects of various formulation parameters on particle size, entrapment efficiency and drug loading capacity. *J Pharm Negative Results* 2014;5(1):8-12. doi: 10.4103/0976-9234.136775

20. Shah NV, Seth AK, Balaraman R, Aundhia CJ, Maheshwari RA, Parmar GR. Nanostructured lipid carriers for oral bioavailability enhancement of raloxifene: Design and in vivo study. *J Adv Res* 2016;7(3):423-34. doi: 10.1016/j.jare.2016.03.002

21. Garg AK, Sachdeva RK, Kapoor G. Comparison of crystalline and amorphous carriers to improve the dissolution profile of water insoluble drug itraconazole. *Int J Pharm Bio Sci* 2013;4(1):934-48.

22. Kalepu S, Manthina M, Padavala V. Oral lipid-based drug delivery systems – an overview. *Acta Pharm Sin B* 2013;3(6):361-72. doi: 10.1016/j.apsb.2013.10.001

23. Reshmi KP, Zachariah SM, Viswanad V. Formulation and evaluation of novel chromene derivatives as an anti-inflammatory agent used for inflammatory bowel diseases. *Asian J Pharm Clin Res* 2017; 10(2):319-24. doi: 10.22159/ajpcr.2017.v10i2.15696

24. Shammika P, Aneesh TP, Viswanad V. Solubility enhancement of synthesized quinazolinone derivative by solid dispersion technique. *Int J Pharm Sci Rev Res* 2016;41(2):197-206.

25. Divya G, Panonnummal R, Gupta S, Jayakumar R, Sabitha M. Acitretin and aloe-emodin loaded chitin nanogel for the treatment of psoriasis. *Eur J Pharm Biopharm* 2016;107:97-109. doi: 10.1016/j.ejpb.2016.06.019

26. Panonnummal R, Jayakumar R, Sabitha M. Comparative anti-psoriatic efficacy studies of clobetasol loaded chitin nanogel and marketed cream. *Eur J Pharm Sci* 2017;96:193-206. doi: 10.1016/j.ejps.2016.09.007

27. Nimitha VV, Parvathy S, Sreeja C Nair, Vidya Viswanad. Leflunomide loaded solid lipid nanoparticle in rheumatoid arthritis. *Int J Pharm Technol* 2017;9(2):29681-706.

24

Chemical Enhancer: A Simplistic Way to Modulate Barrier Function of the Stratum Corneum

Tasnuva Haque[1], Md Mesbah Uddin Talukder[2]*

[1] Department of Pharmacy, East West University, A/2, Jahurul Islam City Gate, Aftab Nagar Main Rd, Dhaka-1212, Bangladesh.

[2] Department of Pharmacy, BRAC University, 66 Bir Uttam AK Khandakar Road, Dhaka 1212, Bangladesh.

Keywords:
· Barrier function
· Chemical enhancer
· Drug delivery
· Modification of skin
· Stratum corneum

Abstract

Human skin could be a prime target to deliver drugs into the human body as it is the largest organ of human body. However, the main challenge of delivering drug into the skin is the stratum corneum (SC), the outer layer of epidermis, which performs the main barrier function of the skin. Scientists have developed several techniques to overcome the barrier properties of the skin, which include other physical and chemical techniques. The most common and convenient technique is to use special formulation additives (chemical enhancers, CEs) which either drags the drug molecule along with it or make changes in the SC structure, thereby allowing the drug molecule to penetrate in to the SC. The main focus is to deliver drugs in the certain layers of the skin (for topical delivery) or ensuring proper percutaneous absorption (for transdermal delivery). However, skin drug delivery is still very challenging as different CEs act in different ways on the skin and they have different types of interaction with different drugs. Therefore, proper understanding on the mechanism of action of CE is mandatory. In this article, the effect of several CEs on skin has been reviewed based on the published articles. The main aim is to compile the recent knowledge on skin-CE interaction in order to design a topical and transdermal formulation efficiently. A properly designed formulation would help the drug either to deposit into the target layer or to cross the barrier membrane to reach the systemic circulation.

Introduction

Since skin is the largest organ of the body, it could be a potential route to deliver drugs into the body. However, barrier property of the outer layer of the skin (stratum corneum, SC) limits the delivery of all types of drug in skin. Topical and transdermal formulations are delivered through the skin, targeting different layers of the skin and systemic circulation, respectively. Topical formulation delivers therapeutically effective concentration of a compound in the specific layer of the skin, to impart a local effect. As for example, sunscreen targets the outer layer of the skin,[1] topical analgesic aims dermal-epidermal layer to reach cutaneous nociceptors,[2] topical antifungals to viable epidermis,[3] etc. In order to reach the specific layer of the skin and systemic circulation, a drug molecule must cross the SC and this only possible if barrier property of the skin is overcome. Chemical enhancers (CEs) are chemical agents which modify the SC barrier function and thereby allow molecules to penetrate into the skin. However, the penetration abilities of CEs changes as different CE interact with drug or skin differently. This article aims to summarize the recent findings on some commonly used CEs so that their incorporation into the formulation can develop more effective topical or transdermal or cosmetic products.

Anatomy of skin

Skin has primarily three layers – epidermis (outer layer), dermis (middle layer) and subcutaneous tissue (bottom layer) (Figure 1).[4] Epidermis contains five different cell strata. From outside to inside, these are stratum corneum (SC), stratum lucidum, stratum granulosum, stratum spinosum and stratum basale. The dermis consists of collagen fibrils and elastic connective tissues.[5] This layer also contains mast cells, macrophages, lymphocytes and melanocytes.[6] Immune and inflammatory responses are provided by the mast cells.[7] Blood vessels, nerves and skin appendages (sweat and sebaceous glands) are also present in this layer. Because of the structural composition, this layer does not offer the same resistance to drugs as the SC. However, reduced permeation of lipophilic drugs may be observed in this layer.[7] In the dermis, there are some sensory receptors such as thermoreceptors which sense temperature, nociceptors which sense pain and some mechanoreceptors which sense touch and pressure. The mechanoreceptors consist of Messiner's corpuscles and Pacinian corpuscles which recognize light touch and pressure, respectively[6] (Figure 1). The subcutaneous tissue is the inner layer containing fat cells interconnected by collagen and elastin fibres. This layer produces and stores large quantities of fat. It also protects the body from mechanical shock and stores large quantities of calories.[5,7]

There are several appendages present in the dermis and epidermis of human skin, such as eccrine and apocrine sweat glands, sebaceous glands, hair follicles and nails (Figure 1).

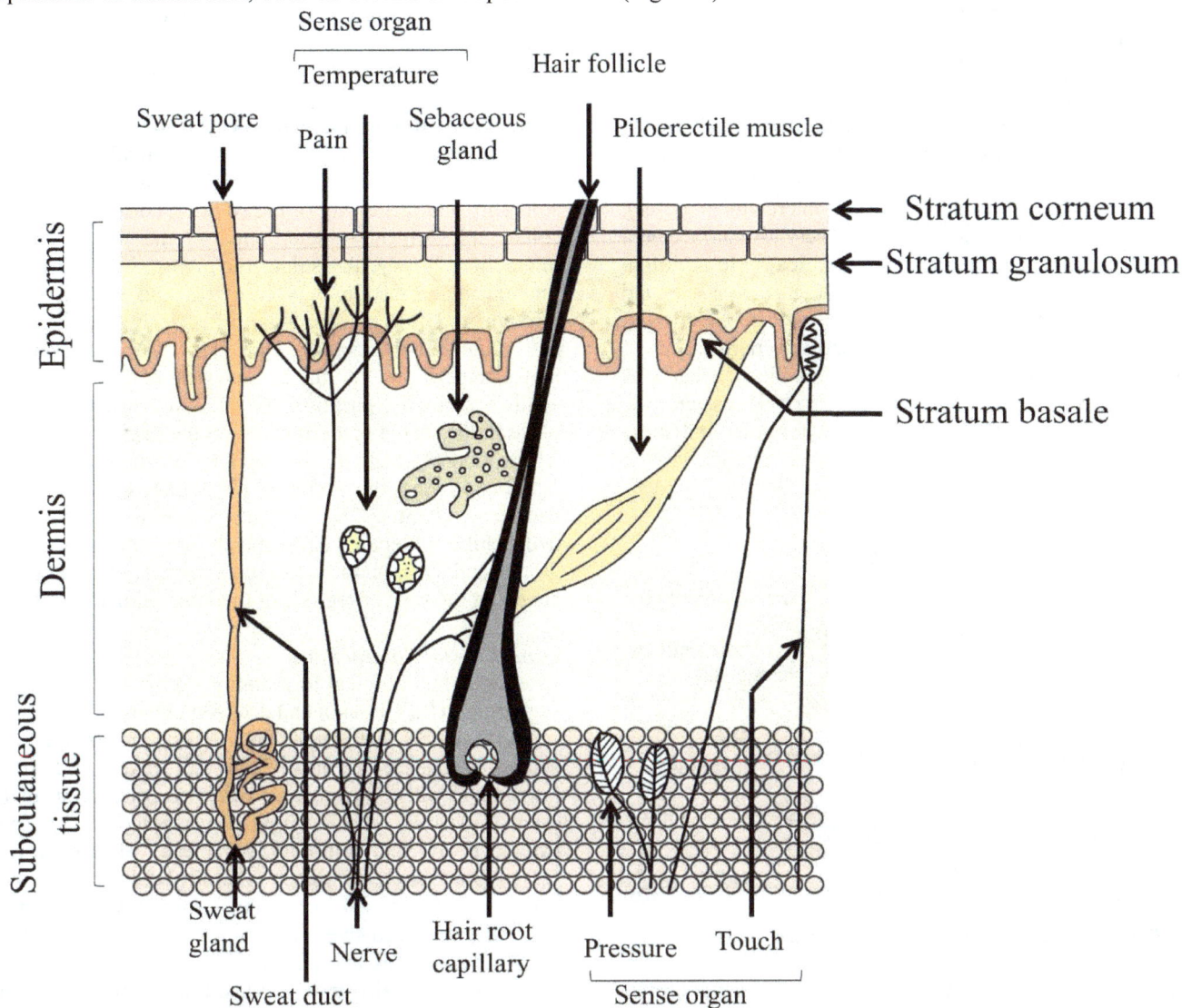

Figure 1. Structure of human skin

Stratum corneum (SC), the main barrier of the skin

The SC is the outermost layer of epidermis having a heterogeneous structure and composed of 70 to 80% protein (keratin) and lipid.[7] It provides the main barrier function of the skin. The SC is composed of 10 to 15 layers of compressed corneocytes present in the SC.[5,8] Between the SC corneocytes different types of lipids are present.[9] If the SC is picturized as a brick wall, the corneocytes are the 'bricks' present in a 'mortar' (or intercellular lipid matrix).[10] Desmosomes are the connectors between the corneocytes. The corneocyte is surrounded by a protein-lipid polymeric envelope.[7] The corneocytes are rigid because of the envelope.[11] The intercellular space between corneocytes is filled with multiple lipid lamellae. The lamellae consist of ceramides, cholesterol, cholesterol esters, cholesterol sulphate and free fatty acids.[7,12] The lipid lamellae are arranged horizontally to the surface of the corneocytes.[13,14]

Intercellular lipids act as shields to prevent water loss from the body.[15] If the lipid from the SC is extracted, the lipid from the SC enhanced the water loss faster compared with non-extracted skin.[16] Thus, intercellular lipid lamellae are very important for the barrier function of the SC and also help in cohesion between corneocytes.[17] The SC also contains approximately 15 to 20% water mainly associated with keratin[7] and a small amount in the polar head group of the intercellular space.[18] The lower water loss and higher barrier function of the SC is because of the unique composition, especially due to the intercellular lipids and corneocyte envelope.[18,19] The epidermis undergoes a differentiation process in which generation of the SC takes place. The process starts at the stratum basale and cells migrate upwards to the SC and it usually takes 2 to 3 weeks.[6]

Routes of permeation in the SC

Diffusion is the principle mechanism by which the permeation of a permeant across human skin takes place.[20] A solute can diffuse through the skin by three main routes: the transappendageal route, the intracellular and intercellular route (Figure 2). Permeation through the transappendageal route is known as the permeation via the hair follicles, sebaceous and sweat glands. Appendageal transport provides an easier path of diffusion in parallel to the transepidermal route (intra- and intercellular routes). However, the skin appendages have very low surface area (only 0.1% of the total skin surface area).[21] In addition, permeation of drugs is not direct in the sweat and sebaceous glands. Sweat moves in the reverse direction of the permeant in sweat gland. Moreover, permeation of only hydrophilic molecules is not possible in sebaceous glands as it has lipid-rich sebum.[22] However, the transappendageal route can be vital for ions and large polar molecules which do not freely cross the SC.[23-25]

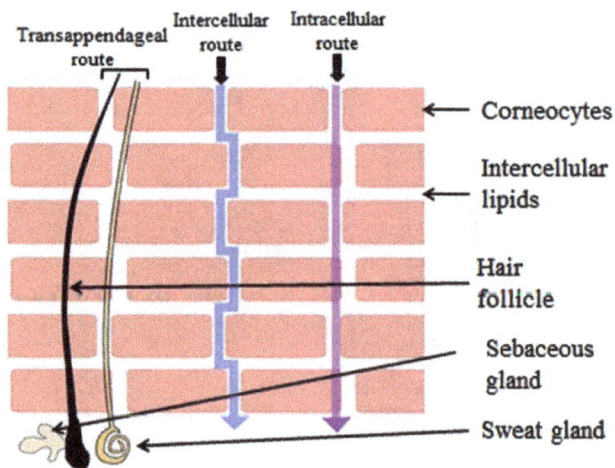

Figure 2. Routes of penetration of a molecule across the SC

Transepidermal pathway is the route which includes intra- and intercellular permeation. If the SC structure is considered as 'brick and mortar', the intracellular is the shortest route through the layers of corneocytes and its surrounding intercellular lipid matrix. When such penetration takes place in a tortuous way via the intercellular lipid matrix, it is called the intercellular route. At first it was believed that hydrophilic drugs preferentially diffuse through the intracellular region and hydrophobic drugs through the intercellular matrix[21]. In both cases, the compound has to penetrate the intercellular lipid. However, later it was found that the intercellular route was the predominant pathway for permeation of most drugs through the human SC.[26-29] Diffusion of a penetrant through the intracellular route requires undergoing via a series of partitioning and diffusion stages in and out of the relatively hydrophilic corneocytes, lipid envelope surrounding the corneocytes and the intercellular matrix. Whereas, the penetrant needs to take a tortuous route consisting of alternating structures of bilayers (containing both aqueous and lipid domains) in the intercellular route. In this route of permeation, a

penetrant passes through a 50-times longer path length compared with the total thickness of the SC. A penetrant also has to undergo sequential partition and diffusion through the aqueous and lipid domains of the intercellular matrix.[22]

Permeation of drug molecule across the skin

The percutaneous absorption of a solute involves a series of transport processes which is mainly determined by the solubility and diffusivity of the solute. The solubility of a solute in a solvent is determined by the solvent-solute interaction. Firstly, the solute requires to be solubilised into the outermost lipid layer of SC and then diffuses through it. These processes are affected by the CE-skin and solute-skin interactions. During this process the solute may also permeate into the corneocytes. In the next stage, again a series of partition followed by diffusion takes place in the viable epidermis and in the papillary dermis. Absorption of solute by the capillary plexus followed by distribution into the systemic circulation occurs in the papillary dermis. Being the prominent pathway, hydrophilic molecules permeate through the polar head groups and hydrophobic molecules permeate via the lipid chains of the bilayer regions of the intercellular route.[30]

Drug-CE-skin interactions

After applying a topical formulation on the surface of the skin, drug - CE, CE -skin and drug-skin interactions[30] may occur. Drug-CE interactions have effects on the rate and extent of release of drug from the solvent. CE-skin interactions either increase or decrease penetration of a drug across the skin.[31] Drug-CE interaction may be explained by the solubility parameter. Higher drug-solvent interaction (or higher solubility of the drug in the solvent) will be evident if the solubility parameter difference between these two is low.[30] However, if the drug molecule has a higher affinity for the CE it may remain preferentially in the CE and low permeation of the drug will be observed.[20] Solvent-skin interaction will be discussed in section 3 of this article. Drug-skin interaction is mainly affected by the physicochemical properties (molecular weight, log P, melting point and solubility parameter) of the drug. Drug-solvent-skin interactions may be explained by the 'push-pull' effect (Figure 3).[32]

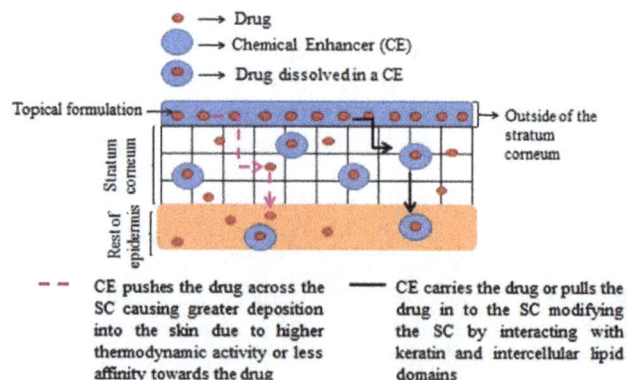

Figure 3. Interaction of CEs with the stratum corneum ('Push-pull'-effect).

'Push' effects are of two types. If the solubility parameter difference between drug and CE is high, attraction of drug will be lower towards the CE and the drug will be easily escaped into the skin from the CE.[30,32] Drugs having higher affinity for the CE, it will be held firmly by the CE and will not allow to penetrate through the SC.[20]Additionally, by increasing the thermodynamic activity, the drug will be pushed into the SC by the CE.[20,32,33] The 'pull' effect explains that CEs change the SC by structural transformation and therefore, increase the solubility of the drug into the SC or drag the drug molecule while diffusing through the skin.[32,33]

Modification of the SC to enhance drug penetration

There are physical and chemical methods to enhance the penetration of a drug in the skin. Physical enhancers involve iontophoresis, sonophoresis, phonophoresis, magnetophoresis, electroporation, thermophoresis, radiofrequency, needleless injection, microneedle etc. Both techniques involve alter the SC in such a way so that drug can penetrate the SC and reach the target site. Here, the effect of different classes of CE on skin will be discussed elaborately.

Chemical enhancers (CEs)

'CEs are pharmacologically inactive compounds which partition and diffuse into the skin and interact with SC components'. They are generally regarded as safe.[34] CEs increase the permeation of drugs by interacting with the intracellular route, interacting in the intercellular route and by modifying the solubility or partition of the SC. In the intercellular route, the solute can interact with the polar head group,in the aqueous regions of intercellular bilayers and interacting in the lipid regions of intercellular bilayers. The skin penetration abilities of selected CEs are discussed below:

Water

Water is the most common and safe penetration enhancer which is used for transporting both drug and cosmetic materials into the skin. Hydrating the skin or using moisturisers can be easiest way to deliver hydrophilic molecules effectively. The water content of the SC is usually 5 to 10%, which can be increased up to 50% under occlusive condition.[35] In 1987, Barry reported that water molecule acts in both inter and intra-cellular pathways to enhance the permeation of both hydrophilic and lipophilic drugs.[36] In case of intracellular region, in dry condition, the SC provides significant barrier to drug molecules because of the presence of several hydrogen bonding group. Since the SC becomes hydrated, the proteinaceous region takes up water. The arrangement of protein of that region becomes disordered and water starts competing for the hydrogen binding sites on the protein, and therefore, reduces the interaction between them. In this way, permeation of molecule through the intracellular pathway increases.[36,37] Barry also stated that water molecule binds with the polar head group and forms a small hydration shell in the lipid bilayer region via hydrogen bonding.

This leads to loosening of lipid packing and extending hydrophilic domain.[36] However, later studies found that water does not cause a massive lipid disorder,[38] it may cause slight disordering of a small population of the SC lipid.[39] Water also found not to swell lipid bilayer but can be present in very small quantities in the polar head group of the lipid bilayer region.[18] The excess amount of water the SC absorbs may be present in the corneocytes (intracellular region) or may be present as a separate phase in the intercellular region.[18,40]

Alcohols

In short chain alcohols, ethanol is the most widely used and studied CE for skin drug delivery in topical and transdermal formulations. Ethanol is also used in such formulations to aid solubility of poorly water soluble drugs or as a cosolvent.[41] At low concentration, ethanol displaces the bound water in the polar head group and disrupts the lipid-polar head/membrane interfacial region. This leads to increase in the interfacial area. At high concentration, ethanol extract lipid and proteins from the SC and thus forms pores in the SC0.[18,42] Ethanol helps penetrating the drug by increasing the solubility in the formulation and by altering the solubility parameter of the SC towards the drug. The residence time of ethanol on skin is short due to its volatile nature.[43] Therefore, higher thermodynamic activity of the drug dissolved in ethanol pushes the drug molecule into or across the SC. In addition, ethanol rapidly penetrates the SC by the mechanisms stated above, which also pulls the drug molecule along with it through the SC.[42] Recently, Moghadam et al. reported no change in short and long lamellar spacing of the SC structure by ethanol. The authors suggested that the penetration enhancing property of ethanol might be due to the solvent's ability to solubilise drug molecule into the SC.[44]

Fatty or long chain alcohol showed a parabolic relationship with the permeation of melatonin with the carbon chain length of saturated fatty alcohol. Melatonin permeation was found to increase up to chain length of 10 carbons (decanol) and then decreases. Decanol caused highest permeation enhancement for melatonin.[45] Lipid extraction was the mechanism of enhancing the permeation of drug for D-hexanol and D-octanol. However, D-decanol was not found to disrupt the lipid content.[46]

Amides

Azone

Azone (Laurocapram) is the first compound which was specially developed as a penetration enhancer.[35] Azone contains a seven membered polar head group attached with its 12 carbon chain.[43] It mainly reduces diffusional resistance of a drug into the SC.[43] Because of this structure, it is inserted into the lipid bilayer region with the seven-membered polar group in the polar plane and the dodecyl chain in the lipid region. In this way, it disrupts the highly ordered lipid packing of the lipid bilayer.[18,35] Azone has been found to increase permeation of hydrophilic, hydrophobic and some peptides. This CE is effective at low concentration (1 to 5%).[35] Azone imparts its penetration enhancing property more efficiently in conjunction with propylene glycol (PG) rather than alone. Azone only modifies the intercellular region; however, PG acts in the intracellular pathway. Therefore, combination of these two CEs efficiently delivered a number of drug molecule.[36] Although Azone has been investigated as a CE for over 25 years,[35] still it is not used in any commercial formulation.[43]

Esters
Alkyl and benzoic acid esters
Ethyl acetate has been found to increase permeation of levonorgestrel. However, its exact mechanism of action is not confirmed yet.[43] Another ester compound, octyl salicylate (OS) is used as a sunscreen at a concentration up to 5%. OSAL is also found to enhance the penetration of fentanyl and testosterone.[43,47,48] Being a lipophilic solvent, OS previously found to alter the highly ordered lipid bilayer region of the SC converting the gel phase of the lipid lamellae to a liquid phase. However, recent studies did not reveal any lipid distortion result in the SC.[49,50] It has been postulated that OS remains in the lipid gel phase as a 'pool' rather than interacting with the lipids and therefore enhance the diffusivity of the compound.[43]

Fatty acid esters
This group includes isopropyl myristate (IPM), propylene glycol monocaprylate (PGMC), Propyleneglycolmonolaurate (PGML).

IPM
IPM is the most widely investigated fatty acid ester. IPM found to impart fluidisation and hampers the order of lipid lamellae. However, later it was reported that IPM inserted into lipophilic region anchoring its isopropyl group in the polar region and hence interact with the lipid region.[51] In a recent study it has been reported that because of its branched structure and highly mobile terminal isopropyl group, IPM did not mix with other SC lipid. This is why IPM perturbed and disordered the assembly of lipid lamellae.[52] IPM was also found to cause phase segregation and lipid extraction from the SC.[52] In a very recent study, neat IPM was found to be present in higher quantities in the skin and therefore, aided higher retention of anthramycin in the skin rather than permeation.[53]

PGMC is the fatty acid ester which showed enhanced drug permeation alone[54-57]sometimes and mostly in combination with diethyleneglycolmonoethyl ether (Transcutol®, TC).[58,59] However, it was found to deposit inside the SC, retaining higher quantities of drug.[60] Recently, Haque et al. sowed that similar to IPM, PGMC retains in the skin in higher quantities which also helps to retain higher quantities of drug dissolve in it.[53] Takahashi et al. found that PGMC reduces the resistance to drug diffusion across the skin by interfering the SC lipid packing. Whereas, no extraction of lipid was evident.[60] Moghimipur et al. found contradicting results on

mechanism of action of PGMC. Fourier transform infrared spectroscopy (FTIR) studies showed SC lipid extraction or fluidisation by PGMC. On the other hand, Differential Scanning Calorimetry (DSC) indicated bilayer cohesion by PGMC. Because of the opposite effects, authors concluded that penetration enhancement effect of PGMC was low.[55] Moghimipur et al. also reported that PGMC interacted mostly with the SC keratins and modifies the skin lipid.[55]

PGML
PGML is recently used to delivery drug percutaneously in transdermal formulation. Like PGMC, PGML found to increase drug penetration.[59,61] Haque et al. showed that when anthramycin was applied on human skin in pure PGML, retention of small amount of PGML in the skin enhanced the drug permeation significantly.[53] However, much enhanced permeation was observed along with hydrophilic enhancers, such as propylene glycol (PG) and TC.[62-65] Parisi et al. showed that combining PGML with PG in 50:50 ratio increased the skin retention of hexamidinediisethionate in significant quantities.[66] The mechanism of action of the PGML is not clearly stated in the literature. However, it may work in the similar way as PGMC.

Ether alcohol
Transcutol® (TC)
TC is a hydrophilic CE with the similar solubility parameter as the skin [10.62 $(cal/cm^3)^{1/2}$].[67] TC is used as a penetration enhancer in both topical and transdermal formulations. TC has been found to increase the flux and retention of drugs.[33,68-71] Recently, Haque et al. showed that TC as a solvent penetrated and retained in the human skin in highest quantities compared with other selected hydrophilic solvents. Therefore, a moderate amount of drug was permeated and accumulated in the skin with the help of TC. TC clearly showed 'pull' effect aiding higher absorption of drug molecule.[53] The main mechanism of this solvent to enhance permeation is to increase the partition parameter of the drug into the skin. This may be because of the close solubility parameter of TC with skin. TC has been reported to present inside the SC as intraceutaneous depot. TC being a hydrophilic molecule, is inserted into the aqueous region between the polar head group and induce swelling of the bilayer region without altering the bilayer structure. Therefore, the swollen lipids hold the drugs soluble in the SC. In this way, TC aids to accumulate drugs in the SC (Pull effect).[68,72,73] Due to its hydrophilicity and hydrophobicity, it was suggested to interact with the intracellular lipids of the other layers of epidermis and dermis. The barrier function of the SC was not altered by TC.[72] However, recently Moghadam et al. suggested that slight disorder in the lamellar structure of the SC caused by TC, which leads to membrane fluidity.[44] Caon et al. showed that skin permeation of ioniaside in TC was reduced but skin retention was increased and the statement goes well with the 'ranscutaneous depot' theory. The authors also conducted DSC and FTR

experiments with rat skin after the permeation study. DSC analysis showed that skin lipid disruption was not caused by TC but slight membrane fluidisation. FTR analysis also confirmed that TC increased the order of both lipid and protein domains of the skin.[74]

Fatty acids
Oleic acid (OA)

OA is an unsaturated lipophilic C fatty acid that is commonly associated with enhanced penetration of polar to fairly polar molecules.[75] OA has been used in both topical and transdermal formulations due to its desirable properties. OA causes temporary and reversible disruption of the SC lipids, increasing fluidisation and diffusivity of the skin. This theory was reinforced in a study using spectrometric and calorimetric measurements which showed that OA increased lipid fluidity and permeant flux in porcine skin.[76] Due to the bent structure of OA, it disrupts the ordered orientation of lipid region and increase the fluidity. The mechanism of action of OA is similar to Azone. However, OA did not found to disturb the structure very drastically.[36] More specifically, the kinked nature of OA (bent *cis* configuration) has mainly been associated with the separation of SC lipid regions, which reduces barrier function of the SC. However, despite the advantages of OA, dermal side effects of unsaturated fatty acids have been reported.[77] These can be overcome by modification of the carboxylic terminal, which reduces the acidic nature of the fatty acid allowing safe use.[78]

The existence of OA as a separate phase within SC lipids was revealed in a study conducted on porcine SC using Fourier Transform Infrared spectroscopy (FT-IR). Results showed that OA interacted with the SC lipids by reducing the lipid transition temperature (T_m), and by increasing the "conformational freedom of lipid alkyl chains" higher than their T_m. OA may cause some sort of permeable defect within the SC that enhances diffusion of permeants. This leads to increased permeability[75] and diffusion coefficient in Fick's law. More recently, a study was conducted using urea, caffeine and diclofenac sodium, in the presence of OA as a CE. In that study OA showed a significant effect on the SC, especially in the model membrane with the higher ratio of phytosphingosine-based ceramide.[79] Recently, Atef et al. showed a time dependent enhancement of OA permeation in rat skin in terms of spectral change in Raman Spectroscopy.[80]

Glycols
Propylene glycols (PG)

PG has been used as a cosolvent in topical and transdermal products since long. It is a well-established topical CE. It acts as a CE not only by on its own but also in combination with a number of other CEs. PG mainly increases drug permeation by improving the partition properties of drugs in to the SC. It solvates the α-keratin and therefore reduce drug-tissue binding.[36] Bouwstra et al. conducted Small-angle X-ray scattering (SAXS) and differential thermal analysis (DTA) of the SC after pre-treating with PG. DTA

results showed that PG interacted with the SC lipid. On the other hand, SAXS showed that SC lipids were unaffected by PG. Due to these two contradicting findings, Bouwstra et al. concluded that PG being a hydrophilic molecule, incorporated into the polar head group of the lipid bilayer. Therefore, it increased mean interfacial area per lipid molecule. PG also induced lateral swelling (side by side). In order to compensate the lateral swelling (to maintain the density of the alkyl chain region), the chain length of the lipids were decreased. Therefore, no change in the SAXS was observed after pre-treatment with PG.[81] Recently, Moghadam et al. and Furuishi et al. conducted several experiments on PG and found no significant skin lipid alteration by PG.[44,82] Therefore, Moghadam et al. suggested improvement of skin partitioning is the main mechanism of PG to enhance permeation.[44] In addition, Mohammed et al. showed that PG increased transepidermal water loss (TWEL) and KLK 7 protease activity in the skin, therefore reduce the barrier property of the SC.[83] PG was shown to be less penetrating molecule to the human skin compared with TC. In case of hydrophilic molecule, it imparts its skin penetration effects by both 'push' and 'pull' effects.[53] Atef et al. showed that in Raman Spectrum, after applying PG on rat skin, the intensity of PG peak (at 840 cm-1) decreased with time in comparison with the skin peaks. The authors concluded that the decrease in PG peak intensity is the indication of increased diffusion of PG in the skin.[80]

Pyrrolidones
N-methyl-2-pyrrolidone (NMP) and 2-pyrrolidone (2P)

NMP and 2P are the pyrrolidones which have been investigated mostly for years.[42] Both of the CEs are dissolved in water in all proportions. The CEs found to enhance the permeation of both hydrophilic and lipophilic compounds.[42] DSC studies conducted by Barry showed that these two CEs partition in the corneocyte region (intracellular region) at low concentration and affect the intercellular region at high concentration. These molecules produces a solvation shell around the polar head group, loosens the tight packing of the lipid bilayer and induce lipid fluidity.[36] However, Trommer et al. suggested that comparatively hydrophilic pyrrolidones work by acting on the polar region and hydrophobic pyrrolidones (such as NMP) work on the lipophilic region.[35] However NMP was found to cause erythema, swelling, skin irritation, thickness of skin etc.[84] In addition, the clinical use of these molecules was restricted due to its skin cytotoxic properties.[43]

Sulphoxides
Dimethyl sulphoxides (DMSO)

DMSO is an aprotic solvent. Because of its special structure, it has broad solvent properties. Like pyrrolidones, DMSO interacts with keratin when applied in low concentration (20%). Due to its small molecular size, the compound can easily penetrate the region of protein subunit. DMSO then displaces the protein-water and hampers the native configuration of the protein (by interfering with hydrogen bonding and hydrophobic interactions). Therefore, drug/compounds get sufficient loose or flexible areas to penetrate through the SC. However, skin's impermeable characteristics restores immediately after removing DMSO as the solvent passes out the skin very quickly and gradual removal of protein-DMSO by competitive bonding with cellular water.[36] In the intercellular region, at higher concentration (above 60%), DMSO produces a large solvation shell around the lipid polar head group by displacing water from the polar group. Hence, it loosens the lipid packing more severely compared with water. This leads to increase the aqueous region in the intercellular pathway and helps to promote the permeation of hydrophilic compounds.[36] In a recent study, DMSO was found to change the highly ordered gel phase of Ceremide 2 into loosely packed liquid crystalline phase at greater than 0.4 mole fraction concentration. It has been also shown that DMSO replaced the water from the interface at higher concentration. It also induced lateral swelling by increasing area per lipid in the lipid bilayer region.[85]

Surfactants

Topical and transdermal formulation contains surfactants in order to increase the solubility of a compound in the formulation. Sodium lauryl or dodecyl sulphate (SLS) (anionic surfactant). Anionic surfactants, such as SLS acts on the skin by affecting both intra- and intercellular pathways.[36] For this reason, irritation and skin damage are very common with this type of surfactant.[35,43] SLS swells the SC and the swollen keratin can absorb more water and help to penetrate drug molecule. Additionally, SLS also unfolds and extends the alpha keratin and opens up the polar pathway for permeating the drug molecule.[36] A recent study revealed that SLS interacts with lipids and is incorporated there to create a lamellar structure.[44]

The cationic surfactants include amines, alkylimidazolines, alkoxylated amines, and quaternary ammonium compounds (or Quats). Cationic surfactants disorders SC lipid organisation more drastically than anionic and non-ionic surfactant. It mainly affects the lateral packing of the SC lipid.[44] Therefore, molecules of this group are more effective as chemical enhancers than anionic and non-ionic ones.[35] However, as this group cause skin irritation, further use in dermal formulation is not encouraged.[43]

The primary non-ionic surfactants used for cosmetics include alcohols (cetyl or stearyl alcohol), alkanolamides, esters, and amine oxides. Non-ionic surfactants disordered the SC less radically compared with ionic surfactants.[44] This is why, these surfactants are less irritating to the skin and comparatively less effective as penetration enhancer than the other types and therefore, regarded as safe.[42]

Terpenes

Terpenes are found in essential oils.[42] These are lipophilic compounds which mainly act on the lipid pathway of the SC. Since it produces less skin irritation, it is regarded as safe.[35] Smaller terpenes are found to enhance drug permeation more effectively than larger terpenes. Furthermore, polar terpenes (menthol, 1,8-cineole, etc.) improve the penetration of hydrophilic and non-polar terpenes (D-limolene) improve the penetration of hydrophobic molecules in the SC. D-limolene, 1,8 cineole hampers the arrangement of the SC lipid. On the other hand, nerolidol, a sesquiterpene strengthens the lipid bilayer may be by incorporating into the bilayer.[42] However, Moghadam et al. investigated different terpenes and terpenoids and found that nerol disrupted the lipid lamellae more drastically than other types of molecules. The hydroxyl group and the alkene of the molecule may donate hydrogen bond and disrupt the interaction between the existing hydrogen bond between the ceramide groups of the lipid bilayer.

Phospholipids

The use of phospholipids as penetrations enhancer has been widely studied as a vesicle or liposomes. However, there are fewer studies of this molecule as non-vesicular chemical enhancers. Because of its lipophilic characteristics, it occludes the SC and increase the hydration of the skin. Therefore, penetration of a drug molecule is enhanced. As a vesicle it is incorporated or fused into the SC lipid and liberates the molecule in the solvent in which it was poorly soluble. Thus thermodynamic activity as well as drug permeation were increased.[42]

Cyclodextrines

Cyclodextrins are not typical enhancers as they cannot penetrate the SC. They form inclusion complexes of hydrophobic drugs and improve their aqueous solubility. However, several studies showed penetration enhancement of certain drugs when cyclodextrin was used in combination with lipophilic enhancers (fatty acids, azone etc.).[35]

Discussion

The various sites of action of different types of CE are as follows:

The intracellular route is the polar route where keratin fibrils are present. Aprotic solvents [for example, dimethyl sulfoxide (DMSO)], pyrrolidone, surfactants interact with the keratin and may disrupt the ordered arrangement in corneocytes. Openings may be formed because of the extensive interactions. Therefore, higher permeability coefficients and fluxes can be observed.[24]

In the intercellular region, CEs may act in three ways. By interaction with the polar head groups, they modify the hydrogen-bonding and ionic forces. As a result, the packing order of the polar head group in the aqueous region may be distressed. This disturbance fluidises the lipid region which also allows polar CEs to diffuse into the aqueous region and increase the volume of water between the lipid layers.[34]

Some CEs act directly in the aqueous region present between the polar head groups. CEs or solvents [for example, propylene glycol (PG), DMSO, Transcutol®

(TC), ethanol (EtOH), pyrrolidones] increase the solubilising property (or change the solubility parameter) of this region so that drug can partition readily into the SC. CEs also act within the alkyl chain (lipid region) of the lipid bilayer by disturbing the lipid packing and enhancing the fluidity of the lipid chains. There are some CEs (DMSO, alcohols, etc.) which may also cause lipid extraction.[24,34] Table 1 summarises the site of action of various types of CE in skin.

Table 1. A summary of reported mechanism of action of commonly used topical and transdermal CEs

Site of action	CE
Interact with corneocytes or keratin	Water[36,37], PGMC[55], NMP, 2P[36], DMSO[36], SLS[36]
Near polar head groups of the lipid bilayer region	Water[18,36], ethanol (at low concentration), NMP, 2P[36], DMSO[36,85]
Extraction of intercellular lipids	Ethanol (high concentration)[18,42], D-hexanol and D-octanol[46], IPM[52]
Disruption of highly ordered lipid packing of SC bilayer region	Azone[18,35], OS[49,50], IPM[52], PGMC[60], OA[77], DMSO[85], Nerol[44]
Present as a 'pool' in the lipid region of the bilayer structure of the SC	OS[43] Phospholipids[42]
Phase separation	IPM[52]
Creates a lamellar structure after incorporating into the lipid phase	SLS[44]
Slight disordering in the lamellar arrangement of the SC	TC[44]
Increase the solubility or partitioning parameter of the drug into the SC	Ethanol[44], TC, PG[36,44]

Conclusion

Several approaches have been taken to enhance penetration of drug molecules across the SC. However, chemical enhancers have been found to be the most efficient and simplest ones. In addition, the chemical enhancers improve the permeation of the molecules in the skin in a most cheap and effective way. Except for some established CEs, the in depth mechanism of action of most of the CEs are poorly understood until now. In this article, we have summarized the studies conducted till now on different CEs. CEs induce structural transformations and enhance drug permeation across the SC by interacting with the major permeation pathway (intercellular region). Some CEs or combination of CEs show dual action, that is, by altering the partition parameter of the skin and by interacting with either the intra-or intercellular regions. 'Pull- Effect' is the result of penetration enhancing properties of either a single of combined CE(s). The mechanism of action of some CEs in molecular levels has been included in this article as well. Though, in case of some CEs contradicting mechanism of actions were suggested, the information would still be a basis to do further studies to confirm the exact mechanism of action. Still we need further studies to have a concrete understanding on the CEs. However, the summarized information on CEs would be useful for the formulation scientists to develop simple topical and transdermal formulations with improved permeation or penetration of a compound.

Ethical Issues

Not applicable

Conflict of Interest

There is no conflict of interest.

References

1. Haque T, Crowther JM, Lane ME, Moore DJ. Chemical ultraviolet absorbers topically applied in a skin barrier mimetic formulation remain in the outer stratum corneum of porcine skin. *Int J Pharm* 2016;510:250-4. doi: 10.1016/j.ijpharm.2016.06.041.

2. D'Arcy Y. Targeted topical analgesics for acute pain. PainMedicine News; 2015 [cited 2016 25 November]; Available from: http://www.painmedicinenews.com/Review-Articles/Article/12-14/Targeted-Topical-Analgesics-For-Acute-Pain/28992/ses=ogst.

3. Güngör S, Erdal MS, Aksu B. New formulation strategies in topical antifungal therapy. *J Cosmet Dermatol Sci Appl* 2013;3:56-65. doi: 10.4236/jcdsa.2013.31A009

4. McGrath JA, Eady RAJ, Pope FM. Anatomy and organization of human skin. In: Burns T, Breathnach S, Cox N, Griffiths C, editors. Rook's textbook of dermatology. 7th ed. Blackwell Publishing, Inc.; 2008. p. 45-128.

5. Katz M, Poulsen BJ. Absorption of drugs through the skin. In: Brodie BB, Gillete J, editors. Handbook of experimental pharmacology. Berlin, Heidelberg, New York: Springer- Verlag; 1971. p. 103-74.

6. Wood EJ, Bladon PT. The human skin. Great Britain, Australia, USA: Camelot Press; 1985.

7. Benson HAE. Skin structure, function, and permeation. In: Benson HAE, Watkinson AC, editors. Topical and transdermal drug delvery: Principles and practice. New Jersey: Jhon Wiley & Sons, Inc.; 2012. p. 3-22.

8. Christophers E. Cellular architecture of the stratum corneum. *J Invest Dermatol* 1971;56(3):165–9.

9. Elias PM, Cooper ER, Korc A, Brown BE. Percutaneous transport in relation to stratum corneum

structure and lipid composition. *J Invest Dermatol* 1981;76(4):297-301.

10. Michaels AS, Chandrasekaran SK, Shaw JE. Drug permeation through human skin: Theory and in vitro experimental measurement. *Aiche J* 1975;21(5):985-96. doi: 10.1002/aic.690210522

11. Elias PM. Structure and function of the stratum corneum permeability barrier. *Drug Dev Res* 1988;13(2-3):97-105. doi: 10.1002/ddr.430130203

12. Wertz PW, Downing DT. Stratum corneum: Biological and biochemical considerations. In: Hadgraft J, Guy RH, editors. Transdermal drug delivery: Developmental issue and research initiatives. New York: Marcel Dekker, Inc.; 1989. p. 1-22.

13. Bouwstra J, Pilgram G, Gooris G, Koerten H, Ponec M. New aspects of the skin barrier organization. *Skin Pharmacol Appl Skin Physiol* 2001;14 Suppl 1:52-62. doi: 10.1159/000056391

14. Pilgram GSK, Pelt AME-v, Bouwstra JA, Koerten HK. Electron diffraction provides new information on human stratum corneum lipid organization studied in relation to depth and temperature. *J Invest Dermatol* 1999;113(3):403-9. doi: 10.1046/j.1523-1747.1999.00706.x

15. Golden GM, Guzek DB, Kennedy AE, McKie JE, Potts RO. Stratum corneum lipid phase transitions and water barrier properties. *Biochem* 1987;26(8):2382-8.

16. Blank IH. Factors which influence the water content of the stratum corneum. *J Invest Dermatol* 1952;18(6):433-40.

17. Swartzendruber DC, Wertz PW, Kitko DJ, Madison KC, Downing DT. Molecular models of the intercellular lipid lamellae in mammalian stratum corneum. *J Invest Dermatol* 1989;92(2):251-7.

18. Suhonen TM, Bouwstra JA, Urtti A. Chemical enhancement of percutaneous absorption in relation to stratum corneum structural alterations. *J Control Release* 1999;59(2):149-61.

19. Potts RO, Francoeur ML. The influence of stratum corneum morphology on water permeability. *J Invest Dermatol* 1991;96(4):495-9.

20. Higuchi T. Physical chemical analysis of percutaneous absorption process from creams and ointments. *J Soc Cosmet Chem* 1960;11(11):85-97.

21. Scheuplein RJ, Blank IH. Permeability of the skin. *Physiol Rev* 1971;51(4):702-47. doi: 10.1152/physrev.1971.51.4.702

22. Morrow DIJ, McCarron PA, Woolfson AD, Donnelly RF. Innovative strategies for enhancing topical and transdermal drug delivery. *Open Drug Deliver J* 2007;1:36-59. doi: 10.2174/1874126600701010036

23. Scheuplein HJ, Blank IH, Brauner GJ, MacFarlane DJ. Percutaneous absorption of steroids. *J Invest Dermatol* 1969;52(1):63-70. doi: 10.1038/jid.1969.9

24. Benson HAE. Transdermal drug delivery: Penetration enhancement techniques. *Curr Drug Deliv* 2005;2:23-33.

25. Hueber F, Wepierre J, Schaefer H. Role of transepidermal and transfollicular routes in percutaneous absorption of hydrocortisone and testosterone: In vivo study in the hairless rat. *Skin Pharmacol* 1992;5(2):99–107.

26. Albery WJ, Hadgraft J. Percutaneous absorption: In vivo experiments. *J Pharm Pharmacol* 1979;31(1):140-7.

27. Potts RO, Guy RH. Predicting skin permeability. *Pharm Res* 1992;9(5):663-9.

28. Nemanic MK, Elias PM. In situ precipitation: A novel cytochemical technique for visualization of permeability pathways in mammalian stratum corneum. *J Histochem Cytoche* 1980;28(6):573-8. doi: 10.1177/28.6.7190175

29. Boddé HE, van den Brink I, Koerten HK, de Haan FHN. Visualization of in vitro percutaneous penetration of mercuric chloride; transport through intercellular space versus cellular uptake through desmosomes. *J Control Release* 1991;15(3):227-36. doi: 10.1016/0168-3659(91)90114-S

30. Roberts MS, Cross SE, Pellett MA. Skin transport. In: Walters KA, editor. Dermatological and transdermal formulation. New York, Basel: Marcel Dekker, Inc.; 2002. p. 89-183.

31. Benson HA, Sarveiya V, Risk S, Roberts MS. Influence of anatomical site and topical formulation on skin penetration of sunscreens. *Ther Clin Risk Manag* 2005;1(3):209-18.

32. Kadir R, Stempler D, Liron Z, Cohen S. Delivery of theophylline into excised human skin from alkanoic acid solutions: A "push-pull" mechanism. *J Pharm Sci* 1987;76(10):774-9.

33. Mura P, Faucci MT, Bramanti G, Corti P. Evaluation of transcutol as a clonazepam transdermal permeation enhancer from hydrophilic gel formulations. *Eur J Pharm Sci* 2000;9:365–72. doi: 10.1016/S0928-0987(99)00075-5

34. Lane ME, Santos P, Watkinson AC, Hadgraft J. Passive skin permeation enhancement. In: Benson HAE, Watkinson AC, editors. Topical and transdermal drug delivery principle and practice. New Jersey: Wiley-Blackwell; 2012. p. 24-42.

35. Trommer H, Neube RHH. Overcoming the stratum corneum: The modulation of skin penetration. *Skin Pharmacol Physiol* 2006;19:106–21. doi: 10.1159/000091978

36. Barry BW. Mode of action of penetration enhancers in human skin. *J Control Release* 1987;6:85-97. doi: 10.1016/0378-5173(95)04108-7

37. Gwak HS, Oh IS, Chun IK. Transdermal delivery of ondansetron hydrochloride: Effects of vehicles and penetration enhancers. *Drug Dev Ind Pharm* 2004;30(2):187–94. doi: 10.1081/DDC-120028714

38. Mak VW, Potts R, Guy R. Does hydration affect intercellular lipid organization in the stratum corneum? *Pharm Res* 1991;8(8):1064-5.

39. Gay CL, Guy RH, Golden GM, Mak VH, Francoeur ML. Characterization of low-temperature (i.E., < 65

degrees c) lipid transitions in human stratum corneum. *J Invest Dermatol* 1994;103(2):233-9.

40. Van Hal DA, Jeremiasse E, Junginger HE, Spies F, Bouwstra JA. Structure of fully hydrated human stratum corneum: A freeze-fracture electron microscopy study. *J Invest Dermatol* 1996;106(1):89-95.

41. Trommer H, Neubert RH. Overcoming the stratum corneum: The modulation of skin penetration. A review. *Skin Pharmacol Physiol* 2006;19(2):106-21. doi: 10.1159/000091978

42. Williams AC, Barry BW. Penetration enhancers. *Adv Drug Deliv Rev* 2004;56(5):603-18. doi: 10.1016/j.addr.2003.10.025

43. Lane ME. Skin penetration enhancers. *Int J Pharm* 2013;447(1-2):12-21. doi: 10.1016/j.ijpharm.2013.02.040

44. Moghadam SH, Saliaj E, Wettig SD, Dong C, Ivanova MV, Huzil JT, et al. Effect of chemical permeation enhancers on stratum corneum barrier lipid organizational structure and interferon alpha permeability. *Mol Pharm* 2013;10(6):2248-60. doi: 10.1021/mp300441c

45. Andega S, Kanikkannan N, Singh M. Comparison of the effect of fatty alcohols on the permeation of melatonin between porcine and human skin. *J Control Release* 2001;77(1-2):17-25.

46. Dias M, Naik A, Guy RH, Hadgraft J, Lane ME. In vivo infrared spectroscopy studies of alkanol effects on human skin. *Eur J Pharm Biopharm* 2008;69(3):1171-5. doi: 10.1016/j.ejpb.2008.02.006

47. Santos P, Watkinson AC, Hadgraft J, Lane ME. Formulation issues associated with transdermal fentanyl delivery. *Int J Pharm* 2011;416(1):155-9. doi: 10.1016/j.ijpharm.2011.06.024

48. Santos P, Watkinson AC, Hadgraft J, Lane ME. Influence of penetration enhancer on drug permeation from volatile formulations. *Int J Pharm* 2012;439(1-2):260-8. doi: 10.1016/j.ijpharm.2012.09.031

49. Casal HL, Mantsch HH. Polymorphic phase behaviour of phospholipid membranes studied by infrared spectroscopy. *Biochim Biophys Acta* 1984;779(4):381-401.

50. El Maghraby GM, Campbell M, Finnin BC. Mechanisms of action of novel skin penetration enhancers: Phospholipid versus skin lipid liposomes. *Int J Pharm* 2005;305(1-2):90-104. doi: 10.1016/j.ijpharm.2005.08.016

51. Brinkmann I, Muller-Goymann CC. An attempt to clarify the influence of glycerol, propylene glycol, isopropyl myristate and a combination of propylene glycol and isopropyl myristate on human stratum corneum. *Pharmazie* 2005;60(3):215-20.

52. Engelbrecht TN, Deme B, Dobner B, Neubert RH. Study of the influence of the penetration enhancer isopropyl myristate on the nanostructure of stratum corneum lipid model membranes using neutron diffraction and deuterium labelling. *Skin Pharmacol Physiol* 2012;25(4):200-7. doi: 10.1159/000338538

53. Haque T, Rahman KM, Thurston DE, Hadgraft J, Lane ME. Topical delivery of anthramycin i. Influence of neat solvents. *Eur J Pharm Sci* 2017;104:188-95. doi: 10.1016/j.ejps.2017.03.043

54. Takahashi K, Komai M, Kinoshita N, Nakamura E, Hou XL, Takatani-Nakase T, et al. Application of hydrotropy to transdermal formulations: Hydrotropic solubilization of polyol fatty acid monoesters in water and enhancement effect on skin permeation of 5-fu. *J Pharm Pharmacol* 2011;63(8):1008-14. doi: 10.1111/j.2042-7158.2011.01308.x

55. Moghimipour E, Salimi A, Zadeh BSM. Effect of the various solvents on the in vitro permeability of vitamin b12 through excised rat skin. *Trop J Pharm Res* 2013;12(5):671-7.

56. Gwak HS, Kim SU, Chun IK. Effect of vehicles and enhancers on the in vitro permeation of melatonin through hairless mouse skin. *Arch Pharm Res* 2002;25(3):392-6.

57. Lee J, Chun I. Effects of various vehicles and fatty acids on the skin permeation of lornoxicam. *J Pharm Invest* 2012;42(5):235-41. doi: 10.1007/s40005-012-0035-2

58. Gwak HS, Chun IK. Effect of vehicles and penetration enhancers on the in vitro percutaneous absorption of tenoxicam through hairless mouse skin. *Int J Pharm* 2002;236(1-2):57-64.

59. Cho YA, Gwak HS. Transdermal delivery of ketorolac tromethamine: Effects of vehicles and penetration enhancers. *Drug Dev Ind Pharm* 2004;30(6):557-64. doi: 10.1081/ddc-120037486

60. Takahashi K, Sakano H, Yoshida M, Numata N, Mizuno N. Characterization of the influence of polyol fatty acid esters on the permeation of diclofenac through rat skin. *J Control Release* 2001;73(2-3):351-8.

61. Lee KE, Choi YJ, Oh BR, Chun IK, Gwak HS. Formulation and in vitro/in vivo evaluation of levodopa transdermal delivery systems. *Int J Pharm* 2013;456(2):432-6. doi: 10.1016/j.ijpharm.2013.08.044

62. Kim KH, Gwak HS. Effects of vehicles on the percutaneous absorption of donepezil hydrochloride across the excised hairless mouse skin. *Drug Dev Ind Pharm* 2011;37(9):1125-30. doi: 10.3109/03639045.2011.561352

63. Jung SY, Kang EY, Choi YJ, Chun IK, Lee BK, Gwak HS. Formulation and evaluation of ubidecarenone transdermal delivery system. *Drug Dev Ind Pharm* 2009;35(9):1029–34. doi: 10.1080/03639040902755205

64. Choi JS, Cho YA, Chun IK, Jung SY, Gwak HS. Formulation and evaluation of ketorolac transdermal systems. *Drug Deliv* 2007;14(2):69-74. doi: 10.1080/10717540600640336

65. Chiang C-M, Cleary GW, inventors; Cygnus Therapeutic Systems, assignee. Skin permeation enhancer compositions, and methods and transdermal systems associated herewith patent 5,053,227. 1991.

66. Parisi N, Paz-Alvarez M, Matts PJ, Lever R, Hadgraft J, Lane ME. Topical delivery of hexamidine. *Int J Pharm* 2016;506(1-2):332-9. doi: 10.1016/j.ijpharm.2016.04.069

67. Liron Z, Cohen S. Percutaneous absorption of alkanoic acids ii: Application of regular solution theory. *J Pharm Sci* 1984;73(4):538-42.

68. Chadha G, Sathigari S, Parsons DL, Jayachandra Babu R. In vitro percutaneous absorption of genistein from topical gels through human skin. *Drug Dev Ind Pharm* 2011;37(5):498-505. doi: 10.3109/03639045.2010.525238

69. Puglia C, Bonina F, Trapani G, Franco M, Ricci M. Evaluation of in vitro percutaneous absorption of lorazepam and clonazepam from hydro-alcoholic gel formulations. *Int J Pharm* 2001;228(1-2):79-87.

70. Prasanthi D, Lakshmi PK. Effect of chemical enhancers in transdermal permeation of alfuzosin hydrochloride. *ISRN Pharm* 2012;2012:965280. doi: 10.5402/2012/965280

71. Shah PP, Desai PR, Patlolla R, Klevans L, Singh M. Effect of combination of hydrophilic and lipophilic permeation enhancers on the skin permeation of kahalalide f. *J Pharm Pharmacol* 2014;66(6):760-8. doi: 10.1111/jphp.12206

72. Panchagnula R, Ritschel WA. Development and evaluation of an intracutaneous depot formulation of corticosteroids using transcutol as a cosolvent: In-vitro, ex-vivo and in-vivo rat studies. *J Pharm Pharmacol* 1991;43(9):609 14.

73. Ritschel WA, Panchagnula R, Stemmer K, Ashraf M. Development of an intracutaneous depot for drugs. Binding, drug accumulation and retention studies, and mechanism of depot. *Skin Pharmacol* 1991;4(4):235-45.

74. Caon T, Campos CE, Simoes CM, Silva MA. Novel perspectives in the tuberculosis treatment: Administration of isoniazid through the skin. *Int J Pharm* 2015;494(1):463-70. doi: 10.1016/j.ijpharm.2015.08.067

75. Ongpipattanakul B, Burnette RR, Potts RO, Francoeur ML. Evidence that oleic acid exists in a separate phase within stratum corneum lipids. *Pharm Res* 1991;8(3):350-4.

76. Golden GM, McKie JE, Potts RO. Role of stratum corneum lipid fluidity in transdermal drug flux. *J Pharm Sci* 1987;76(1):25-8.

77. Sintov A, Ze'evi A, Uzan R, Nyska A. Influence of pharmaceutical gel vehicles containing oleic acid/sodium oleate combinations on hairless mouse skin, a histological evaluation. *Eur J Pharm Biopharm* 1999;47(3):299-303.

78. Ben-Shabat S, Baruch N, Sintov AC. Conjugates of unsaturated fatty acids with propylene glycol as potentially less-irritant skin penetration enhancers. *Drug Dev Ind Pharm* 2007;33(11):1169-75. doi: 10.1080/03639040701199258

79. Ochalek M, Podhaisky H, Ruettinger HH, Neubert RH, Wohlrab J. Sc lipid model membranes designed for studying impact of ceramide species on drug diffusion and permeation, part iii: Influence of penetration enhancer on diffusion and permeation of model drugs. *Int J Pharm* 2012;436(1-2):206-13. doi: 10.1016/j.ijpharm.2012.06.044

80. Atef E, Altuwaijri N. Using raman spectroscopy in studying the effect of propylene glycol, oleic acid, and their combination on the rat skin. *AAPS PharmSciTech* 2018;19(1):114-22. doi: 10.1208/s12249-017-0800-7

81. Bouwstra JA, de Vries MA, Gooris GS, Bras W, Brussee J, Ponec M. Thermodynamic and structural aspects of the skin barrier. *J Control Release* 1991;15(3):209-20. doi: 10.1016/0168-3659(91)90112-Q

82. Furuishi T, Kato Y, Fukami T, Suzuki T, Endo T, Nagase H, et al. Effect of terpenes on the skin permeation of lomerizine dihydrochloride. *J Pharm Pharm Sci* 2013;16(4): 551-63

83. Mohammed D, Hirata K, Hadgraft J, Lane ME. Influence of skin penetration enhancers on skin barrier function and skin protease activity. *Eur J Pharm Sci* 2014;51:118-22. doi: 10.1016/j.ejps.2013.09.009

84. Åkesson B. Concise international chemical assessment document 35: N-methyl-2-pyrrolidone. Geneva: World Health Organization, 2001.

85. Notman R, den Otter WK, Noro MG, Briels WJ, Anwar J. The permeability enhancing mechanism of dmso in ceramide bilayers simulated by molecular dynamics. *Biophys J* 2007;93(6):2056-68. doi: 10.1529/biophysj.107.104703

25

Fabrication and Characterization of Gliclazide Nanocrystals

Nagaraju Ravouru[1]*, **Rajeswari Surya Anusha Venna**[1], **Subhash Chandra Bose Penjuri**[2], **Saritha Damineni**[3], **Venkata Subbaiah Kotakadi**[4], **Srikanth Reddy Poreddy**[2]

[1] *Institute of Pharmaceutical Technology, Sri Padmavathi Mahila University, Tirupati, Andhra Pradesh, India.*
[2] *Department of Pharmaceutics, MNR College of Pharmacy, Sangareddy, Telangana, India.*
[3] *Department of Pharmaceutics, Sultan-ul-Uloom College of Pharmacy, Hyderabad, Telangana, India.*
[4] *Research Scientist, DST Purse Centre, S.V. University, Tirupati, Andhra Pradesh, India.*

Keywords:
· Dissolution rate
· Gliclazide
· Particle size
· Sonoprecipitation
· Zeta potential

Abstract
Purpose: The main aim of the present investigation was to enhance the solubility of poorly soluble Gliclazide by nanocrystallization.
Methods: In present investigation gliclazide nanocrystals were prepared by sonoprecipitation using Pluronic F68, Poly Vinyl Alcohol (PVA), Poly ethylene Glycol 6000 (PEG), Poly Vinyl Pyrrolidine (PVP K30) and Sodium Lauryl Sulphate (SLS) as stabilizers. Fourier Transform Infrared Spectroscopic study (FTIR), Differential Scanning Calorimetry (DSC) and X ray diffraction (XRD) studies were conducted to study the drug interactions. Size and zeta potential of the nanocrystals were evaluated. *In vitro* and *in vivo* studies of nanocrystals were conducted in comparison to pure gliclazide.
Results: The Gliclazide nanocrystals (GN) showed mean particle size of 131±7.7 nm with a zeta potential of -26.6 mV. Stable nanocrystals were formed with 0.5% of PEG 6000. FTIR, DSC and XRD studies of nanocrystals showed absence of interactions and polymorphism. SEM photographs showed a change in morphology of crystals from rod to irregular shape. There is an increase in the saturation solubility and the percentage drug release from formulation GN5 (Optimized Gliclazide Nanocrystals) was found to be 98.5 in 15 min. In the *in vivo* study, GN5 nanocrystals have reduced the blood glucose level to 296.4±4.26 mg/dl in 12 hr. The nanocrystals showed lower t_{max} and higher C_{max} values as compared to pure gliclazide.
Conclusion: The prepared nanocrystals of gliclazide were stable without any drug polymer interactions. Increase in the dissolution of nanocrystals compared to pure gliclazide and significant reduction in blood glucose level *in vivo* indicated better bioavailability of the nanocrystals. Therefore, it is concluded that nanocrystal technology can be a promising tool to improve solubility and hence dissolution of a hydrophobic drug.

Introduction

According to Biopharmaceutical classification system drugs are categorized into 4 classes, each class having its own rate limiting factor affecting its bioavailability. At present most of the drugs (approximately 70%) in the development pipelines belongs to class II and have rate of dissolution as limiting factor for the absorption due to poor solubility.[1]

Though different approaches are available to improve the rate of dissolution, drug nanocrystals are preferred over the other. Nanocrystals are particles with nanometric dimension made from 100% drug; typically they are stabilized by surfactants or polymeric stabilizers.[2] Nanocrystals also exhibit other advantages like increased saturation solubility and dissolution velocity which can be attributed to higher effective surface area and excellent adhesion to biological surfaces by which not only the bioavailability can be improved but the variations in the bioavailability can be reduced, an advantage which cannot be attained by microcrystals.[1,3]

Bottom-up process results in nanocrystals with small particle size and narrow size distribution compared to top-down process but have the main limitation of uncontrolled particle growth.[4] Usage of an external ultrasonic wave force has been proved to make more intense mass transfer, increase in rate of molecular diffusion and lesser induction time of crystallization, enhancement in the nucleation rate, leading in reduction of crystal size, hindrance of agglomeration and regulation of the crystal size distribution.

Gliclazide is a 2nd generation sulphonylurea, which shows less prevalence of hypoglycemia, low rate of secondary failure and has a potential for slowing the progression of diabetic retinopathy. Hence, gliclazide used as drug of choice in long term for the control of NIDDM. Gliclazide is a BCS class II drug having low

Corresponding author: Nagaraju Ravouru, Tel: +919440179194, Email: profnagaraju@gmail.com aqueous solubility, which resulted in poor dissolution rate and intersubject variability of its bioavailability. So, in the present study nanocrystallization of gliclazide by sonoprecipitation method is employed to enhance the solubility, thereby to increase its bioavailability.[5]

Materials and Methods
Gliclazide was kindly provided by Dr. Reddy's laboratories, Hyderabad, India. Chemicals and reagents used were of analytical grade and were purchased from Merck, Mumbai, India.

Preparation of gliclazide nanocrystals
Gliclazide nanocrystals were prepared by the combination of precipitation and ultrasonication (sonoprecipitation) using probe sonicator. Gliclazide was dissolved in DMSO to form an organic drug solution of concentration 30 mg/ml. Two ml of drug solution was added to the stabilizer solution (at a ratio of 1:20 v/v) fixed under the probe which was immersed 10 mm in the liquid which leads the wave transferring downwards and upwards (Hielscher Ultrasonics GmbH., Germany) at an ultrasonic power input of 200 W and an amplitude of 40% for 15 min. The ultrasonic sound burst was set to 0.5 sec with a pause of 0.5 sec between two bursts. During the preparation process the temperature was maintained by using an ice-water bath. The formed nanodispersion was concentrated by centrifugation at 15,000 rpm for 20 min using a cooling centrifuge (Remi Instruments ltd, India) and the product was vacuum filtered and air dried.[6]

Particle size analysis
The average particle size of gliclazide nanocrystals was determined by light scattering technique (Nano Partica SZ-100-Z, Horiba Ltd., Japan). The dried nanocrystals were diluted with water before measurement and analyzed at scattering angle of 90°C.[7]

Particle shape and morphology
The shape and morphology of gliclazide and optimized formulation was determined using scanning electron microscopy (SEM) (Zeiss EVO MA 15). Nanocrystals were placed on a glass slide and kept under vacuum. The nanocrystals were coated with a thin gold layer using a sputter coater unit. The scanning electron microscope was operated at 15 kV acceleration voltage.[7]

Zeta potential
The zeta potential was measured by photon correlation spectroscopy instrument (Malvern, UK) at 25°C.[7]

Fourier transform infrared spectroscopy
The FTIR spectral measurements were taken at ambient temperature using a Shimadzu, Model 8400 (USA). About 2 mg of the crude gliclazide and gliclazide nanocrystals were dispersed in KBr powder and the pellets were made by applying 6000 kg/cm^2 pressure.

FTIR spectra were obtained by powder diffuse reflectance on FTIR spectrophotometer.[7]

Differential scanning calorimetry (DSC)
DSC studies were performed by using DSC-60 calorimeter (Schimadzu Corporation, Japan) to evaluate the molecular structure of crude gliclazide, and gliclazide nanocrystals.[7]

X-Ray powder diffraction
The X-ray powder diffraction (XRPD) studies were carried by using a powder X-ray diffractometer (Rigaku Geigerflex XRD, Co., Japan). XRPD studies were measured at 40 kV and 45 mA. During XRPD studies the range of 2θ angle was used between 5° and 40° at a scan rate and step size of 5°/min and 0.01° respectively.[7]

Saturation solubility
Saturated solution of gliclazide and gliclazide nanocrystals was prepared in 5 ml of water. Saturated solution was centrifuged at 17,000 rpm for 3 hr. Supernatant liquid was collected and the gliclazide concentration was analyzed at 228 nm by using UV spectrophotometer (Schimadzu Corporation, Japan).[8]

Determination of residual solvents concentration
Gas chromatography (Shimadzu GC-14B Chromatograph, Japan) was used to estimate residual DMSO in gliclazide nanocrystals.[9]

Dissolution studies
Dissolution studies of pure gliclazide and gliclazide nanocrystals was carried using USP XXIV-Type II (Electro Lab, Mumbai, India). 900 ml of 0.1 N HCl was used as dissolution medium. 5 ml samples were withdrawn at the end of 10, 20, 30, 40, 50 and 60 min and sink conditions were maintained. The gliclazide content in the samples was analyzed at 228 nm by using UV spectrophotometer (Schimadzu Corporation, Japan).[8,10]

In vivo studies
Pharmacodynamic studies
The anti-diabetic activity of gliclazide nanocrystals was evaluated by alloxan-induced diabetic method. Study protocol was approved by IAEC (Reg. No. IAEC/1434/PO/E/S/11/2015). Male/female wistar rats weighing around 275-350 gm were used for the study. Rats were housed in polypropylene cages at a temperature 25±2°C with 12 hr day and 12 hr night cycle. All animals received standard laboratory diet and water ad libitum. Diabetes was induced in rats by administration of alloxan solution (150 mg/kg) intraperitonially. After a week, diabetic rats with fasting blood glucose of > 300 mg/dl were included in the study for 12 hr. These rats were divided into two groups of six rats in each and treated as below.

Animal grouping for anti-diabetic studies
The animals were divided into two groups (six animals in each group) for anti-diabetic studies.

Group I: Diabetes induced and gliclazide pure drug administered animals

Group II: Diabetes induced and gliclazide nano crystals administered animals

Pure gliclazide and gliclazide nanocrystals (Dose: 2 mg/kg) was given by using oral feeding needle. Blood samples (0.1 ml) were collected through retro-orbital plexus under ether anesthesia at regular intervals for 12 hours. The blood glucose levels were determined using the commercial glucose kit. Comparative *in vivo* blood glucose level in alloxan-induced diabetic rats after oral administration of pure gliclazide and gliclazide nanocrystals were evaluated.[11,12]

Pharmacokinetic studies
Pharmacokinetic study protocol was approved by the IAEC (Reg. No. IAEC/1434/PO/E/S/11/2015). The oral pharmacokinetics of pure gliclazide and gliclazide nanocrystals was assessed in wistar rats. Animals were fasted overnight with free access to water for 12 hr before dosing. A dose equivalent to 2 mg/kg of pure gliclazide and gliclazide nanocrystals was given by using oral feeding needle. 0.1 ml of blood was collected from each rat through retro-orbital plexus under ether anesthesia at 1, 2, 4, 6, 8, 10 and 12 hr and the plasma was separated from blood by centrifuging at 2500 rpm for 10 min and stored under refrigerated conditions prior to assay on the same day. Assay of the gliclazide in plasma was estimated by HPLC method. The pharmacokinetic parameters were calculated using WinNonlin software.[13,14]

Results and Discussion
Preparation of gliclazide nanocrystals
Crystal formation includes particle nucleation, molecular growth of the particle and agglomeration/ aggregation of the particles, and their rate determines the particle size and size distribution.[4,5] The driving force of the crystal formation is supersaturation, which determines the particle nucleation rate and also the diffusion-controlled growth rate of the crystal. The crystal growth depends on the rate of supersaturation, higher the rate of supersaturation leads to faster crystal growth.

Solvent and anti solvent
Nucleation of a drug molecule is faster when it is dissolved in good solvent, because availability of more monomers in solvent phase for nucleation. So, DMSO was selected as a good solvent for gliclazide. In DMSO gliclazide showed nucleation at low supersaturation condition. In case of acetone and methanol the solubility of gliclazide is low which may not provide sufficient supersaturation.[4] Water is selected as anti solvent due to the low solubility of gliclazide. Moreover, if the drug molecules having crystalline properties water is used as anti-solvent in most of the studies.[15] DMSO: Water (1:20

ratio) was used to attain better particle size. With an increase in anti-solvent to solvent ratio the size of the crystal gradually decreases due to increase in the degree of supersaturation.[16,17] At this antisolvent to solvent ratio (1:20), the nucleation rate is high and at the same time higher solvent phase instigate the particle growth, which leads to increase in the particle size.

Effect of drug concentration
Gliclazide concentration in the solvent was selected to be 30 mg/ml as increase in concentration of the gliclazide may also lead to the increase in the particle size of the crystals. Higher the supersaturation, the faster will be the crystal growth which may be due to higher drug concentration, higher diffusion-controlled growth and higher agglomeration rate.[4,5]

Effect of temperature
Temperature plays major role of particle size in crystallization. At a higher temperature, solubility of gliclazide increased which leads to lower rate of nucleation. Which may be due to reduction in the level of supersaturation. So, less crystal nuclei will be available for crystal growth and leads to formation of larger crystals.[18] After nucleation, surface of the crystal will grow in a molecular way by two major pathways; 1. Movement of solute molecules from solution to the surface of the crystal diffusion, convection and combination of diffusion and convection. 2. Addition of molecules into the crystal lattice by surface integration (surface reaction process). At higher temperature faster crystal growth rate will occur due to higher diffusion and increased reaction kinetics at the interface. So, 3°C was selected as suitable crystallization temperature to get small particle with narrow particle size distribution.[4,5]

Effect of ultrasonication
Ultrasonication converts thermodynamically unstable matter into a more stable form by single/multiple application of energy, followed by thermal relaxation. Lowering of energy can be achieved by conversion of the solid from a less ordered to a more ordered lattice structure (an amorphous state to a crystal form). Alternatively, lowering of energy can be achieved by reducing the surface energy at the solid liquid interface by using surfactant molecules.[18] During the crystallization process, ultrasound/sonication enhances the mixing and provides uniform conditions. Ultrasonication improves the mass transfer and enhances the molecular diffusion which leads to reduction in the crystallization time and enhancement in nucleation rate. This process helps to reduce the crystal size, agglomeration and narrow particle size distribution.[18] Precipitation may occur in amorphous forms which were usually unstable and tends to transform into stable crystalline forms by the application of external energy.[18]

Effect of stabilizer on particle size

Simple precipitation method has a limitation of uncontrolled nucleation crystal growth and spontaneous agglomeration, thus small particles need to be stabilized by surfactant or/and protective polymer. PEG 6000, Pluronic F68, PVPK30, PVA and SLS were screened as stabilizers for preparing gliclazide nanocrystals. The particle size and zeta potential are taken as basis for the selection of the best stabilizer. PEG 6000 allows the production of crystals with mean particle diameter of 128.6 nm and low particle size distribution of 7.7 nm (Table 1). Mean particle size of nanocrystals produced by all other stabilizers was beyond 128.

Table 1. Particle size distribution of gliclazide nanocrystals in different stabilizers

Stabilizer	Particle size (nm)	Zeta Potential (mV)
Pluronic F68	249.1 ± 28.7	-16.7
PVA	197.6 ± 18.6	-2.9
PEG 6000	128 ± 7.7	-26.6
PVPK 30	765.4 ± 27.6	-11.8
SLS	681.1 ± 19.3	-5.6

Mean ± SD, (n=3)

Effect of stabilizer on zeta potential

Particle charge is one of the factors determining their physical stability. The higher is the electronic repulsion between the particles and the higher is the physical stability. As a rule of thumb, particles with zeta potential above 30 mV (absolute value) are physically stable. Particles with a potential above 60 mV show excellent stability. Particles below 20 mV are of limited stability; below 5 mV they undergo pronounced aggregation. In case of steric stabilizers zeta potential of about 20 mV was still sufficient to stabilize the system completely as the adsorption of a steric stabilizer layer leads to drop in the measured zeta potential, which is however not an indication of a reduced electrostatic repulsion. The adsorption layer of the steric stabilizer shifts the plane, at which the zeta potential is measured at away from the particle surface. Consequently, the measured zeta potential is lower. From the zeta potential analysis, it was found that PEG 6000 resulted in surface charge of -26.6 mV (Table 1) which is sufficient for stabilization of nanocrystals. Though PVA resulted in particle size nearer to the PEG 6000 formulation, they were found to have low zeta potential which is not sufficient enough for the stabilization of nanoparticles.

Effect of stabilizer concentration

A suitable stabilizer concentration should be used for each drug to achieve smaller particle size. The crystal growth was shielded by the sorption of stabilizers. The amount/concentration of stabilizer should be abundant for full coverage of the crystal surface to provide adequate steric repulsion between the crystals.

Inadequate surface coverage by stabilizer leads to rapid crystal growth and agglomeration. While high concentration of stabilizer will hinder the transmission of ultrasonic vibration and the diffusion between solvent and the anti-solvent during precipitation which may be due to enhanced viscosity. To optimize the minimum concentration of PEG 6000 which could produce smallest stable gliclazide nanocrystals possible with higher dissolution rate, the concentration of stabilizer is varied in the formulations (Table 2).

Table 2. Composition of different nanocrystal formulations

	GN1	GN2	GN3	GN4	GN5
Gliclazide (mg)	30	30	30	30	30
DMSO (ml)	1	1	1	1	1
PEG 6000 (%)	0.05	0.1	0.25	0.5	1
Water (ml)	20	20	20	20	20

Particle shape and morphology

The morphology of nanocrystals formed by precipitation is altered by stabilizers used and drug concentration, so, SEM imaging was performed. From the images (Figure 1) it was found that nanocrystals are in irregular shape with uniform size while pure gliclazide was long cylindrical and non-uniform.

Fourier transform infrared spectroscopy

FTIR spectra showed characteristic peaks that belong to gliclazide in nanocrystals (Figure 2) without any shifting in bands indicating that chemical structure of gliclazide was preserved in the nanocrystal formulation and the preparation method employed or stabilizer had no effect on the stability of gliclazide. It further shows that there were no chemical interactions. The new bands found in the FTIR spectra of nanocrystals may be due to the stabilizer (PEG 6000).

Differential scanning calorimetry

The gliclazide coarse powder exhibited a single endothermic peak at 172°C. The thermogram of nanocrystals showed characteristic endothermic peak corresponding to that of pure gliclazide with slight change in crystallinity due to change in melting point 167°C (Figure 3). No additional peaks are found in thermogram which indicates the absence of polymorphic changes in gliclazide nanocrystals.[19-21]

X-ray powder diffraction (XRPD)

During the precipitation process there is possibility of formation of amorphous or crystal compounds. In order to know the nature of the compound XRPD analysis was performed. As shown in the Figure 4, the XRPD pattern of the pure drug was very similar to that of the nanocrystalline compound, with characteristic peaks at diffraction angles between 10-11, 14.5-15.5, 16.5-19, 20.8-22.5, 25-26, 26.5-27.5, this indicate that crystallinity is retained in the nanocrystals with the same intensity as in gliclazide raw crystals. Conservation of the crystal structure/lattice of the drug in the formulation is very important for stability of the compound.

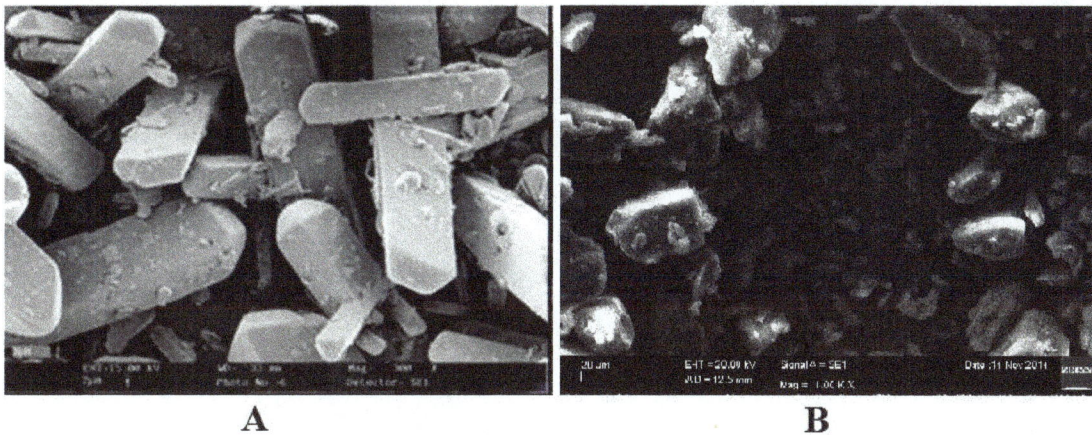

Figure 1. SEM images of A. Pure gliclazide B. Gliclazide nanocrystals

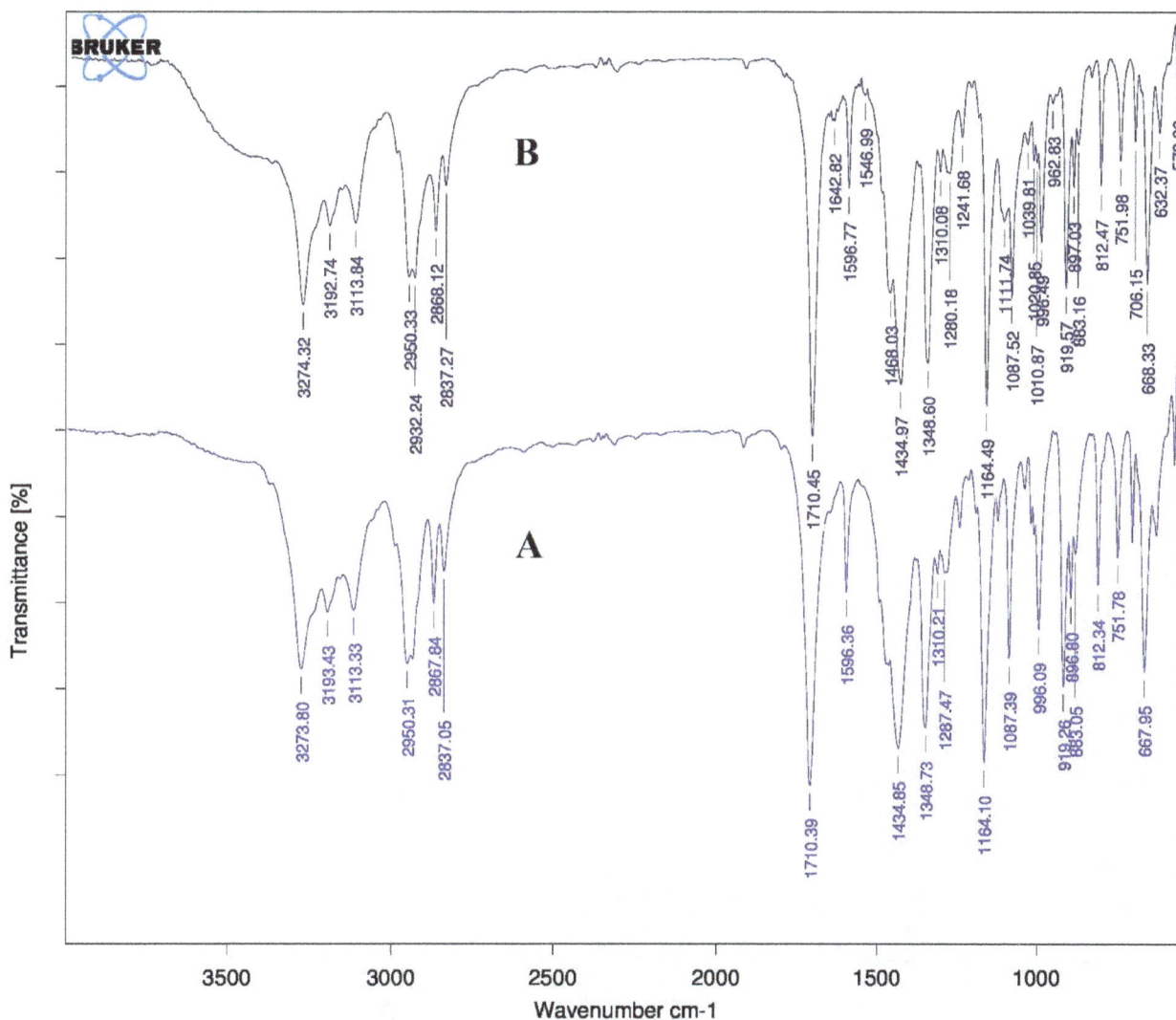

Figure 2. FTIR spectra of A. Pure gliclazide, B. Gliclazide nanocrystals

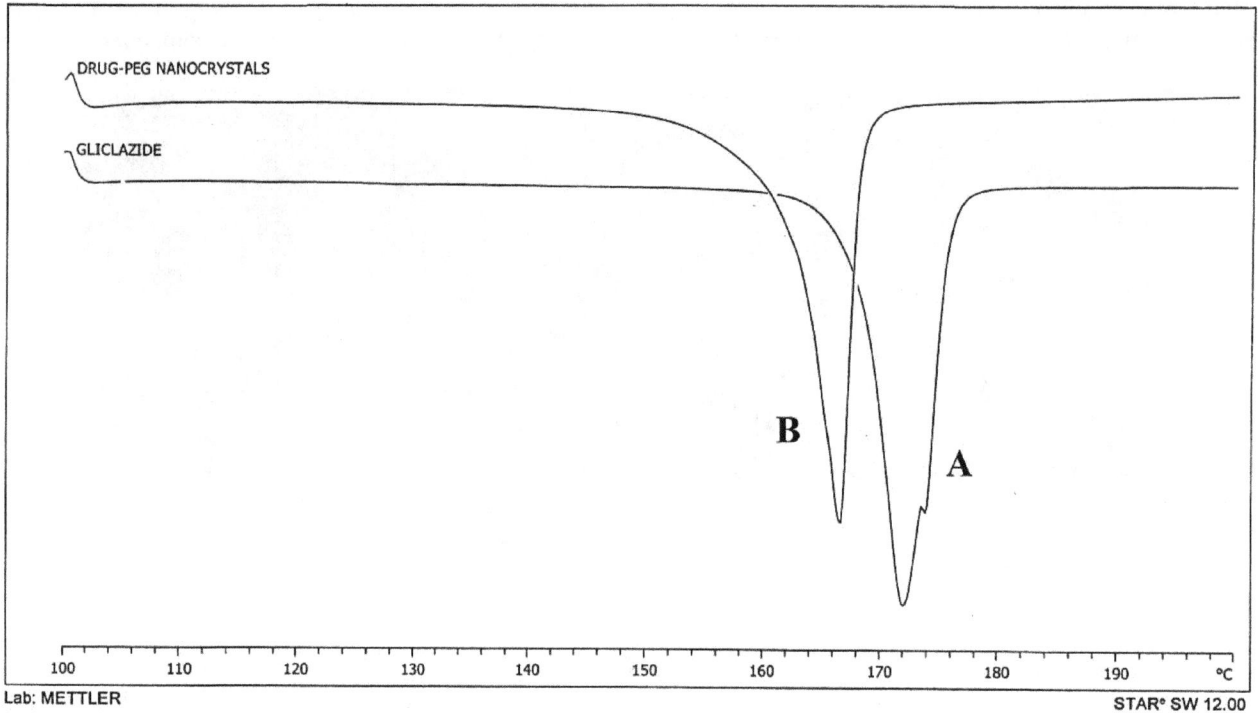

Figure 3. DSC thermograms of A. Pure gliclazide, B. Gliclazide nanocrystals

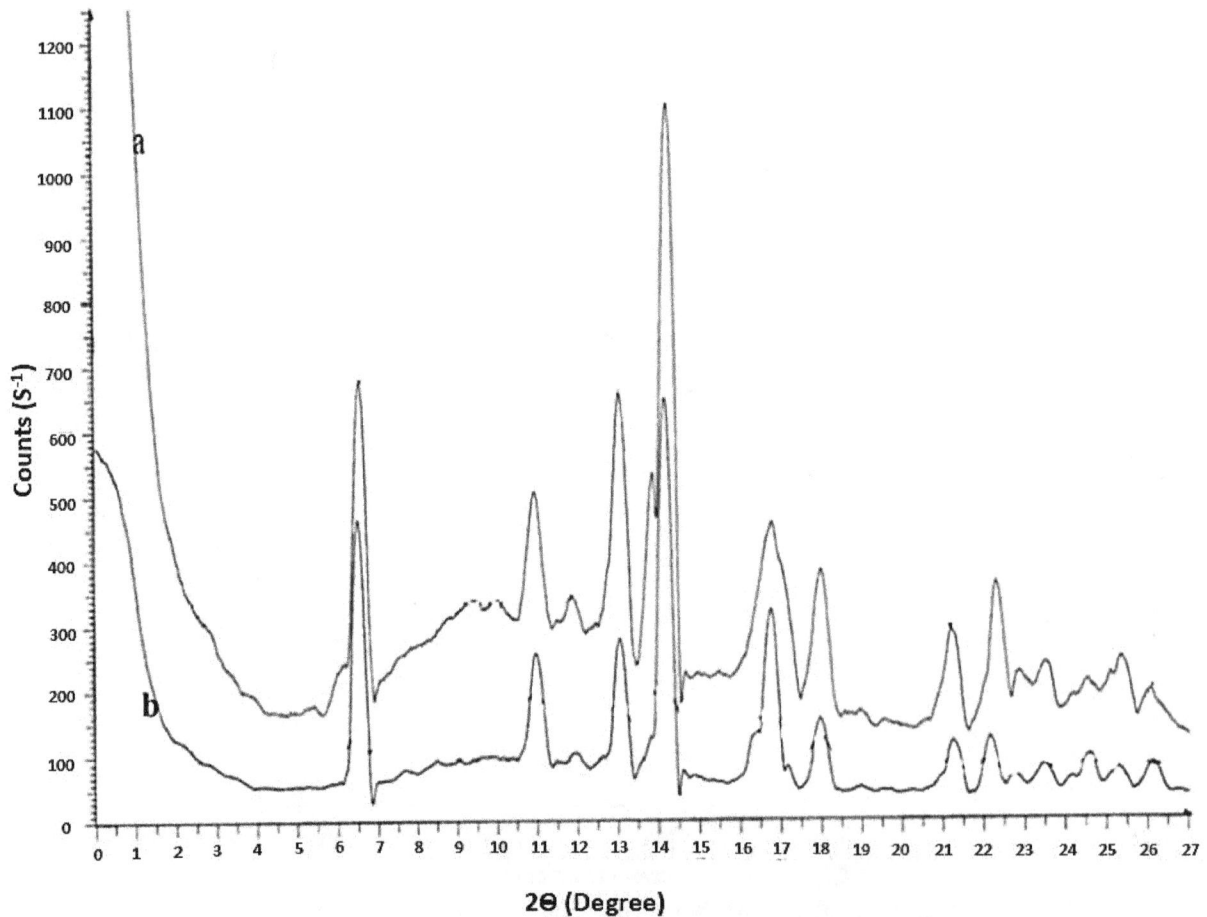

Figure 4. XRD spectra of A. Gliclazide pure drug, B. Gliclazide nanocrystals

Saturation solubility

Nanonisation has an extra effect when compared to micronisation. Nanonisation increases the surface area and saturation solubility of drugs. The solubility of drugs with normally depends on temperature and the solvent. The saturation solubility of a drug is a function of particle size. Due to strong curvature of the particles will enhance saturation solubility which may be due to increase in dissolution pressure. An increase in saturation solubility leads to enhancement of dissolution rate and formation of a supersaturated solution. This leads to increase in the concentration gradient between lumen of the gut and blood. This would enhance the drug diffusion from nanocrystals, promoting the better absorption. The saturation solubility of the formulations was determined with different concentrations of PEG 6000. It was found that there was an increase in the solubility of the gliclazide with an increase in the concentration of PEG 6000. The increase in solubility of the drug can be attributed both to the particle size and the stabilizer concentration (Table 3). The increased saturation solubility of the drug leads to an improvement in the solubility as well as bioavailability.[7]

Table 3. Saturation solubility data of pure gliclazide and nanocrystals

Formulation	Solubility (gm/lit)
Pure Gliclazide	0.022 ± 0.03
GN1	0.4 ± 0.01
GN2	0.512 ± 0.08
GN3	0.69 ± 0.3
GN4	0.75 ± 0.83
GN5	0.8 ± 0.5

Mean ± SD, (n=3)

Residual solvents concentration

The concentration of DMSO was found to be 791 ppm. According to guidelines for residual solvents Q3C (ICH), DMSO is class 3 solvent (solvent with low toxic potential), thus the limits of 5000 ppm is acceptable without justification.

Dissolution studies

The percentage release of gliclazide from pure drug was only 31.31±2.89 in 15 min while GN4 and GN5 showed 81.25±3.22 and 98.5±1.35 in 15 min (Figure 5) respectively which are having a high concentration of stabilizer. An increase in the concentration of stabilizer helped in better stabilization of nanocrystals and also an enhancement in dissolution of the drug was observed. Rate of dissolution was found to be higher for the nanocrystals produced with stabilizer concentration of 0.5% and 1% (GN4 & GN5). GN1, GN2 and GN3 (stabilizer concentration less than 0.5%) showed less improvement in dissolution rate which can be attributed to inefficient stabilization of nanocrystals and crystal growth resulting in high particle size. The rate of dissolution of nanocrystals (GN5) was found to be increased 3 times in comparison to the gliclazide raw crystals. Gliclazide nanocrystals (GN5) showed faster release so it was selected for further *in vivo* studies.

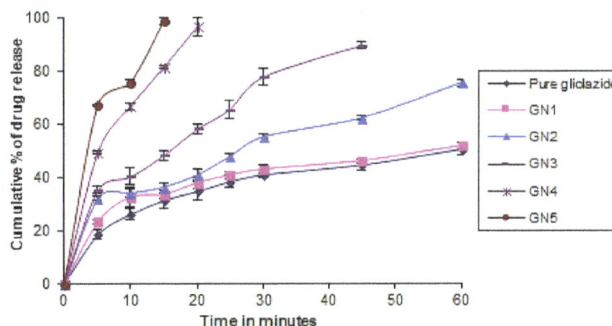

Figure 5. Dissolution profiles of pure gliclazide and gliclazide nanocrystals

In vivo studies

Pharmacodynamic study was performed in diabetes induced rats. In diabetic rats, it was found that pure gliclazide and GN5 have reduced the blood glucose level to 296.4±4.26 mg/dl and 182.31±2.52 mg/dl respectively at the end of 12 hours (Figure 6). The decrease in glucose levels reflects an increase of gliclazide in the blood levels as a result of the drug dissolution and absorption.[13]

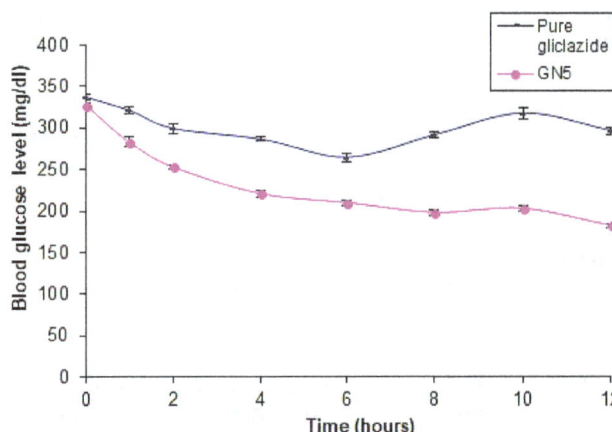

Figure 6. Comparative *in vivo* blood glucose level in diabetic rats after oral administration of pure gliclazide and GN5

The absorption of gliclazide from nanocrystals was faster indicated by its low t_{max} value (2.12±3.29 hours) in comparison with pure gliclazide which may be due to increased solubility. The C_{max} value of gliclazide nanocrystals was comparatively higher than the pure gliclazide which might be due to better absorption. The $t_{1/2}$ and MRT values of the gliclazide from powder and nanocrystals were found to be approximately 6 hours. This suggests that the drug stays in the body for a longer duration of time before being eliminated. AUC of gliclazide from nanocrystals was found to be significantly higher than the pure gliclazide (Table 4) which indicates an improvement in bioavailability of gliclazide from nanocrystals.

Table 4. Pharmacokinetic parameters of gliclazide in normal rats

Parameter	Oral administration	
	Pure gliclazide	Gliclazide nanocrystals (GN5)
C_{max} (µg/ml)	34.78±3.22	50.52±4.33
t_{max} (hr)	2.7±4.58	2.12±3.29
$t_{1/2}$ (hr)	6.79±2.24	6.18±3.80
MRT (hr)	6.12±1.24	6.73±1.80
$AUC_{0-\infty}$ (hr.µg/ml)	217.24± 63.19	392.76±73.38

Mean ± SD, (n=6)

Conclusion

Gliclazide nanocrystals formulated by sonoprecipitation showed enhanced dissolution rate. Fourier Infrared Spectroscopy (FTIR), Differential Scanning Calorimetry (DSC) and X ray diffraction (XRD) studies showed that there is no polymorphism or no change in the crystal structure. The gliclazide nanocrystals showed better antidiabetic activity in the rats compared to pure gliclazide due to enhanced solubility and absorption. MRT and AUC of gliclazide nanocrystals were found to be higher than the pure gliclazide which indicates an improvement in bioavailability of gliclazide from nanocrystals.

Acknowledgments

The authors would like to thank Dr. Reddy's laboratories, Hyderabad, India for providing gift sample of gliclazide.

Ethical Issues

The protocol of animal use was in compliance with Committee for the Purpose of Control and Supervision of Experiments on Animals, India.

Conflict of Interest

The authors declare no conflict of interests.

References

1. Gao L, Liu G, Ma J, Wang X, Zhou L, Li X. Drug nanocrystals: *In vivo* performances. *J Control Release* 2012;160(3):418-30. doi: 10.1016/j.jconrel.2012.03.013
2. Muller RH, Gohla S, Keck CM. State of the art of nanocrystals--Special features, production, Nanotoxicology aspects and intracellular delivery. *Eur J Pharm Biopharm* 2011;78(1):1-9. doi: 10.1016/j.ejpb.2011.01.007
3. Bansal S, Bansal M, kumaria M. Nanocrystals: Current Strategies and Trends. *Int J Res Pharm Biomed Sci* 2012;3(1):407-19.
4. Sinha B, Muller RH, Moschwitzer JP. Bottom-up approaches for preparing drug nanocrystals: Formulations and factors affecting particle size. *Int J Pharm* 2013;453(1):126-41. doi: 10.1016/j.ijpharm.2013.01.019
5. Xia D, Quan P, Piao H, Piao H, Sun S, Yin Y, et al. Preparation of stable nitrendipine nanosuspensions using the precipitation-ultrasonication method for enhancement of dissolution and oral bioavailability. *Eur J Pharm Sci* 2010;40(4):325-34. doi: 10.1016/j.ejps.2010.04.006
6. Schultheiss N, Newman A. Pharmaceutical Cocrystals and Their Physicochemical Properties. *Cryst Growth Des* 2009;9(6):2950-67. doi: 10.1021/cg900129f
7. Basavaraj KN, Ganesh KD, Hiren MB, Veerendra KN, Manvi FV. Design and Characterization of Nanocrystals of Lovastatin for Solubility and Dissolution Enhancement. *J Nanomed Nanotechnol* 2011;2(2):1-7. doi: 10.4172/2157-7439.1000107
8. Detroja C, Chavhan S, Sawant K. Enhanced Antihypertensive Activity of Candesartan Cilexetil Nanosuspension: Formulation, Characterization and Pharmacodynamic Study. *Sci Pharm* 2011;79(3):635-51. doi: 10.3797/scipharm.1103-17
9. Takeuchi A, Yamamoto S, Narai R, Nishida M, Yashiki M, Sakui N, et al. Determination of dimethyl sulfoxide and dimethyl sulfone in urine by gas chromatography-mass spectrometry after preparation using 2,2-dimethoxypropane. *Biomed Chromatogr* 2010;24(5):465-71. doi: 10.1002/bmc.1313
10. Varshosaz J, Tavakoli N, Enteshary S. Enhancement of anti-diabetic effects of gliclazide using immediate release Tablets in streptozotocin-induced Diabetic and normal rats. *Farmacia* 2013;61(4):820-35.
11. Prajapati SK, Tripathi P, Ubaidulla U, Anand V. Design and development of gliclazide mucoadhesive microcapsules: *in vitro* and *in vivo* evaluation. *AAPS PharmSciTech* 2008;9(1):224-30. doi: 10.1208/s12249-008-9041-0
12. Venkidesh R, Pal DK, Mohana LS, Saravanakumar A, Mandal SC. Antidiabetic activity of Smilax chinensis L. extract in streptozotacin-induced diabetic rats. *Int J Phytopharm* 2010;1(2):16-21.
13. Pal D, Nayak AK. Development, Optimization, and Anti-diabetic Activity of Gliclazide-Loaded Alginate-Methyl Cellulose Mucoadhesive Microcapsules. *AAPS PharmSciTech* 2011;12(4):1431-41. doi: 10.1208/s12249-011-9709-8
14. Du B, Shen G, Wang D, Pang L, Chen Z, Liu Z. Development and characterization of glimepiride nanocrystal formulation and evaluation of its pharmacokinetic in rats. *Drug Deliv* 2013;20(1):25-33. doi: 10.3109/10717544.2012.742939
15. Zhang JY, Shen ZG, Zhong J, Hu TT, Chen JF, Ma ZQ, et al. Preparation of amorphous cefuroxime axetil nanoparticles by controlled nanoprecipitation method without surfactants. *Int J Pharm* 2006;323(1-2):153-60. doi: 10.1016/j.ijpharm.2006.05.048
16. Wang Z, Chen JF, Le Y, Shen ZG. Preparation of ultrafine beclomethasone dipropionate drug powder by antisolvent precipitation. *Ind Eng Chem Res* 2007;46(14):4839-45. doi: 10.1021/ie0615537
17. Zhang ZB, Shen ZG, Wang JX, Zhao H, Chen JF, Yun J. Nanonization of megestrol acetate by liquid

precipitation. *Ind Eng Chem Res* 2009;48(18):8493-9. doi: 10.1021/ie900944y

18. Matteucci ME, Hotze MA, Johnston KP, Williams RO 3rd. Drug nanoparticles by antisolvent precipitation: mixing energy versus surfactant stabilization. *Langmuir* 2006;22(21):8951-9. doi: 10.1021/la061122t

19. Pu X, Sun J, Wang Y, Wang Y, Liu X, Zhang P, et al. Development of a chemically stable 10-hydroxycamptothecin nanosuspensions. *Int J Pharm* 2009;379(1):167-73. doi: 10.1016/j.ijpharm.2009.05.062

20. Du B, Li XT, Zhao Y, A YM, Zhang ZZ. Preparation and characterization of freeze-dried 2-methoxyestradiol nanoparticle powders. *Pharmazie* 2010;65(7):471-6.

21. Quan P, Xia D, Piao H, Piao H, Shi K, Jia Y, et al. Nitrendipine nanocrystals: its preparation, characterization, and in vitro-in vivo evaluation. *AAPS PharmSciTech* 2011;12(4):1136-43. doi: 10.1208/s12249-011-9682-2

Permissions

All chapters in this book were first published in APB, by Tabriz University of Medical Sciences; hereby published with permission under the Creative Commons Attribution License or equivalent. Every chapter published in this book has been scrutinized by our experts. Their significance has been extensively debated. The topics covered herein carry significant findings which will fuel the growth of the discipline. They may even be implemented as practical applications or may be referred to as a beginning point for another development.

The contributors of this book come from diverse backgrounds, making this book a truly international effort. This book will bring forth new frontiers with its revolutionizing research information and detailed analysis of the nascent developments around the world.

We would like to thank all the contributing authors for lending their expertise to make the book truly unique. They have played a crucial role in the development of this book. Without their invaluable contributions this book wouldn't have been possible. They have made vital efforts to compile up to date information on the varied aspects of this subject to make this book a valuable addition to the collection of many professionals and students.

This book was conceptualized with the vision of imparting up-to-date information and advanced data in this field. To ensure the same, a matchless editorial board was set up. Every individual on the board went through rigorous rounds of assessment to prove their worth. After which they invested a large part of their time researching and compiling the most relevant data for our readers.

The editorial board has been involved in producing this book since its inception. They have spent rigorous hours researching and exploring the diverse topics which have resulted in the successful publishing of this book. They have passed on their knowledge of decades through this book. To expedite this challenging task, the publisher supported the team at every step. A small team of assistant editors was also appointed to further simplify the editing procedure and attain best results for the readers.

Apart from the editorial board, the designing team has also invested a significant amount of their time in understanding the subject and creating the most relevant covers. They scrutinized every image to scout for the most suitable representation of the subject and create an appropriate cover for the book.

The publishing team has been an ardent support to the editorial, designing and production team. Their endless efforts to recruit the best for this project, has resulted in the accomplishment of this book. They are a veteran in the field of academics and their pool of knowledge is as vast as their experience in printing. Their expertise and guidance has proved useful at every step. Their uncompromising quality standards have made this book an exceptional effort. Their encouragement from time to time has been an inspiration for everyone.

The publisher and the editorial board hope that this book will prove to be a valuable piece of knowledge for researchers, students, practitioners and scholars across the globe.

List of Contributors

Mohammadali Torbati
Department of Food Science and Technology, Faculty of Nutrition, Tabriz University of Medical Sciences, Tabriz, Iran

Solmaz Asnaashari
Biotechnology Research Center, Tabriz University of Medical Sciences, Tabriz, Iran

Fariba Heshmati Afshar
Department of Pharmacognosy, Faculty of Pharmacy, Tabriz University of Medical Sciences, Tabriz, Iran

Carolina Harder, Regina Yuri Hashimoto Miura and Sandro Rostelato-Ferreira
Institute of Health Sciences, Universidade Paulista (Unip), Av. Independência 210, 18087-100, Sorocaba, SP, Brazil

Akila Lara de Oliveira and Yoko Oshima-Franco
University of Sorocaba (Uniso), Rodovia Raposo Tavares km 92.5, 18023-000, Sorocaba, SP, Brazil

Andreia Borges Scriboni
Department of Pharmacology, Piracicaba Dental School, State University of Campinas (UNICAMP), Av. Limeira 901, 13414-903, Piracicaba, SP, Brazil

Adélia Cristina Oliveira Cintra
Faculty of Pharmaceutical Sciences, Department of Clinical and Toxicological Analysis and Bromatology, São Paulo University (USP), Via do Café S/N, 14040-903, Ribeirão Preto, SP, Brazil

Raphael Schezaro-Ramos and Rafael Stuani Floriano
Department of Pharmacology, Faculty of Medical Sciences, State University of Campinas (UNICAMP), Rua Tessália Vieira de Camargo 126, 13083-887, Campinas, SP, Brazil

Márcio Galdino dos Santos
Tocantins Federal University (UFT), Av. NS 15, ALC NO14, 109 Norte, 77001-090, Palmas, TO, Brazil.

Karina Cogo-Müller
Faculty of Pharmaceutical Sciences, State University of Campinas (UNICAMP), Rua Cândido Portinari, 200, 13083-871, Campinas, SP, Brazil

Reza Hajihosseini Baghdadabadi
Department of Biology, Payame Noor University, Tehran, Iran

Roghiyeh Pashaei-Asl
Department of Biology, Payame Noor University, Tehran, Iran
Department of Anatomy, Medical School, Iran University of Medical Science, Tehran, Iran
Cellular and Molecular Research Center, Iran University of Medical Sciences, Tehran, Iran

Khodadad Khodadadi
Genetic Theme, Murdoch Children's Research Institute, Royal Children's Hospital, The University of Melbourne, Melbourne, Australia

Fatima Pashaei-Asl
Molecular Biology Laboratory, Biotechnology Research Center, Tabriz University of Medical Sciences, Tabriz, Iran

Gholamreza Haqshenas
Microbiology Department, Biomedical Discovery Institute, Monash University, Melbourne, Australia

Nasser Ahmadian
Transplantation Center, Department of Curative Affairs, Ministry of Health and Medical Education, Tehran, Iran

Maryam Pashaiasl
Drug Applied Research Center, Tabriz University of Medical Sciences, Tabriz, Iran
Department of Anatomical Sciences, Faculty of Medicine, Tabriz University of Medical Sciences, Tabriz, Iran

Cristina Mateescu, Tatiana Onisei and Adina Elena Raducanu
National Office for Medicinal, Aromatic Plants and Bee Products - National Research and Development Institute for Food Bioresources – IBA Bucharest, 6 Dinu Vintila Str., 021102, Bucharest, Romania

Anca Mihaela Popescu
National Office for Medicinal, Aromatic Plants and Bee Products - National Research and Development Institute for Food Bioresources – IBA Bucharest, 6 Dinu Vintila Str., 021102, Bucharest, Romania
Faculty of Applied Chemistry and Materials Science - University Politehnica of Bucharest, 1-7 Polizu Str., 011061, Bucharest, Romania

Gabriel Lucian Radu
Faculty of Applied Chemistry and Materials Science - University Politehnica of Bucharest, 1-7 Polizu Str., 011061, Bucharest, Romania

Sri Handayani
Research Center for Chemistry, Indonesian Institute of Sciences (LIPI), Serpong, Indonesia
Cancer Chemoprevention Research Center, Faculty of Pharmacy, Universitas Gadjah Mada, Yogyakarta, Indonesia

Ratna Asmah Susidarti, Riris Istighfari Jenie and Edy Meiyanto
Cancer Chemoprevention Research Center, Faculty of Pharmacy, Universitas Gadjah Mada, Yogyakarta, Indonesia

Shadi Farsaei
Department of Clinical Pharmacy and Pharmacy Practice, Isfahan Pharmaceutical Sciences Research Center, Isfahan University of Medical Sciences, Isfahan, Iran

Sajad Ghorbani
Department of Clinical Pharmacy and Pharmacy Practice, Isfahan University of Medical Sciences, Isfahan, Iran

Payman Adibi
Department of Gastroenterology, Integrative Functional Gastroenterology Research Center, Isfahan University of Medical Sciences, Isfahan, Iran

Rabinarayan Parhi
GITAM Institute of Pharmacy, GITAM University, Gandhi Nagar Campus, Rushikonda, Visakhapatnam-530045, Andhra Pradesh, India

Parizad Piran
Biotechnology Research Center, Tabriz University of Medical Sciences, Tabriz, Iran

Hossein Samadi Kafil
Infectious and Tropical Diseases Research Center, Tabriz University of Medical Sciences, Tabriz, Iran
Drug Applied Research Center, Tabriz University of Medical Sciences, Tabriz, Iran

Rezvan Safdari and Hamed Hamishehkar
Drug Applied Research Center, Tabriz University of Medical Sciences, Tabriz, Iran

Saeed Ghanbarzadeh
Zanjan Pharmaceutical Nanotechnology Research Center, and Department of Pharmaceutics, Faculty of Pharmacy, Zanjan University of Medical Sciences, Zanjan, Iran

Mojtaba Keshavarz, Majid Reza Farrokhi and Atena Amiri
Shiraz Neuroscience Research Center, Shiraz University of Medical Sciences, Shiraz, Iran

Nazli Namazi
Diabetes Research Center, Endocrinology and Metabolism Clinical Sciences Institute, Tehran University of Medical Sciences, Tehran, Iran
Nutrition Research Center, Faculty of Nutrition, Tabriz University of Medical Sciences, Tabriz, Iran

Mohammad Alizadeh and Elham Mirtaheri
Nutrition Research Center, Faculty of Nutrition, Tabriz University of Medical Sciences, Tabriz, Iran

Safar Farajnia
Drug Applied Research Center, Tabriz University of Medical Sciences, Tabriz, Iran

Hasan Bagherpour Shamloo
Biotechnology Research Center, Tabriz University of Medical Sciences, Tabriz, Iran
Dryland Agricultural Research Institute (DARI), Agricultural Research, Education and Extension Organization (AREEO), Maragheh, Iran

Saber Golkari
Dryland Agricultural Research Institute (DARI), Agricultural Research, Education and Extension Organization (AREEO), Maragheh, Iran

Zeinab Faghfoori
Tuberculosis and Lung Research Center, Tabriz University of Medical Sciences, Tabriz, Iran
Student Research Committee, Faculty of Nutrition, Tabriz University of Medical Sciences, Tabriz, Iran

Ali Akbar Movassaghpour
Hematology and Oncology Research Center, Tabriz University of Medical Sciences, Tabriz, Iran.

Hajie Lotfi and Abolfazl Barzegari
Department of Medical Biotechnology, Faculty of Advanced Medical Science, Tabriz University of Medical Sciences, Tabriz 51664, Iran

Ahmad Yari Khosroushahi
Drug Applied Research Center, Tabriz University of Medical Sciences, Tabriz, Iran
Department of Pharmacognosy, Faculty of Pharmacy, Tabriz University of Medical Sciences, Tabriz, Iran

Tahereh Eteraf-Oskouei and Moslem Najafi
Department of Pharmacology and Toxicology, Faculty of Pharmacy, Tabriz University of Medical Sciences, Tabriz, Iran

Sevda Mikaily Mirak
Student Research Committee, Faculty of Pharmacy, Tabriz University of Medical Sciences, Tabriz, Iran

Swati Jagdale and Saylee Pawar
MAEER's Maharashtra Institute of Pharmacy, MIT campus, Kothrud, Pune (MS) 411038, Savitribai Phule Pune University, India

Saeid Yaripour
Department of Drug and Food Control, Faculty of Pharmacy, Tehran University of Medical Sciences, Tehran, Iran
Department of Pharmaceutical and Food Control, Faculty of Pharmacy, Urmia University of Medical Sciences, Urmia, Iran

Mohammad-Reza Delnavazi and Saeed Tavakoli
Department of Pharmacognosy, Faculty of Pharmacy, Tehran University of Medical Sciences, Tehran, Iran

Parina Asgharian
Drug Applied Research Centre, Tabriz University of Medical Sciences, Tabriz, Iran
Department of Pharmacognosy, Faculty of Pharmacy, Tabriz University of Medical Sciences, Tabriz, Iran

Samira Valiyari
Department of Medical Biotechnology, Pasteur Institute of Iran, Tehran, Iran.

Hossein Nazemiyeh
Research Center for Pharmaceutical Nanotechnology, Faculty of Pharmacy, Tabriz University of Medical Sciences, Tabriz, Iran
Department of Pharmacognosy, Faculty of Pharmacy, Tabriz University of Medical Sciences, Tabriz, Iran

Elham Safarzadeh, Tohid Kazemi, Mona Orangi, Dariush Shanehbandi, Leila Mohammadnejad, Ali mohammadi, Mehrdad Ghavifekr Fakhr and Behzad Baradaran
Immunology Research Center, Tabriz University of Medical Sciences, Tabriz, Iran

Abbas Delazar
Department of Pharmacognosy, Faculty of Pharmacy, Tabriz University of Medical Sciences, Tabriz, Iran

Solmaz Esnaashari
Drug Applied Research Center, Tabriz University of Medical Sciences, Tabriz, Iran

Saeed Sadigh-Eteghad
Neurosciences Research Center (NSRC), Tabriz University of Medical Sciences, Tabriz, Iran

Paulo César Venâncio
Department of Exact Sciences, Technical School of Limeira, Cotil, UNICAMP, Limeira, São Paulo, Brazil

Sidney Raimundo Figueroba, Bruno Dias Nani, Luiz Eduardo Nunes Ferreira, Bruno Vilela Muniz and Francisco Carlos Groppo
Department of Physiological Sciences, Piracicaba Dental School, UNICAMP, Piracicaba, São Paulo, Brazil

Fernando de Sá Del Fiol
Department of Pharmacological Sciences, School of Pharmacy of Sorocaba, UNISO, Sorocaba São Paulo, Brazil

Adilson Sartoratto
Research Center for Chemistry, Biology and Agriculture, CPQBA, UNICAMP, Paulínia, São Paulo, Brazil

Edvaldo Antonio Ribeiro Rosa
Xenobiotics Research Unit, PUC-Paraná, Curitiba, Paraná, Brazil

Shahla Mirzaeei
Pharmaceutical Sciences Research Center, School of Pharmacy, Kermanshah University of Medical Sciences, Kermanshah, Iran
Nano Drug Delivery Research Center, School of Pharmacy, Kermanshah University of Medical Sciences, Kermanshah, Iran

Kaveh Berenjian and Rasol Khazaei
Student Research Committee, School of Pharmacy, Kermanshah University of Medical Sciences, Kermanshah, Iran

Fataneh Narchin, Kambiz Larijani and Abdolhossein Rustaiyan
Department of Chemistry, Science and Research Branch, Islamic Azad University, Tehran, Iran

Samad Nejad Ebrahimi
Department of Phytochemistry, Medicinal Plants and Drugs Research Institute, Shahid Beheshti University, Evin Tehran, Iran

Farzaneh Tafvizi
Department of Biology, Parand Branch, Islamic Azad University, Parand, Iran

Seyedeh Sara Esnaashari, Masood Khosravani and Mahdi Adabi
Department of Medical Nanotechnology, School of Advanced Technologies in Medicine, Tehran University of Medical Sciences, Tehran, Iran

Fatemeh Madani
Department of Medical Nanotechnology, School of Advanced Technologies in Medicine, Tehran University of Medical Sciences, Tehran, Iran
Student's Scientific Research Center, Tehran University of Medical Sciences, Tehran, Iran

Basil Mujokoro
Department of Medical Nanotechnology, School of Advanced Technologies in Medicine, International Campus, Tehran University of Medical Sciences, Tehran, Iran

Farid Dorkoosh
Department of Pharmaceutics, Faculty of Pharmacy, Tehran University of Medical Sciences, Tehran, Iran

Rohanizah Abdul Rahim and Nor Hazwani Ahmad
Advanced Medical and Dental Institute, Universiti Sains Malaysia, 13200 Kepala Batas, Pulau Pinang, Malaysia

Khaldun Mohammad Al Azzam
Preparatory Year Department, Al-Ghad International Colleges for Applied Medical Sciences, Riyadh, Kingdom of Saudi Arabia
Department of Chemistry, Dalhousie University, Halifax, Nova Scotia, Canada

Ishak Mat
Unit Kanser MAKNA-USM, Advanced Medical and Dental Institute, Universiti Sains Malaysia, 13200 Kepala Batas, Pulau Pinang, Malaysia

Seyyed Pouya Hadipour Moghaddam
Department of Pharmaceutics and Pharmaceutical Chemistry, School of Pharmacy, University of Utah, Salt Lake City, UT 84112, USA
Utah Center for Nanomedicine, Nano Institute of Utah, University of Utah, Salt Lake City, UT 84112, USA

Sajjad Farhat and Alireza Vatanara
Department of Pharmaceutics, School of Pharmacy, Tehran University of Medical Sciences, Tehran, Iran

Abed Ghavami, Faezeh Ghalichi and Elyas Nattagh-Eshtivan
Department of Nutrition, School of Nutrition, Tabriz University of Medical Sciences, Tabriz, Iran

Neda Roshanravan
Cardiovascular Research Center, Tabriz University of Medical Sciences, Tabriz, Iran

Shahriar Alipour
Department of Molecular Medicine, Nutrition Research Center, Tabriz University of Medical Sciences, Tabriz, Iran

Meisam Barati
Department of Nutrition, School of Nutrition, Shahid beheshti University of Medical Sciences, Tehran, Iran

Behzad Mansoori
Immunology Research Center, Tabriz University of Medical Sciences, Tabriz, Iran

Alireza Ostadrahimi
Nutrition Research Center, Tabriz University of Medical Sciences, Tabriz, Iran

Yadhu Krishnan, Shilpa Mukundan, Suresh Akhil, Swati Gupta and Vidya Viswanad
Amrita School of Pharmacy, Amrita Institute of Medical Sciences and Research Centre, Amrita Vishwa Vidyapeetham, Kochi – 682041, India

Tasnuva Haque
Department of Pharmacy, East West University, A/2, Jahurul Islam City Gate, Aftab Nagar Main Rd, Dhaka-1212, Bangladesh

Md Mesbah Uddin Talukder
Department of Pharmacy, BRAC University, 66 Bir Uttam AK Khandakar Road, Dhaka 1212, Bangladesh

Nagaraju Ravouru and Rajeswari Surya Anusha Venna
Institute of Pharmaceutical Technology, Sri Padmavathi Mahila University, Tirupati, Andhra Pradesh, India

Subhash Chandra Bose Penjuri and Srikanth Reddy Poreddy
Department of Pharmaceutics, MNR College of Pharmacy, Sangareddy, Telangana, India

Saritha Damineni
Department of Pharmaceutics, Sultan-ul-Uloom College of Pharmacy, Hyderabad, Telangana, India

Venkata Subbaiah Kotakadi
Research Scientist, DST Purse Centre, S.V. University, Tirupati, Andhra Pradesh, India

Index